AF291225

# POSTURE AND PERFORMANCE

## Principles of Training Horses from the Anatomical Perspective

### GILLIAN HIGGINS

with Stephanie Martin

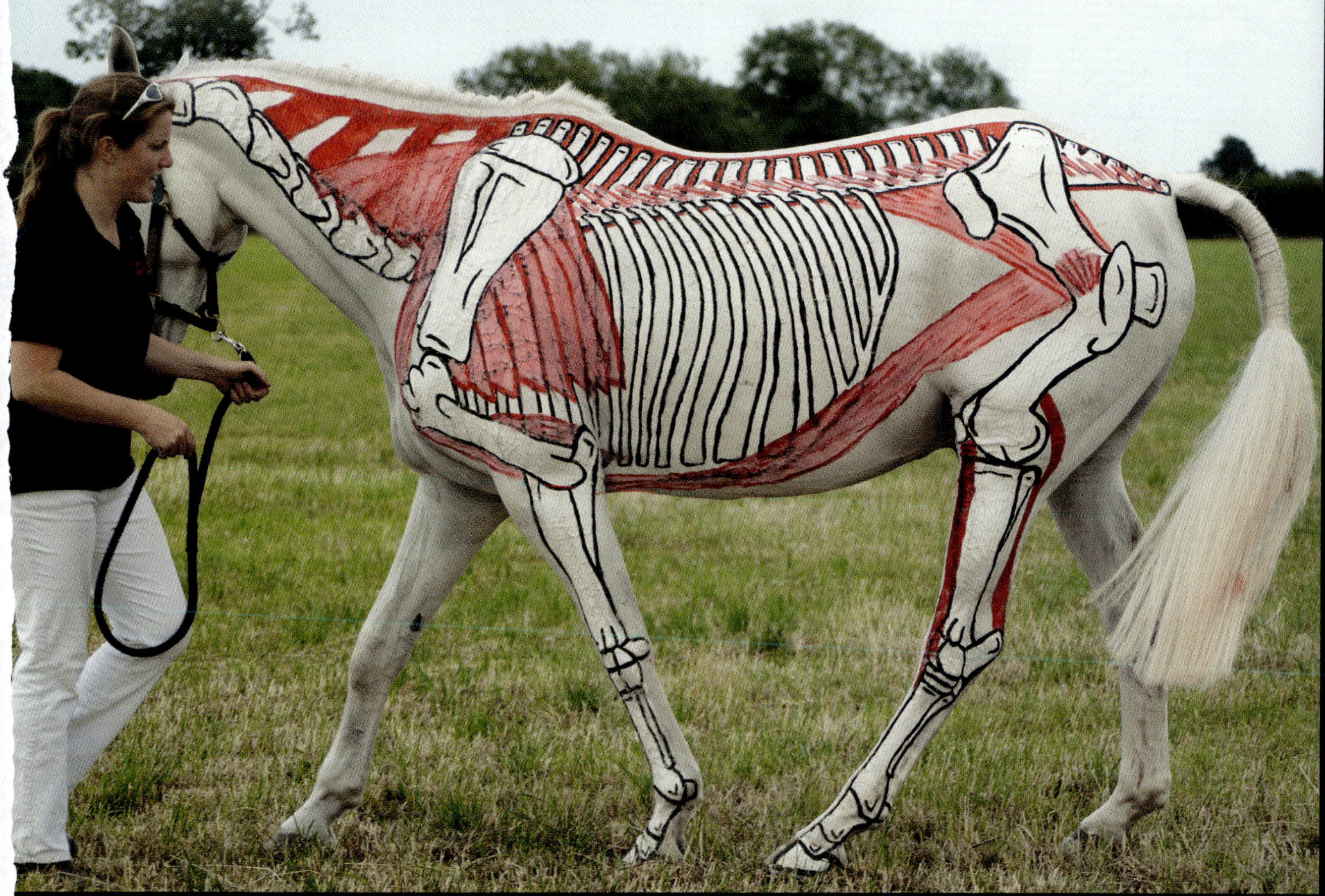

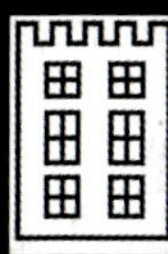

KENILWORTH PRESS

First published in the UK in 2016 by Kenilworth Press,
an imprint of Quiller Publishing Ltd



British Library Cataloguing-in-Publication Data
A catalogue record for this book is available from the
British Library

ISBN 978 1 910016 00 8



All the drawings and diagrams in the book are hand-drawn by
the author except for the arena exercises which are designed
by Gillian Higgins and produced by Carole Vincer.

Designed by Paul Saunders
Printed in China

Disclaimer
This book is not intended to be a training manual but rather
an explanation of functional anatomy, biomechanics and how
the horse moves. Whilst every effort is taken to ensure the
information disseminated is correct, the authors can take no
responsibility for any misinterpretation of the text.

## Kenilworth Press

An imprint of Quiller Publishing Ltd
The Hill, Merrywalks, Stroud, **GL5 4EP**
Tel: 01453 847800   Email: info@quillerbooks.com
Website: www.quillerpublishing.com

Appointed GPSR EU Representative:
Easy Access System Europe Oü, 16879218
Address: Mustamäe tee 50, 10621, Tallinn, Estonia
Contact Details: gpsr.requests@easproject.com,
+358 40 500 3575

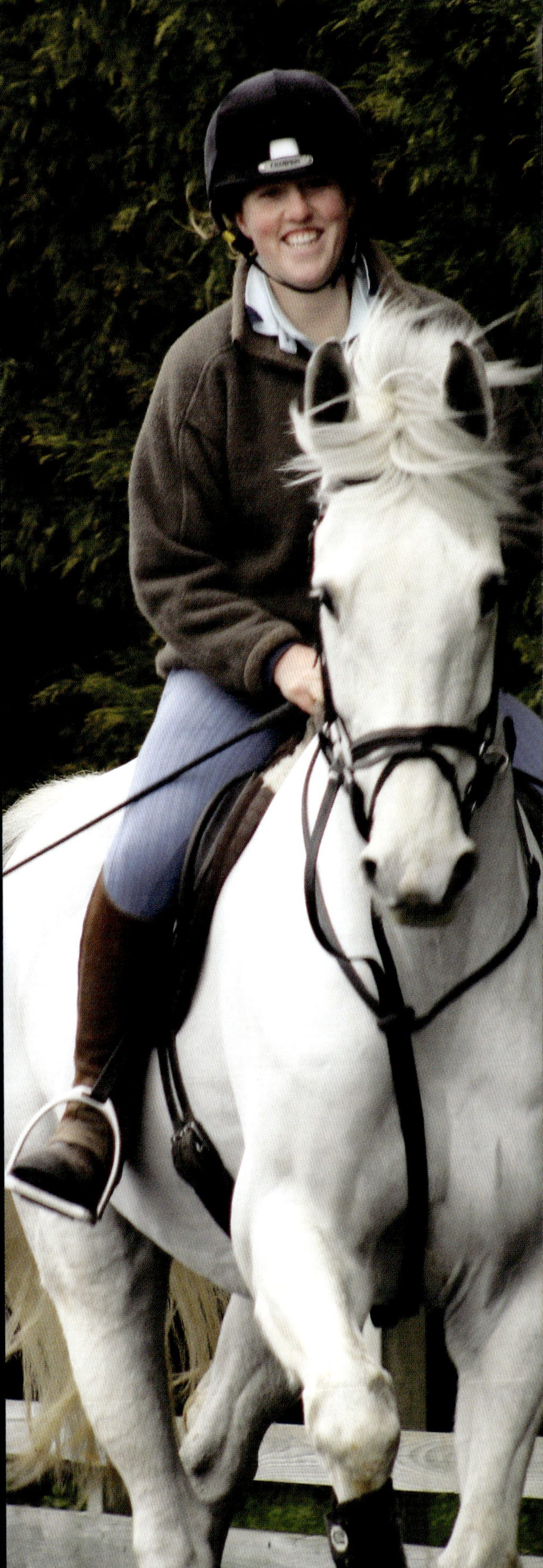

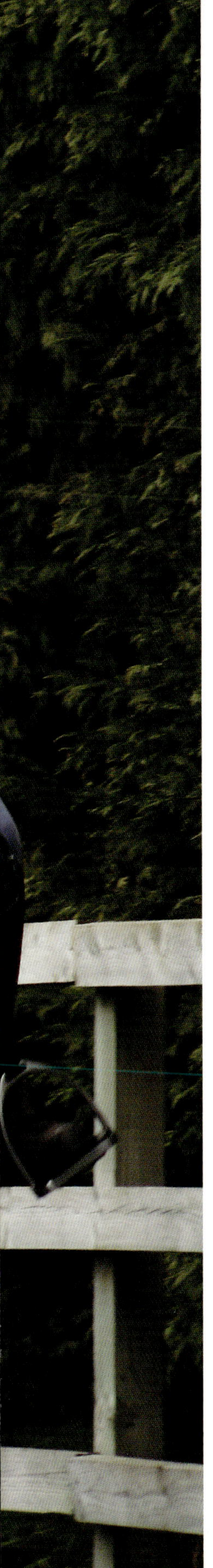

# Contents



## PART 1 The Principles of Training

This section looks at basic anatomy and the principles of training horses from the anatomical perspective, examines the importance of posture and considers both asymmetries and compensation patterns.

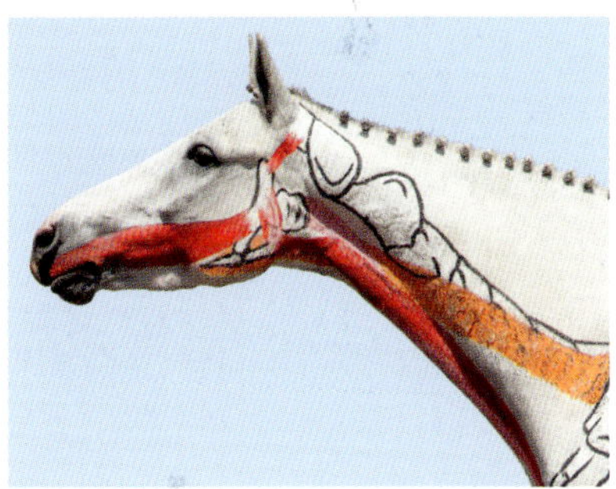



## PART 2 Exercises for Performance

Some suggestions for improving outline, gait, posture, flexibility, core stability and musculoskeletal health.

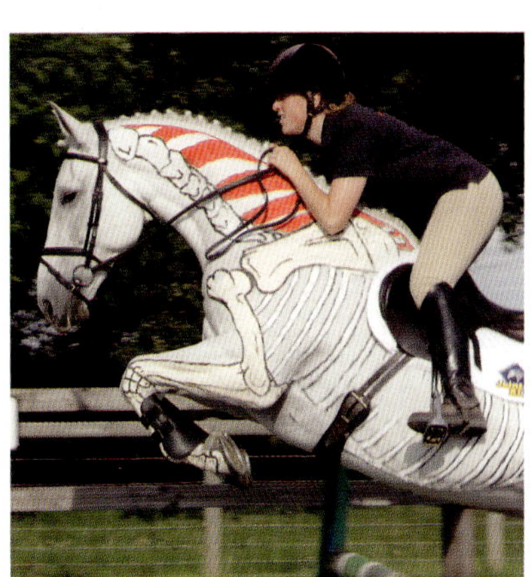

# Acknowledgements

Thank you to the riders Matt Frost, Laura Tomlinson, Molly Brown, Jenny Brown and Nathan Bull. Thank you to everyone at Elms Farm who helped and allowed me to paint their horses. Without them this book would not exist. A very big thank you must go to Adam Kemp who so generously gave his time and technical expertise painstakingly reading through the manuscript. Finally special praise and polos go to my patient, lovable horses Furst Edition and Freddie Fox.

Thanks also to the following who have taken photographs for this book: David Higgins, Helen Richmond, Matthew Roberts, Steve Russell and Alan and Jane Douglas.

## Photograph credits

# About the Authors

**GILLIAN HIGGINS** is an equine and human sports and remedial therapist, British Horse Society Senior Coach and event rider with a passion for equine anatomy and anatomical art. As a leading expert in her field she founded **HORSES INSIDE OUT**. This unique organisation gives riders, trainers, students and therapists a fascinating insight into the training, management, comfort and welfare of their horses through understanding anatomy, physiology and biomechanics. With an enthusiastic style of presentation and the ability to bring her subject to life she is in demand worldwide. Gillian runs courses in anatomy and biomechanics, dissections for therapists, massage and stretching for horse owners as well as day courses for colleges and universities and evening lecture-demonstrations for all. She has written several books and produced two DVDs.

**STEPHANIE MARTIN** has been involved with horses from a very early age and has a particular interest in their welfare. With a keen interest in literature, and a 'way with words', she has written various articles and has played a valuable part in putting together the text for this book.

## Painting Horses

All of the paintings reproduced are designed and painted on the horse by the author. It takes between four and six hours to paint a horse depending on the complexity of the anatomical system. The paint is water-based, non-toxic and completely harmless.

To learn more visit **www.HorsesInsideOut.com**

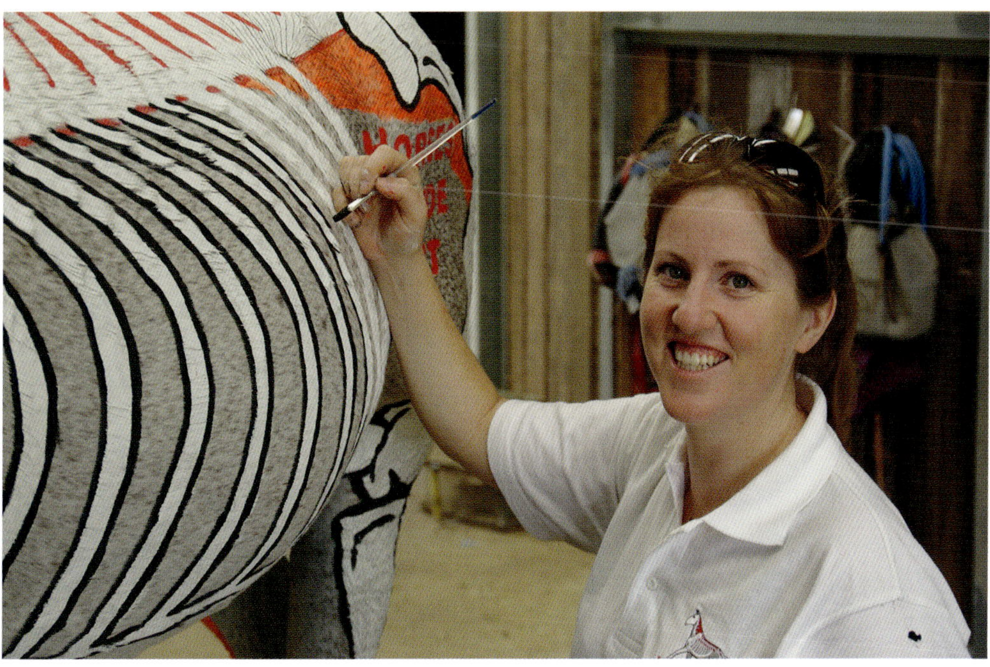

# Useful Terms

**Abduction** – When the leg is taken away from the body.

**Adduction** – When the leg is brought towards or across the body.

**Asymmetrical gait** – A gait in which the limb movements are different on the left and right sides, for example canter and gallop.

**Atrophy** – Wasting away, loss of muscle bulk and function.

**Cadence** – Rhythm combined with impulsion and spring.

**Caudal** – Towards the tail.

**Cranial** – Towards the skull.

**Impact** – The first point at which the hoof makes contact with the ground.

**Impulsion** – Energy.

**Lateral flexion** – Side bend through the spine.

**Myofascia** – Skeletal muscle and its surrounding fascia.

**Neural** – Relating to nerves.

**Overtracking** – When the hind leg is placed in front of the imprint of the fore hoof.

**Proprioception** – Perception of body positioning and spatial awareness.

**Propulsion** – The moment in the stride from mid-stance to where the tip of the hoof digs into the surface to propel the horse forward.

**Protraction** – Where the limb moves forwards in relation to the body: it begins at breakover and ends just before impact.

**Retraction** – Where the limb moves backwards in relation to the body: it begins just before the hoof touches the ground at impact and ends at breakover.

**Rhythm** – Regularity of the steps or strides in each gait.

**Rotation** – The action of rotating around an axis.

**Spinal extension** – Hollowing of the spine, accompanied with a degree of high head and tail carriage.

**Spinal flexion** – Rounding of the spine.

**Stance** – The moment of the stride when the foot is on the ground. There are different parts to stance:

1. *Deceleration* from impact and when the limb is in front of vertical

2. *Loading* when the body weight is loaded onto the limb

3. *Load-bearing* where vertical impact is at its greatest

4. *Breakover* – From when the heel lifts off the ground until the toe leaves and the swing phase begins.

**Stride length** – The distance from the placement of one hoof to where it next falls.

**Swing phase** – The moment of the stride when the foot is off the ground and coming through the air.

**Symmetrical gait** – Gait in which limb movements on one side are repeated on the opposite side half a stride later. Example: trot, pace.

**Tempo** – The speed of the rhythm of the gait.

**Tracking up** – When the hind hoof steps into the imprint of the fore.

**Tuberosity** – A bony protuberance, which provides an area for muscle attachment.

# Foreword

## By **Adam Kemp**

I first met Gillian Higgins in 2012 when we were both invited, independently, to give a presentation at a British Horse Society conference at Hartpury College. I was immediately taken by her boundless enthusiasm for, and deep knowledge of, the relationship between anatomy, biomechanics and training of horses.

I've been training horses and riders for many years with a quest for performance enhancement in both horse and rider. Gillian has really helped me understand the anatomical and biometric possibilities of the horses' physiology and anatomy in my training philosophies.

Understanding what a horse's body is capable of is paramount in designing a training and educational regime to help bring the best out of each individual horse we are lucky enough to train. This book will help you understand what effects each training phase and exercise will have on your horse's body, which will assist you in designing a programme of performance enhancement training to suit his individual needs.

Performance enhancement requires firstly an assessment of your horse's needs, followed by a systematic training regime involving education, gymnastics, and body building. Gillian will help you understand these concepts, and guide you through the practical application of the theory.

Having had a very extensive education in the practicalities of training horses I have found it refreshing and intriguing to learn more about the theories of biomechanics of the equine athlete's capabilities. This knowledge hasn't changed what I believe in or do. What it has done is greatly enhance the enjoyment I get from developing the equine athlete. I believe in maximising the horse's capability through education and physical development. Understanding the physiological implications of this process has served to further my thrill and wonderment of the challenge.

This book will help you understand what you are trying to achieve, and why success in training your horse is somewhat elusive! You will marvel at the success of your training, as much as you will rationalise your failings. Through systematic, educated reasoning you will see why things work, and why things don't.

Training a horse to be the best he can be is one of the most rewarding, and challenging things I've done. Things will go wrong on the way, but remember, you are the intelligent member of the horse/rider combination. He has immense physical strength that will always outdo yours. Your strength is in your head – use it wisely to win him over.

Horses are not machines. Use this book to help you embrace, and be richly rewarded by, this challenge.

Enjoy the book, and enjoy your horse.

Adam Kemp

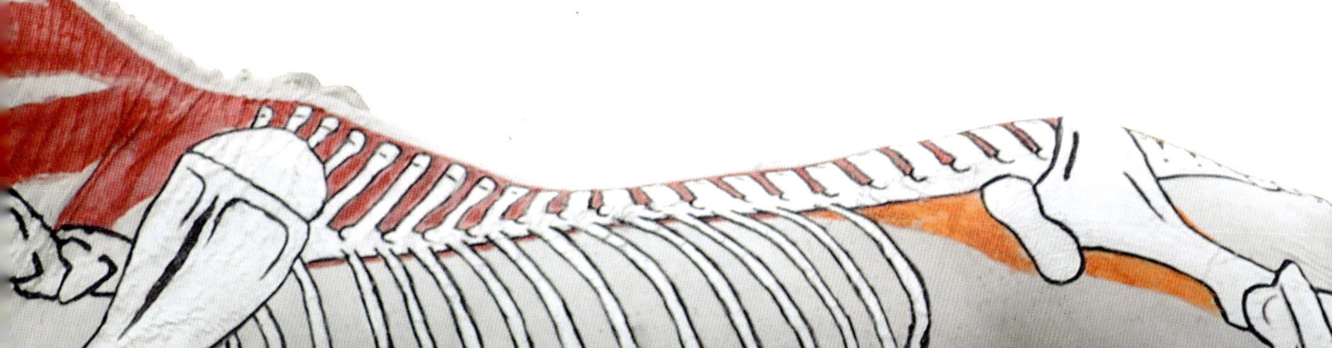

# Introduction

This book is refreshingly different! It shows riders how, by understanding more about anatomy, biomechanics, how their horses function and the principles of training from an anatomical perspective they are in a position to make informed decisions related to riding, training and management. By applying their knowledge they can then maximise their own and their horse's potential, improve their skills, achieve their goals and thus gain more success, satisfaction and enjoyment.

*Posture and Performance* shows riders how to think of themselves as personal trainers to their horses, take care of their musculature and consider every aspect of their well-being in general and their posture in particular. It shows how to train with empathy, sensitivity and always with the best interest of the horse at heart.

Today's horse is an athlete. We are continually pushing him to his physiological limits. We are constantly raising the bar – in some cases literally as well as metaphorically. We expect him to run faster, jump higher and perform increasingly complicated movements often requiring seemingly unattainable feats of skill, strength and balance, all whilst carrying the weight of the rider. To do this he must be fit, agile, relaxed, strong and mentally prepared. As riders, we often train in a gym. Our horses' gym is the arena, field, hill and dale.

The universally recognised German scales of training are a tried and tested training system developed to maximise the horse's natural, physical and mental aptitudes. By following their principles in conjunction with a thorough understanding of anatomy and biomechanics, the rider will enjoy a well-trained, obedient, supple and comfortable horse that is willing to cooperate without resistance in any situation. This applies to all horses regardless of breed or discipline.

The six principles of the training scale are:

- Rhythm and regularity of steps
- Suppleness, relaxation and elasticity of movement
- Contact, acceptance of the bit and aids
- Impulsion
- Straightness and equal contact on both reins
- Collection, increased engagement and balance.

All levels are interdependent and, although each stage should be well established before moving on to the next, they also need to be considered as a whole. *Posture and Performance* is descriptively illustrated, arranged in bite-sized pieces and approaches the subject in an easily digestible format.

This illuminating and unique book is not designed to be a definitive training manual but rather to give food for thought, provide an insight into the anatomical and biomechanical principles of posture and training and to encourage us all to improve our personal skills and achieve the very best for our horses.

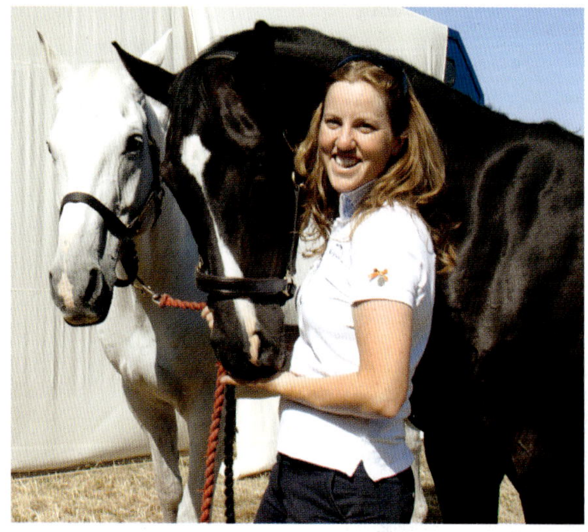

# The Principles of Training

This section looks at basic anatomy and the principles of training horses from the anatomical perspective, examines the importance of posture and considers both asymmetries and compensation patterns.

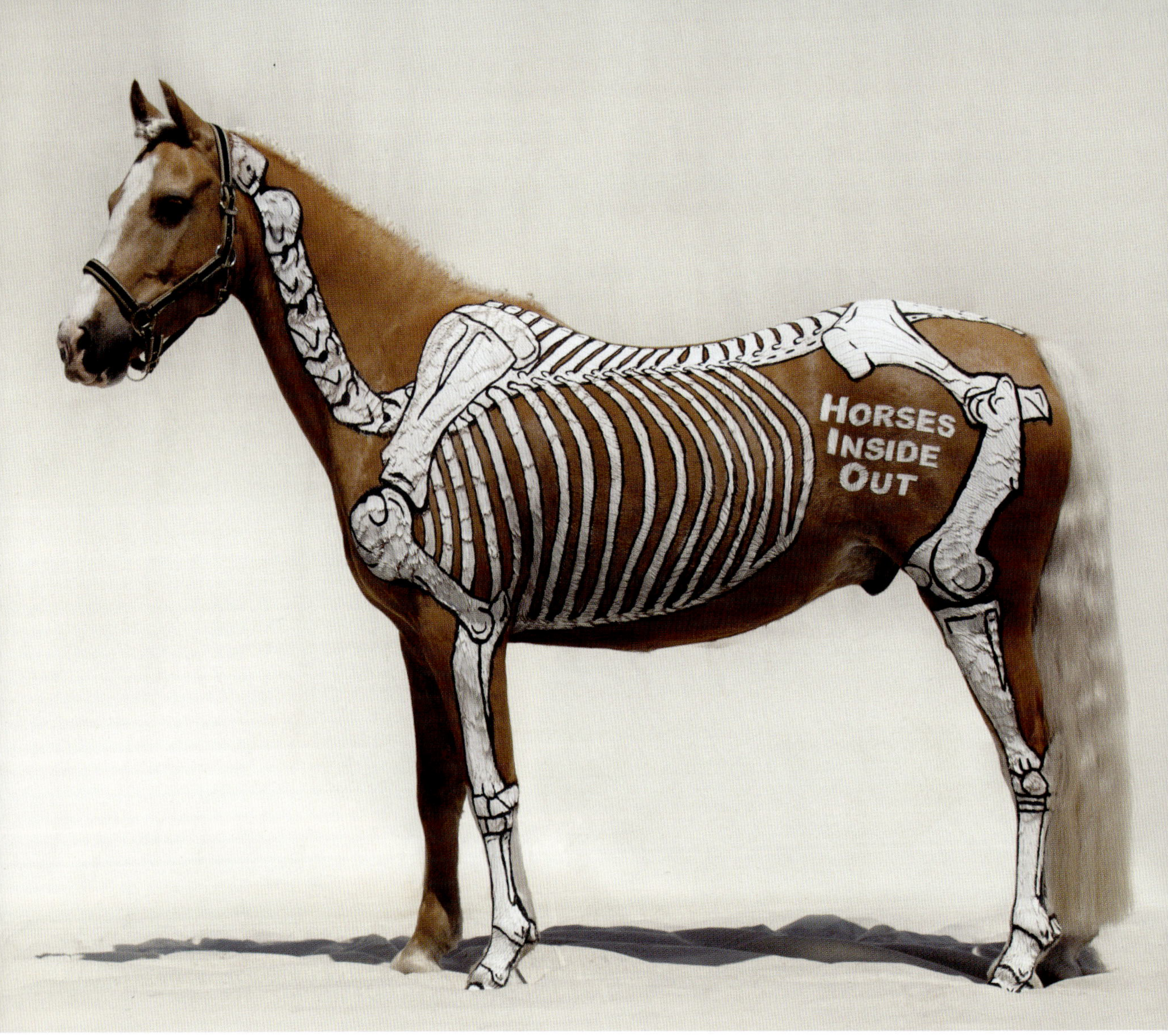



Anatomy is a study of the structure and relationship between all the parts of the body. Knowledge of anatomy is essential for every rider, trainer and equine professional. It allows us to understand the dynamics of movement and encourage the horse to move freely without putting undue stress on joints, tendons, ligaments, or muscles. Understanding anatomy promotes a good rider, trainer, therapist, farrier or saddler to great. It is critical for achieving optimum performance and for understanding the limitations of our horses.

This chapter explores the relationship between the principle aspects of the axial and appendicular skeleton, fascial connections, how muscles function and the importance of muscle chains all related to movement.

# The Spine

The spine is a complicated arrangement of vertebrae, cartilaginous discs, strong ligaments and joints. Forming a bridge between the fore and hindlimbs, it transfers the forces created by the thrust of the hind end, supports the weight of the digestive system and carries the weight of the rider. It is made up of five sections. The shape of the vertebrae, all of which have common features, change at the junction between each section. Each vertebra has areas for muscle and ligament attachments and each has a vertebral canal running through the centre that houses the spinal cord. This transmits messages between the brain and the rest of the body.

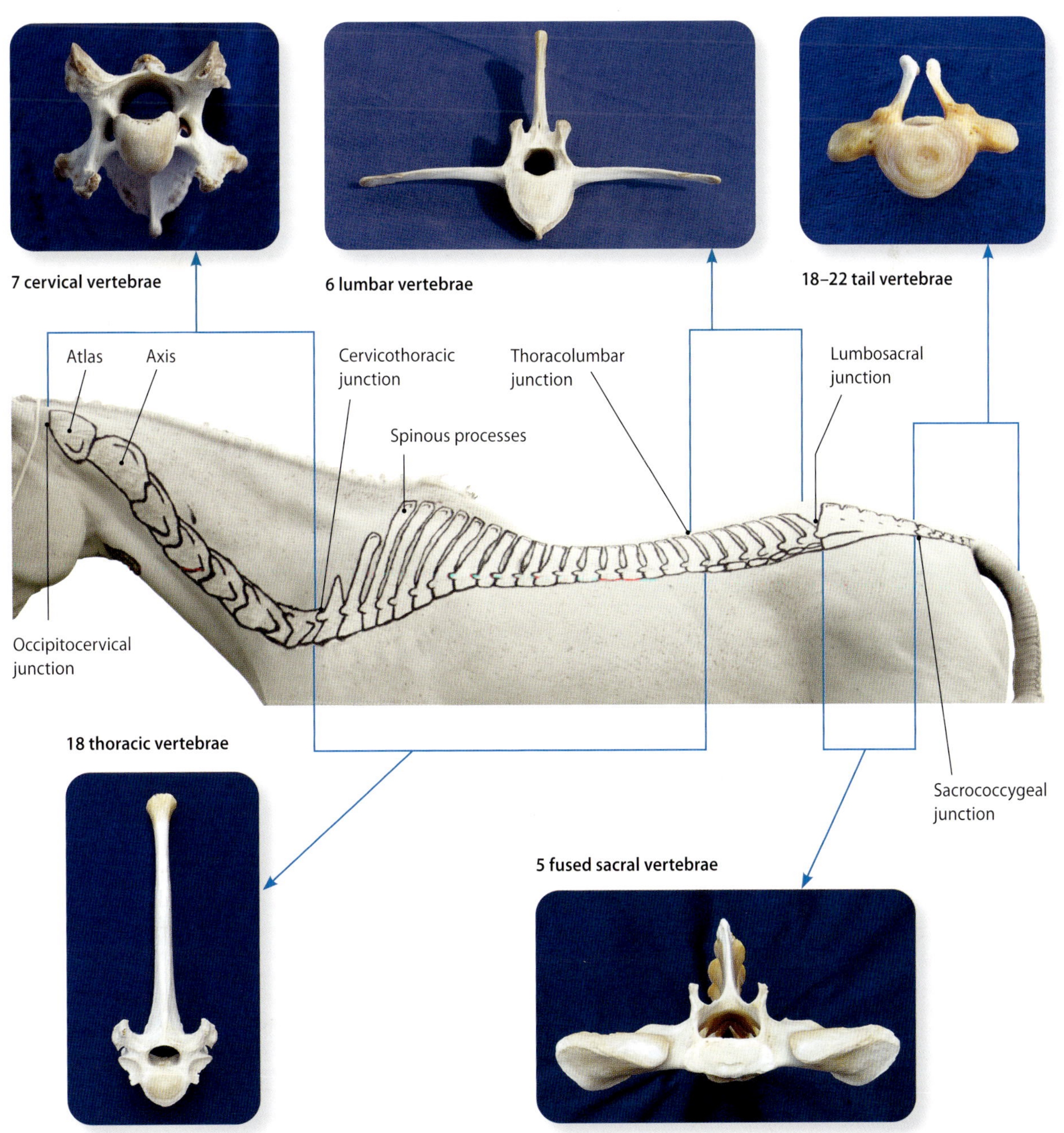

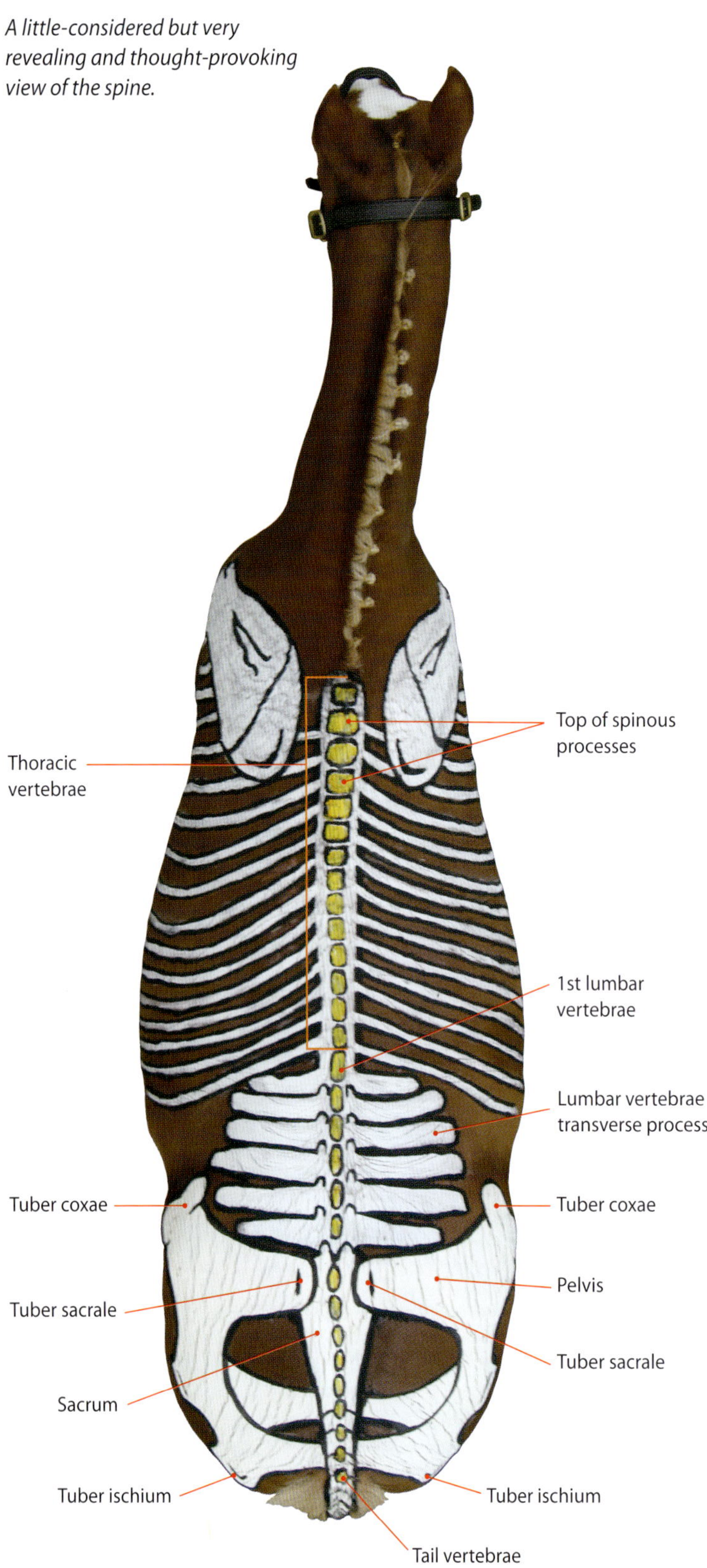



The eighteen pairs of ribs protrude from between each neighbouring thoracic vertebrae. These support the back and contribute to the horse's ability to bend. They consist of:

- Eight true ribs which connect directly into the sternum and are considered to be supporting ribs. There is little movement here.
- Ten false ribs which connect to the sternum via cartilage and connective tissue. As there is more spring in this section they are known as 'breathing ribs'.

Six lumbar vertebrae, characterised by the length and width of the transverse processes, protect underlying organs, provide an area for muscle attachment and increase stability. As the lumbar vertebrae are unsupported by the ribs it is important that the saddle and thus the rider's weight are positioned above the ribs. The thoracolumbar section of the spine is very inflexible with only minor flexion-extension (up and down), lateral (side to side) and rotational movement.

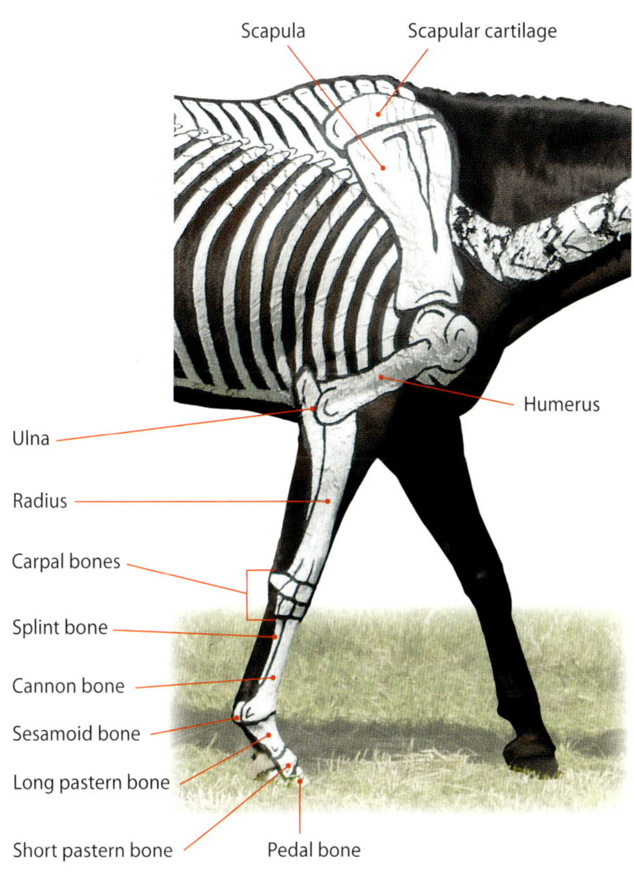


# The Forelimbs

The forelimb, essentially an upright bony column, is connected to the spine via the thoracic sling, a series of muscles and soft tissue which allows the horse to turn and which dissipates concussive forces, particularly when landing from a jump. Its main function is to support weight and contribute to balance, turning and braking.

# The Hindlimbs

The hindlimb is connected to the spine via the pelvis at the sacroiliac joint. The bones in the hindlimbs are large and strong to withstand and create enormous forces. The main function of the powerful hind leg is to create propulsion. The angles, length and alignment of the bones determine the amount of flexibility, forward propulsion, range of movement and thus gymnastic ability. The more acute the angles, the more the horse can compress and the more suited he will be to competitive jumping or high levels of dressage. The horse with more upright, open angles will have less spring and absorb concussion less efficiently.

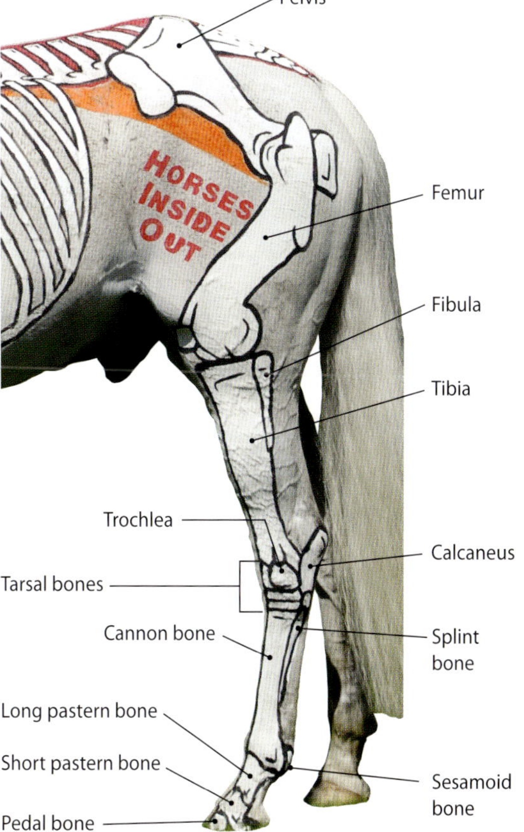

# Muscles

There are hundreds of skeletal muscles in the horse's body. These create movement by applying force to bone via tendons to operate joints. Muscle length, strength and tone determine the degree of skeletal support.

## Muscles work in opposition to each other

Muscles work in pairs. As one muscle, referred to as the agonist, contracts, the opposite one, the antagonist, lengthens. This principle is extended to groups and chains of muscles. The chains affect movement patterns and posture.

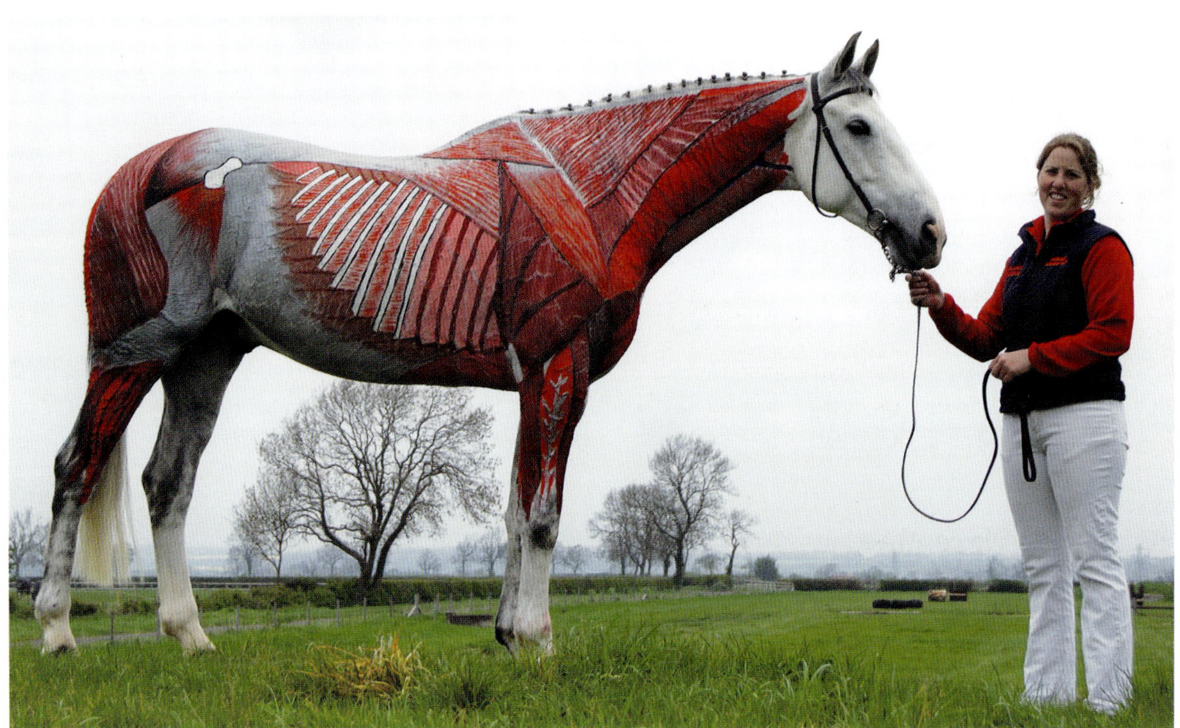

## How muscles contract

Muscle comprises of many strands of tissue called fascicles. An example of these can be seen in red meat or poultry. Within each fascicle are bundles of tens of thousands of thread-like myofybrils, which can contract, relax, and elongate. The myofybrils themselves are made up of millions of microscopic bands of sarcomeres consisting of overlapping thick and thin myofilaments of the contractile proteins actin and myosin.

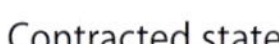


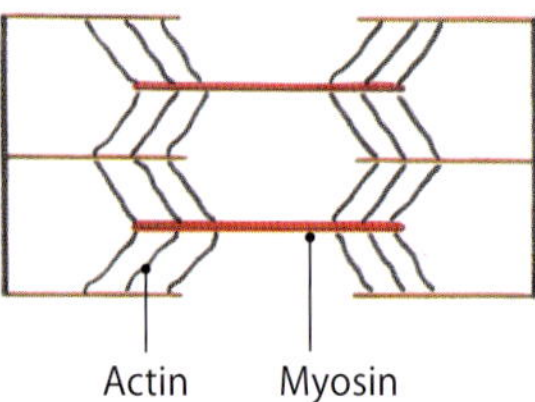


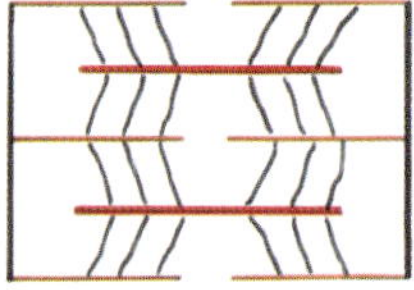


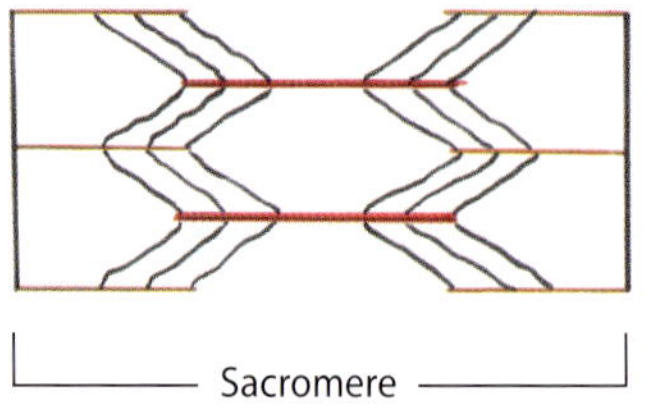


*Arrangement of the actin and myosin filaments in a single sarcomere in a stretched, relaxed and contracted state.*

## Muscle fibre toning and stretching

People who do sit-ups on a regular basis have shortened, more toned stomach muscles. If a muscle or muscle fibre is repeatedly asked to contract, over time the tissue will respond by removing some sarcomeres to reduce the overall length of the myofibrils. This is how muscles become more toned with strengthening exercises. Conversely, when continuously stretched, additional sarcomeres will be added to the myofibrils thus elongating the muscle fibre. This muscle response is also true of horses.

## Muscle fibre recruitment

Muscle fibres are unable to vary the intensity of their contraction. Varying the strength of force relies on the number of muscle fibres recruited by the central nervous system. The more that are recruited the stronger the contraction.

To avoid fatigue, prolong muscular endurance or to counteract damage, the muscle fibres alternate between work and rest. This is rather like a factory

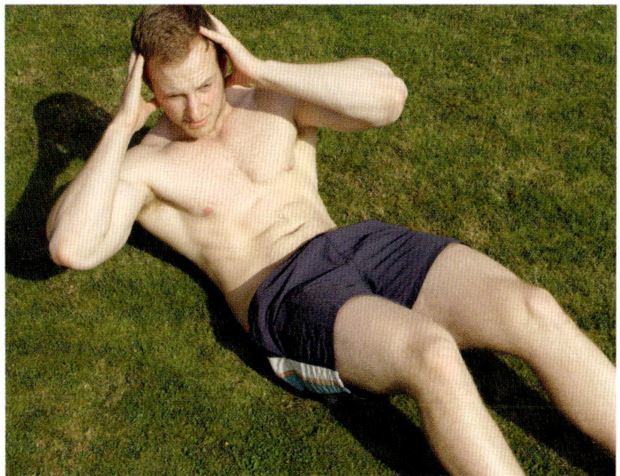

*Performing regular sit-ups creates shortened, more toned stomach muscles.*

shift system! If some fibres are damaged, for example after a bout of hard exercise, the muscle will avoid using them until they have recovered. It is important to allow the muscles time to rest and recover after new or strenuous exercise.

## Types of muscle contraction

There are two types of muscle contraction; isometric and isotonic. Understanding these helps us to train our horses more effectively and sensitively.

### Isometric contractions

These are used when the muscle is working statically to maintain a position. For example when we hold a heavy weight at arm's length or when a horse is required to hold his head in an elevated flexed neck outline. This can be muscularly tiring. To counteract this we need to allow the horse regular breaks to stretch down and relax.

### Isotonic contractions

These create or control movement and can be further divided into:

- **Concentric** muscle contraction, which occurs when the muscle is actively shortened. It is used when initiating propulsion, taking off for a jump, going uphill, accelerating and creating cadence.
- **Eccentric** muscle contraction, which occurs when the muscle is actively lengthened. It is used when braking, during the loading phase of the stride, landing from a jump or going downhill.

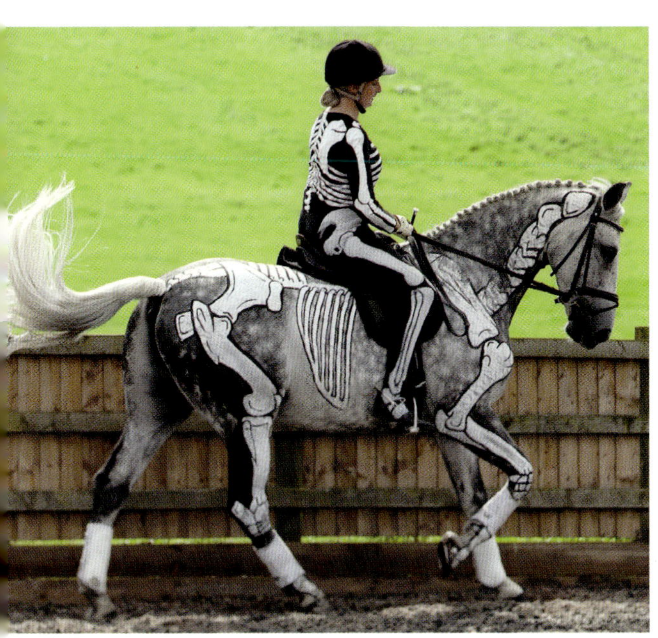

*This horse is using his neck muscles isometrically.*

# Connective Tissue

Connective tissue links and supports all the structures and systems of the body. It is comprised of the protein, collagen and includes fascia, tendons and ligaments.

## Fascia

Fascia, the main components of which are collagen and elastin, is the most abundant material in the body. It is a pliable, web-like, integrated, continuous sheet of tissue that penetrates and links every structure and organ. It surrounds bone in the form of the periosteum and gives muscles shape, structural support and protection. Another function is to allow the transport of nutrients and waste. When fascia, which is 80% water, is hydrated, it is resilient and flexible, allowing its moist layers to glide smoothly past each other without interference. When emotional stress or injury occurs, the fascia may harden, become inflexible and locally dehydrated or disorganised at a cellular level. This causes the layers to adhere together leading to muscular tension, restricted movement patterns and sometimes pain often far removed from the original site of the problem.

## Tendons

Tendons attach skeletal muscle to bone. They are dense fibrous parallel bundles of collagen arranged in long cords that have high tensile strength but limited elasticity. They originate in the parent muscle, and insert into bone. Blood supply to tendons is limited and explains the poor healing capacity. During muscular activity the force generated by the muscle is transmitted to the tendon and then to the bone, thereby initiating movement. As horses have no muscles below the knee, tendons bear the brunt of the workload. Once a tendon or ligament has been damaged, the scar tissue that forms is aligned haphazardly and is less strong.

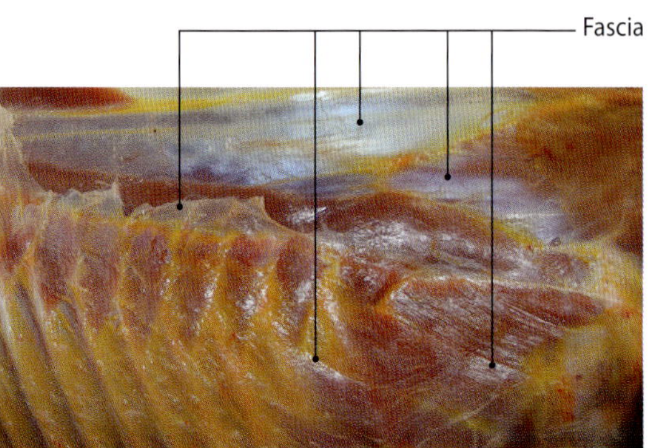


**SCAR TISSUE**

Scar tissue is formed from the excessive amounts of collagen produced as part of the normal healing process following injury. This can be as a result of an external cut or internal injury when muscles, ligaments or tendons are damaged. The initial production of granulation tissue is necessary to provide tensile strength for repair. Unfortunately, owing to poor structural organisation of the collagen, it is less pliable, less flexible and less consistent than the tissue it replaces. In some cases and depending on the severity of the original injury, it can cause restriction and even pain.

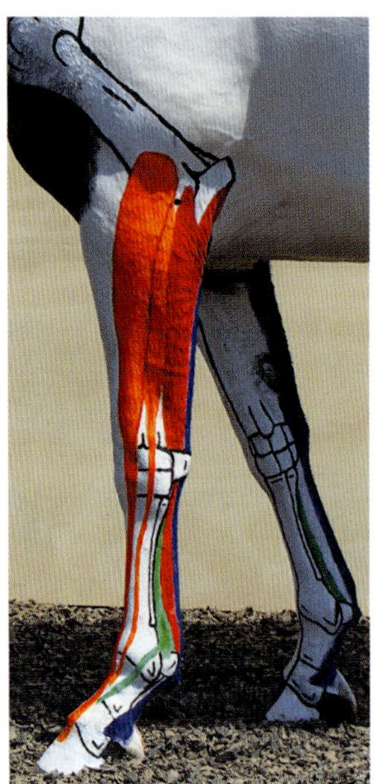

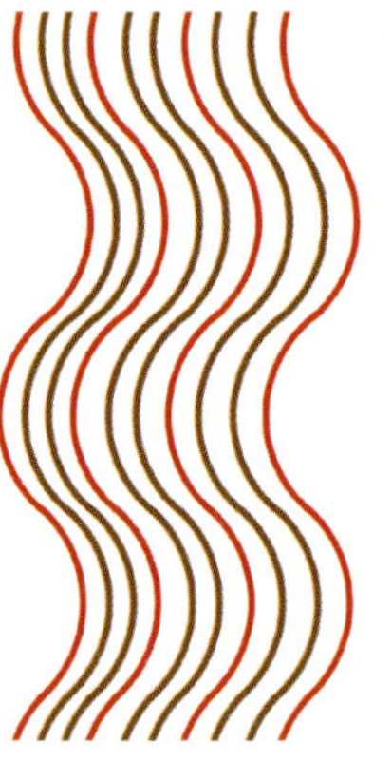

*Healthy tendon tissue with well aligned collagen fibres.*

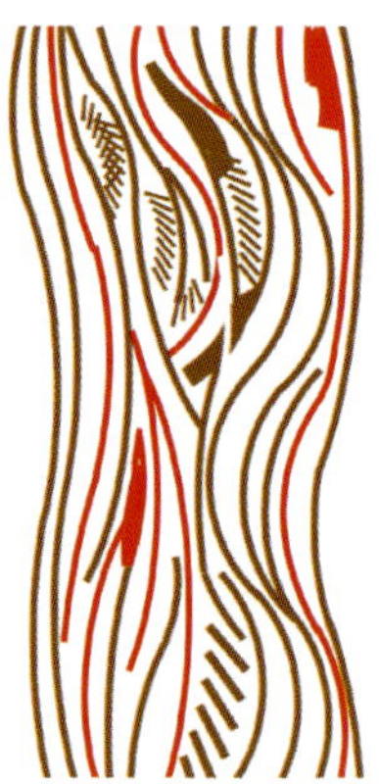

*Damaged tendon tissue with poorly aligned collagen fibres and scar tissue.*

# Ligaments

Ligaments connect bone to bone across joints. They are found throughout the body. They are composed of fibrous bands of connective tissue made up of relatively inelastic white fibres and more elastic yellow fibres that have the ability to stretch. The degree of elasticity within the ligament depends on the amount and type of the fibres, location, function and range of movement within the joint. Ligaments that cross joints where there is more movement require a higher proportion of yellow fibres. The nuchal ligament in the neck for example, requires more stretch than the collateral ligaments that stabilise and prevent lateral movement in the hinge joints of the limbs.

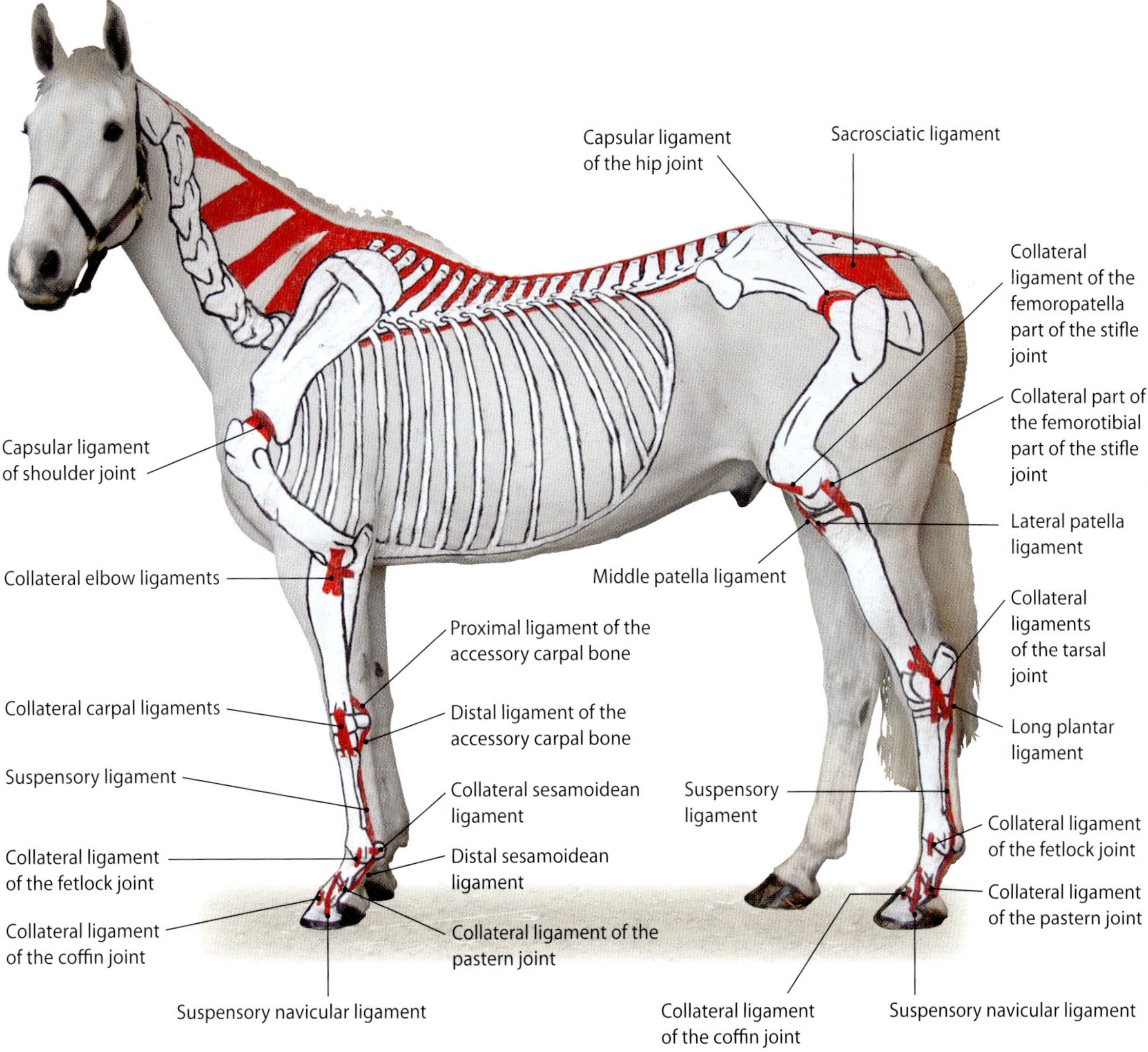

# How Muscle Chains Contribute to Movement

There are many different muscle chains within the horse's body. These work together to create smooth, flowing movement. If there is a constriction in any part of the chain, perhaps from pain, stiffness or lack of strength, this will affect performance. The main chains involved in creating movement include:

## The spinal extensor chain

Strength within this chain is important for power, thrust, expression, cadence and ground coverage. Concentric shortening of the extensor chain results in retraction of the hindlimb and extension of the stifle, hip, lumbosacral junction, back and neck. It helps to push the horse forwards and upwards, raising the forehand. When used eccentrically and isometrically, the extensor chain of muscles also helps to carry weight, maintain flexion in the haunches during the weight-bearing phase, prevent over-flexion in the back and maintain an elevated flexed neck outline. The muscles within this chain are situated above the spine and behind the bones of the hind leg. It can be traced from the hind heel all the way to the skull. This chain works in opposition to the spinal flexor chain. Tension within this chain can inhibit the action of the flexor chain, reduce the ability to round the back and protract the hindlimb.

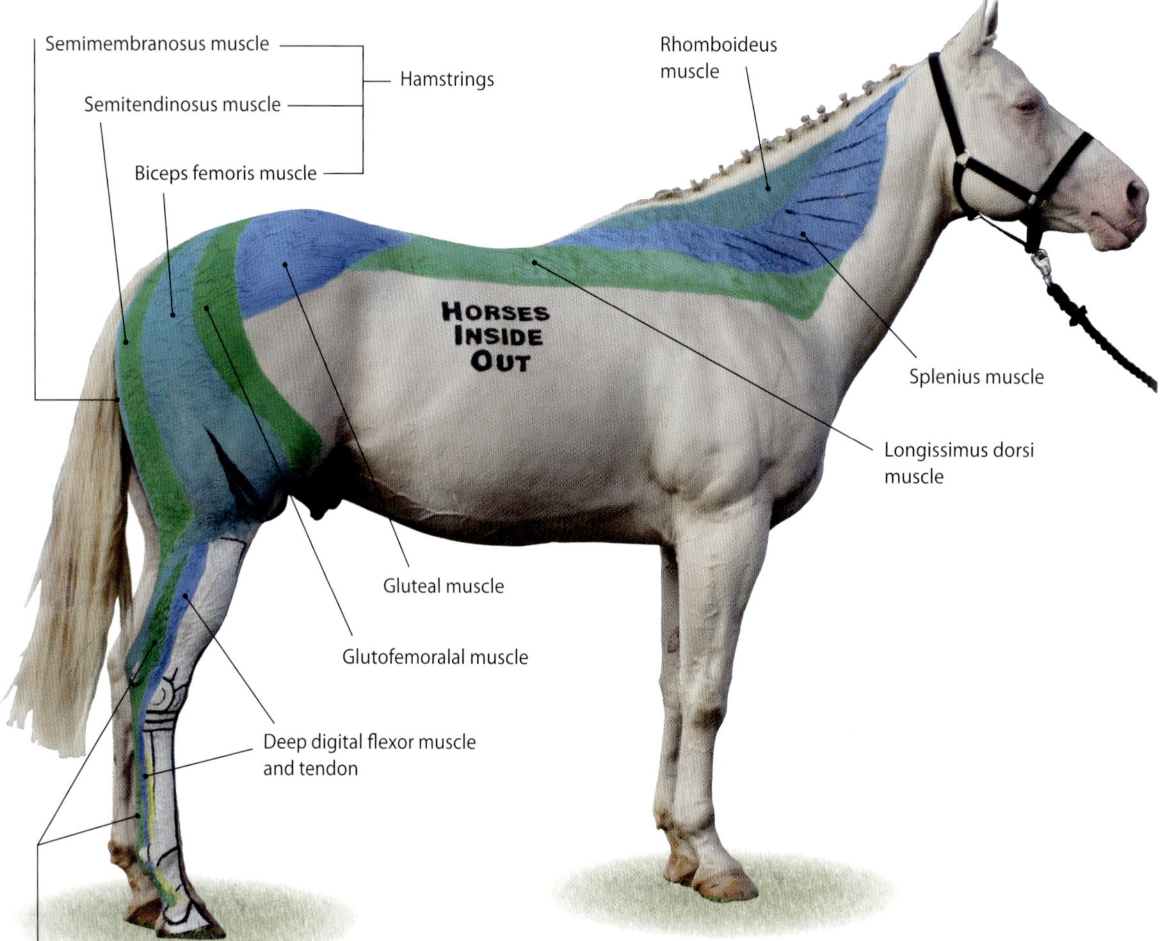


*The spinal extensor chain.*

## The spinal flexor chain

Strength within the flexor chain is important for core stability, supporting good posture and carrying the weight of the rider. Concentric shortening of the flexor chain results in protraction of the hindlimb and flexion of the stifle, hip, lumbosacral junction, back and neck. It helps to round the back and bring the hind leg under the body. Eccentric and isometric contraction of this muscle chain limits extension within the back. The muscles within this chain are situated below the spine and in front of the bones of the hindlimb. It can be traced from the hind toe all the way to the tip of the tongue. This chain works in opposition to the spinal extensor chain. Tension within this chain can reduce the ability to show lengthened strides. Good tone of this chain is vital for good posture.

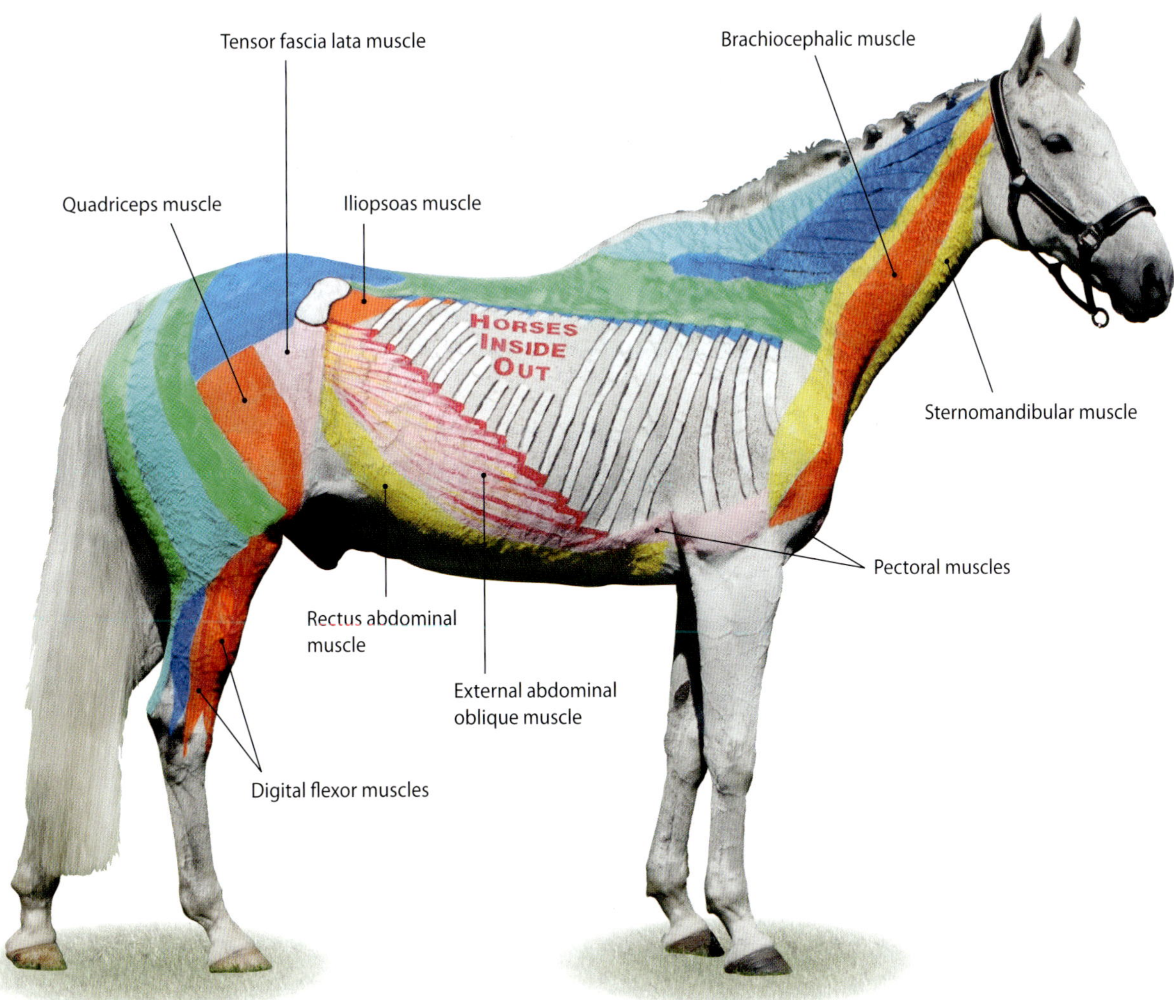



*The spinal flexor chain.*

## Forelimb protraction chain

Strength within this chain is important for developing forelimb expression. Concentric shortening of this chain results in protraction of the forelimb. Most of the muscles are situated in front of the forelimb bones, with the exception of the thoracic part of the trapezius muscle which stabilises the top of the scapula during protraction. This chain, which works in opposition to the forelimb retraction chain, can be traced from the fore toe through to the poll. Tension within this chain can reduce the ability to retract the forelimb resulting in a loss of forelimb power.

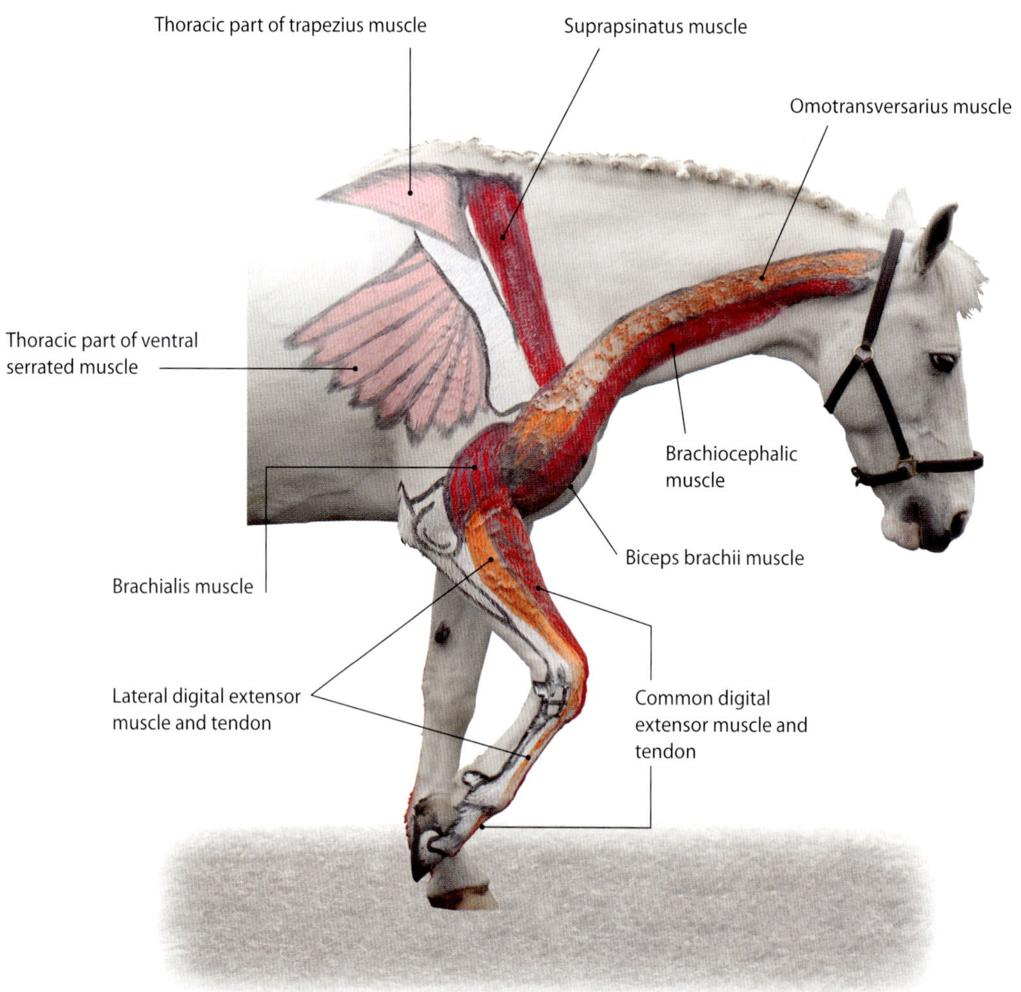


*Forelimb protraction chain.*

## Forelimb retraction chain

Strength within this chain is important for forelimb power, cadence and expression. Concentric shortening of this chain results in retraction of the forelimb and helps to pull the heavy weight of the body over the planted foreleg. Most of the muscles are situated behind the forelimb bones with the exception of the rhomboideus and the cervical part of the trapezius muscle, which stabilise the top of the scapula during retraction. This chain, which works in opposition to the forelimb protraction chain, can be traced from the fore heel through to the lumbosacral region of the back. Tension here can reduce forelimb protraction and expression.

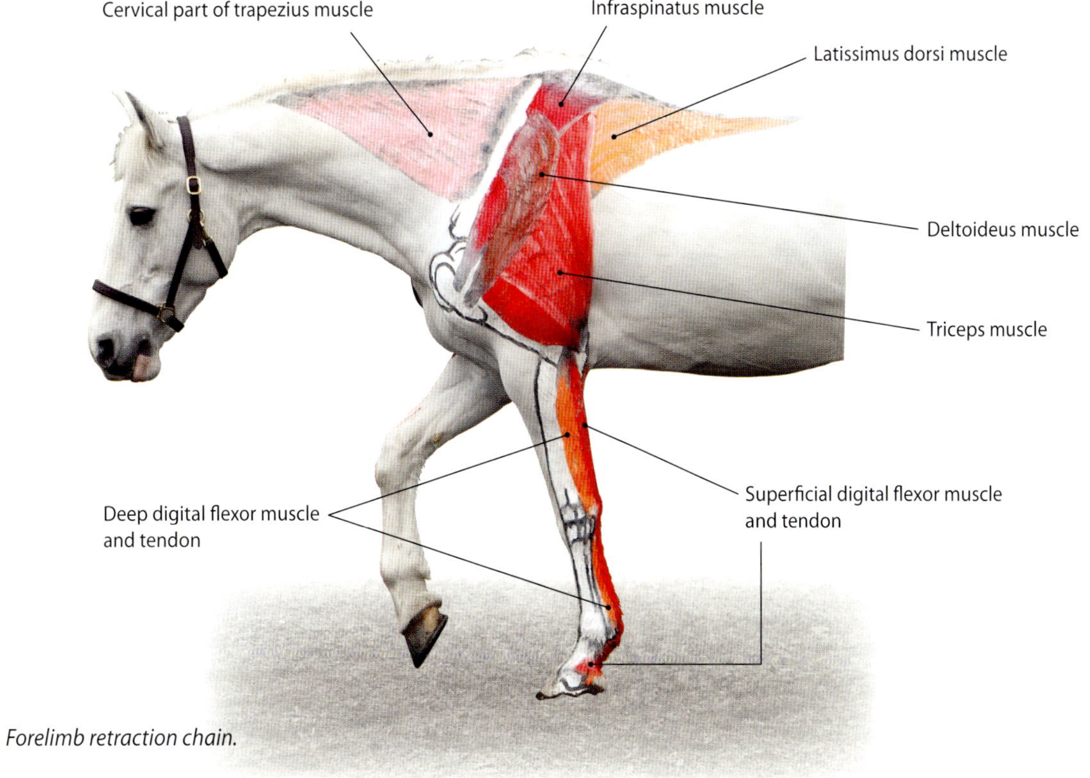


*Forelimb retraction chain.*

## SUMMARY

- The spine forms a bridge between the fore and hindlimbs.
- It transfers the forces created by the thrust of the hind end, supports the weight of the digestive system and carries the weight of the rider.
- The forelimb is connected to the spine by the thoracic sling muscles.
- The hindlimb is connected to the spine via the pelvis at the sacroiliac joint.
- Muscles work in pairs, groups of pairs and chains.
- The fascia surrounds, intertwines and links every muscle, bone, tendon, ligament, nerve, blood vessel and organ in the body forming full body continuity.
- If there is a restriction in any part of a muscle chain it will affect the movement in other areas of the body often far removed from the site of the original problem.

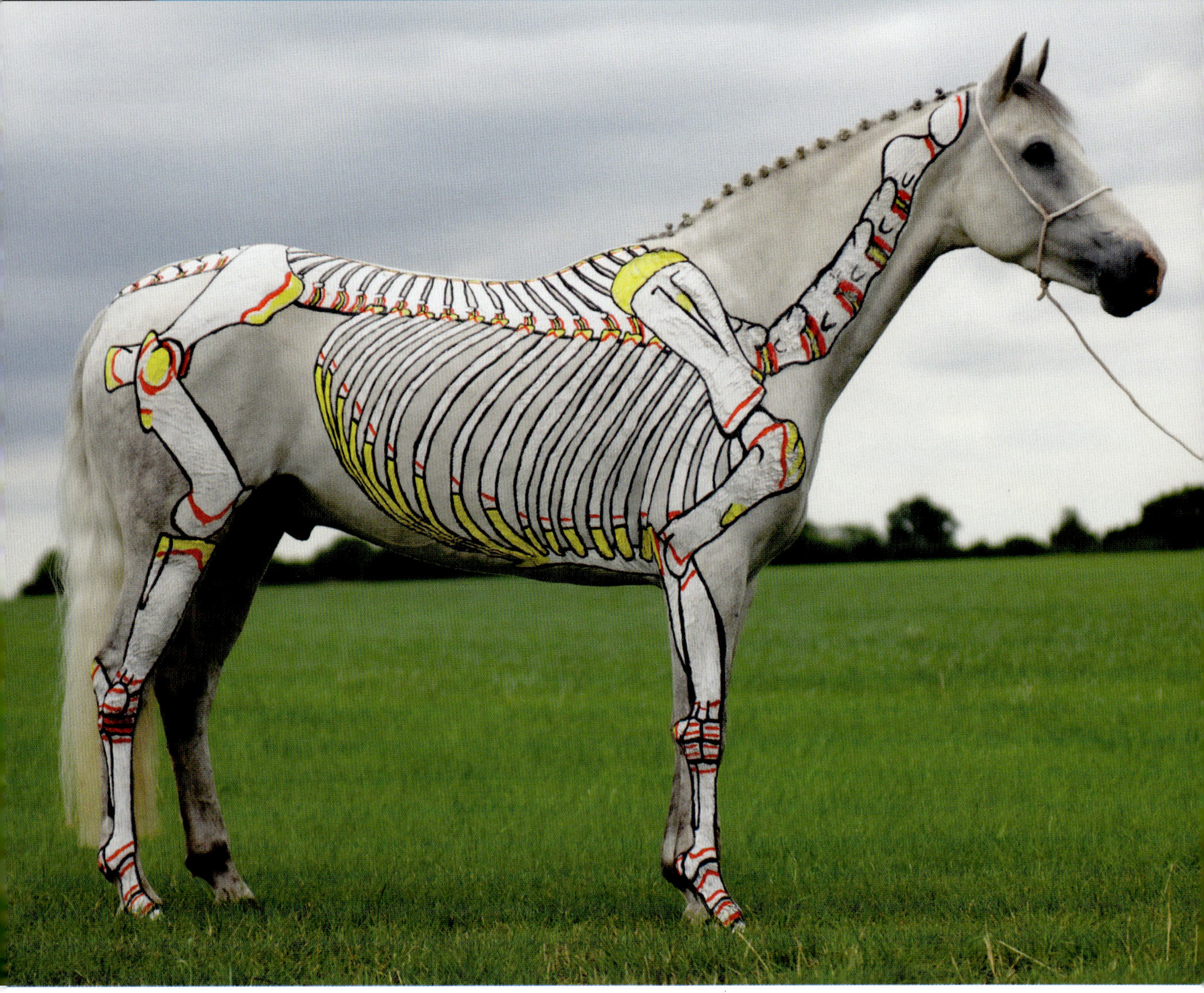

A strong, well-developed skeletal system is essential to ensure optimum structural support, limb soundness and to minimise the loading, strain and concussive forces imposed on bones and joint structures.

There are over 80 growth plates within the spine. These mature between 4 and 7 years. An important aspect of skeletal maturity is the timing and rate of maturation of the growth plates. These mature when the cartilage changes to bone and close from the hoof up. The coffin joint closes at birth, the

*The red lines on this painting indicate the location of growth plates in the horse's skeleton.*

short pastern between birth and 6 months and the scapula and pelvis, which has growth plates on the points of hip (tuber coxae), the peak of croup (tuber sacrale), and points of buttock (tuber ischii), between 5 and 5½ years. The hock does not fully mature until the horse is 4 years old and is often considered a weak link.

## HOW BONES GROW

**B**ones develop from mineralised cartilage which progressively hardens and ossifies as the horse matures. This occurs at the centre (diaphysis) and ends (epiphyses) of the future bone. Between these two points is another (metaphyseal) growth plate which allows the long bones to lengthen as the foal grows. At birth, the foal's skeleton contains approximately 20% of the mature bone mineral content, increasing to approximately 75% by the end of the first year.

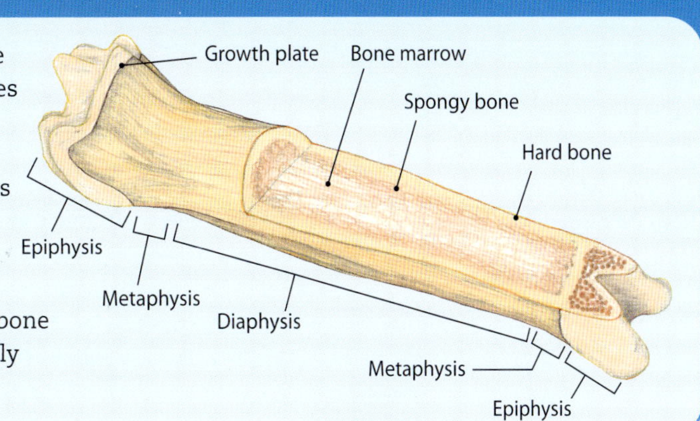


**Age at which forehand growth plates mature**

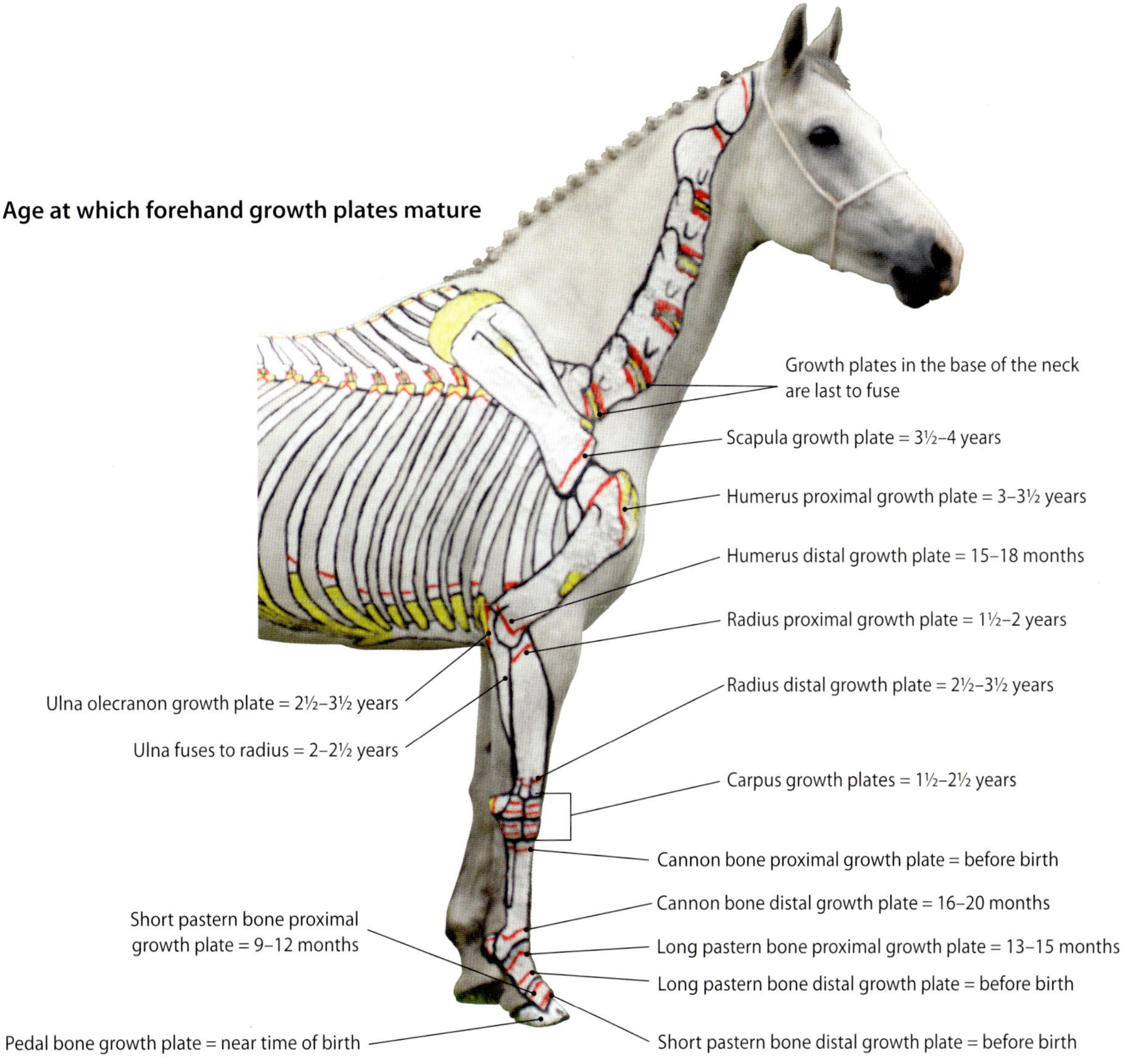

## Age at which hindlimb growth plates mature

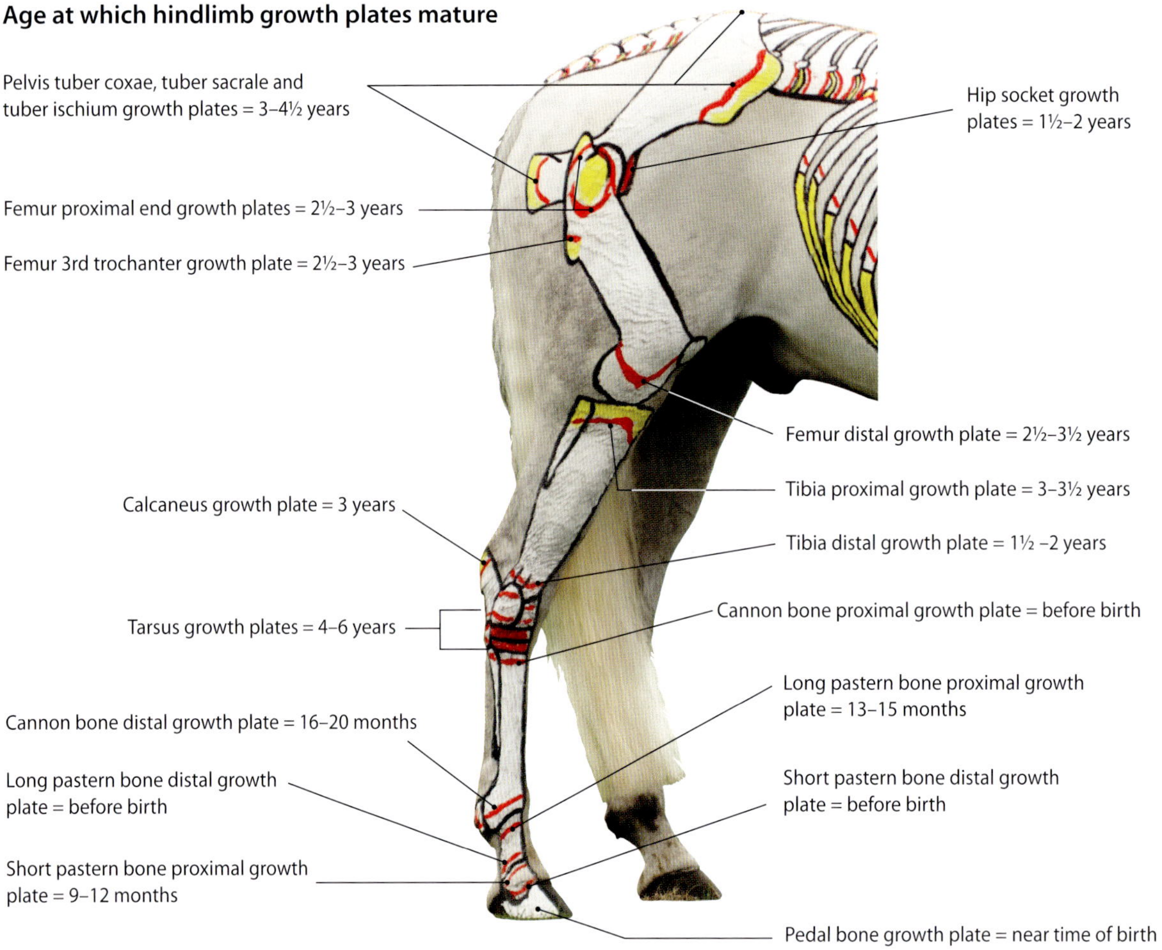

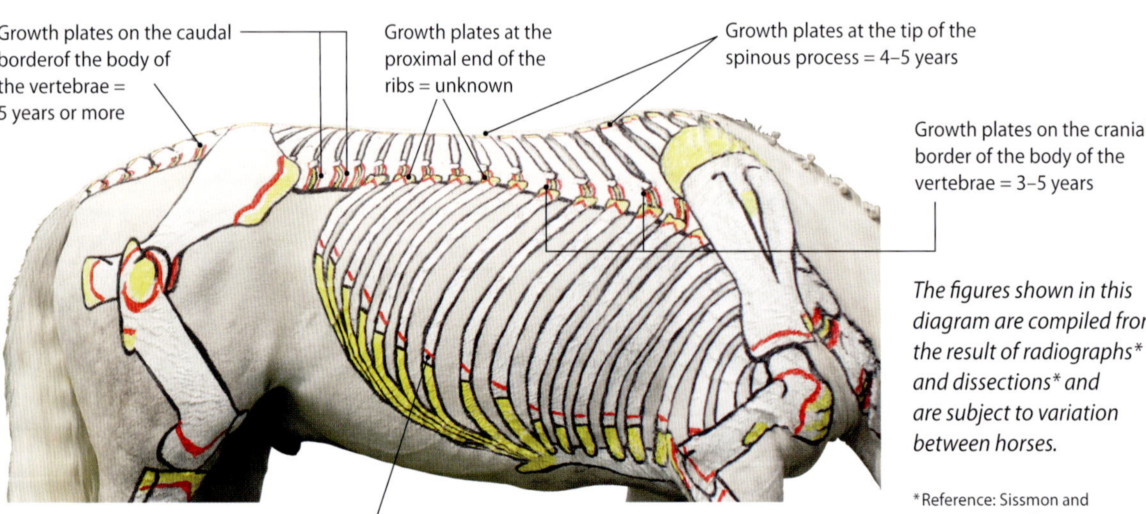


## Age at which axial skeleton growth plates mature



*The figures shown in this diagram are compiled from the result of radiographs* and dissections* and are subject to variation between horses.*

*Reference: Sissmon and Grossman, Dr Deb Bennet, Eric Strand and personal study.

## Sequence of Maturation

Although all horses follow the same pattern of skeletal maturity, nutrition, size and gender can affect the age of maturation. Male horses tend to mature 6 months later than mares and, the larger and better fed the horse, the later the maturation. Although most horses have finished growing in height around 5 years of age, the spine is not fully mature until up to 8 years.

The base of neck is the last area within the spine to fuse. The growth plates in the cervical vertebrae of a large 7-year-old Warmblood dressage horse will almost certainly not have completely fused. This means the neck is not fully skeletally mature and strong until the horse is 8 years old and is an important consideration when flexing the neck or selecting an appropriate outline for the horse's age and stage.

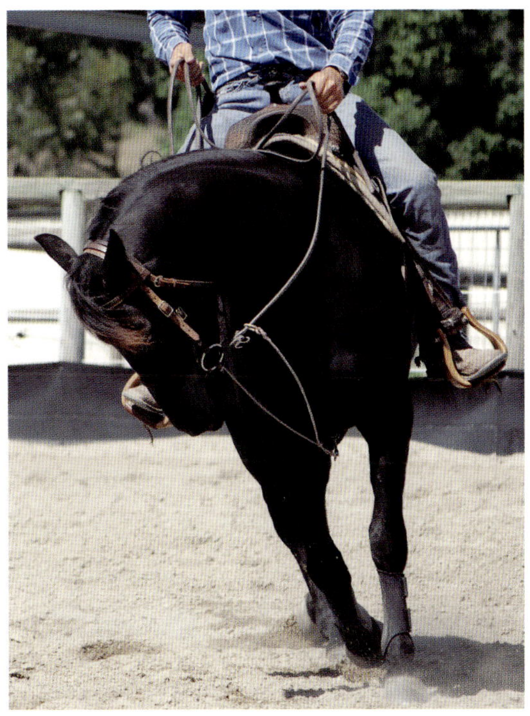

**RIGHT** *This 3-year-old skeletally immature Western horse is being ridden in an inappropriate outline. This will have a detrimental effect on his future posture and musculoskeletal health.*

## Too Much Too Soon!

Forces and impact on immature bones can reach unacceptably high levels in young horses doing too much too soon. The tendency of unsoundness, particularly in young competition horses, can be linked to excessive concussive forces on immature bone and joint structures which struggle to adapt as the horse increases in weight. A horse galloping at speed exerts many times its body weight as force on the lower limb and although the limbs are supported by muscles, tendons and ligaments it is ultimately the bones which bear the brunt of the force.

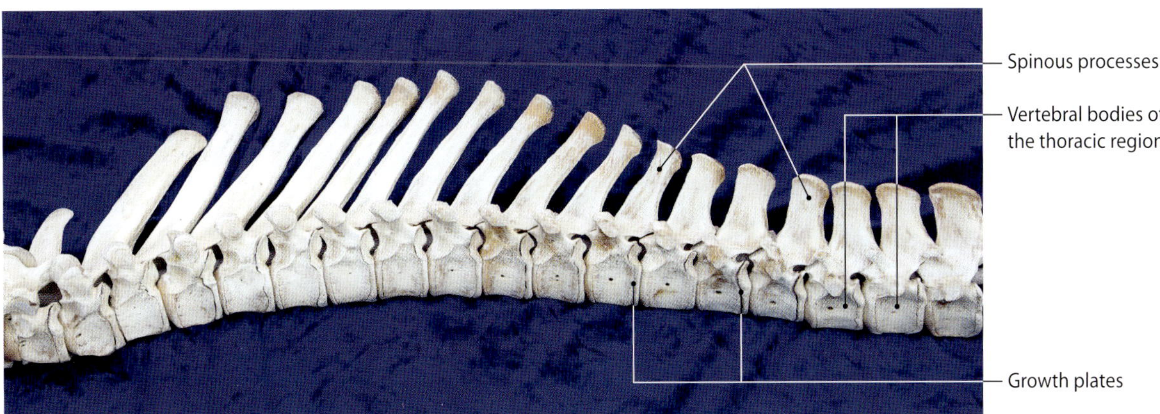


*This spine from a 4-year-old horse clearly shows the immature growth plates running perpendicular to the ground. Carrying excessive weight, being ridden in a poor posture or for unacceptably long periods before these plates close can adversely affect development and lead to problems as the horse matures.*

# Managing Young, Skeletally Immature Horses

Young horses are generally well balanced and move naturally with good posture. As humans intervene freedom of movement is curtailed and the youngster begins his training, this can change and early compensation patterns begin to emerge. These have an influence on how the horse moves, carries himself and performs.

Early influences by human intervention include:
- Restriction of liberty
- Hoof trimming
- Familiarisation with tack
- Dentistry
- Injury and trauma
- Carrying weight.

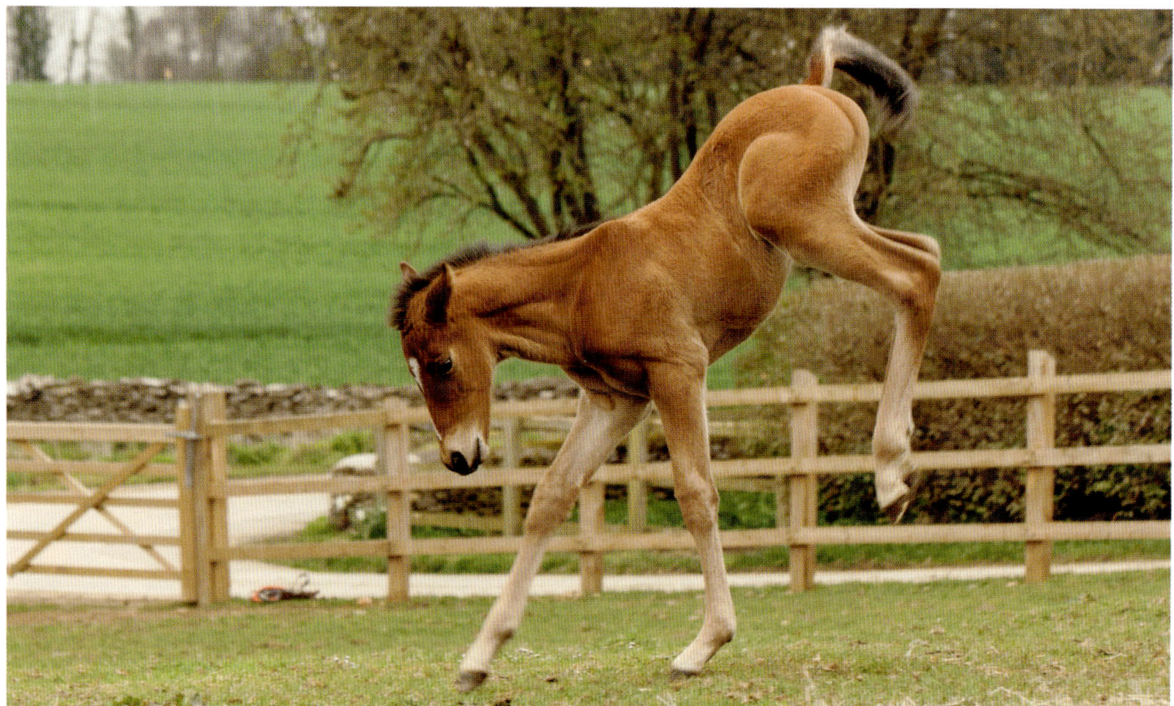

**ABOVE** *It is important that growing horses have access to free field exercise for optimum musculoskeletal development.*

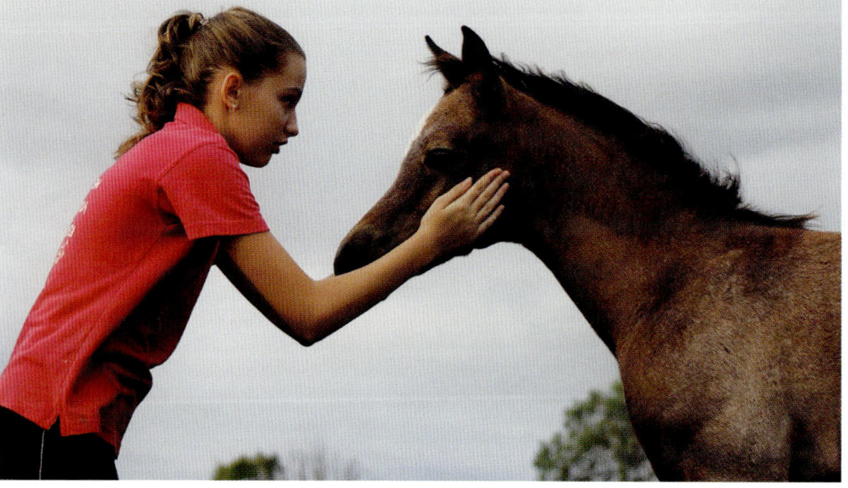

**LEFT** *To foster trust, understanding, cooperation and partnership it is important that every contact with a human is positive and correct.*

There are a significant number of beneficial activities which can be practised before the horse is skeletally mature and which will prepare him for his future work. These include:

- Handling and leading from both sides
- Appropriate 'Pilates' type core strengthening, stretching, posture and balance exercises
- Lungeing and long-reining
- Groundwork exercises
- Pole work
- Loading

- Accepting a light burden
- Mild exercise on a variety of slopes, surfaces and terrain
- Slowly increasing the time handled or worked to build muscular and cardiovascular fitness.

Racehorses and some horses used for futurity competitions are started before they are skeletally mature, sometimes between 18 and 24 months, but for most horses not destined for this type of competition 4 is a safer and more sensible age to start placing weight on the back.

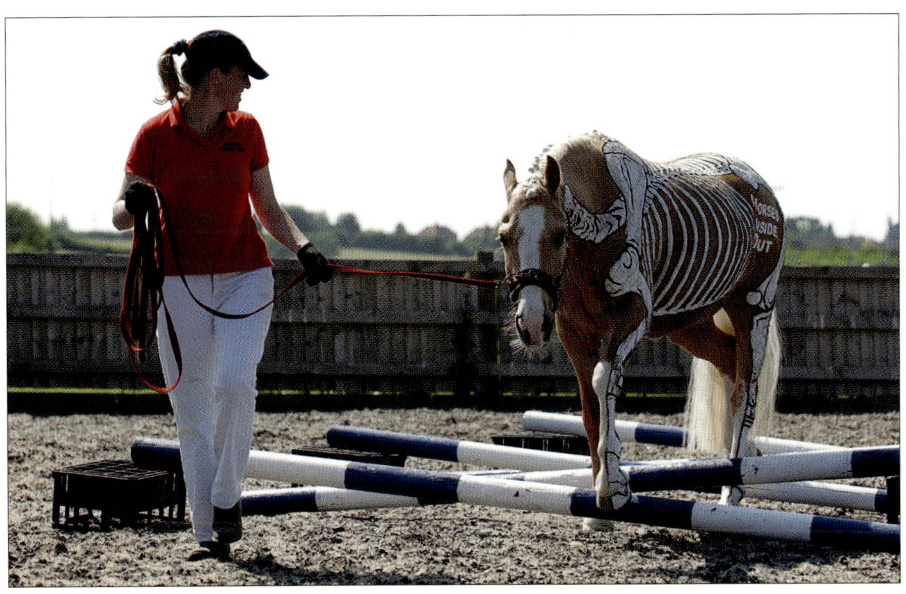


**LEFT** *Build up muscular strength slowly. Only work for very short periods of time (10 minutes is enough to start with). As a rule of thumb work a 4-year-old no more than four times a week and a 5-year-old five times per week.*

## SUMMARY

- The later we can start riding our horses and the more preparation and conditioning we can do beforehand the better.
- When starting a young horse it is important to ensure he constantly works in a good posture.
- Avoid expecting the horse to carry too much weight for too long or too often.
- Avoid working him when he is tired.
- Understanding the maturation of growth plates can help reduce the strain we put on joints, enable us to train more sympathetically and make informed decisions about the type of movements we ask of our horses, how often and for how long we train.

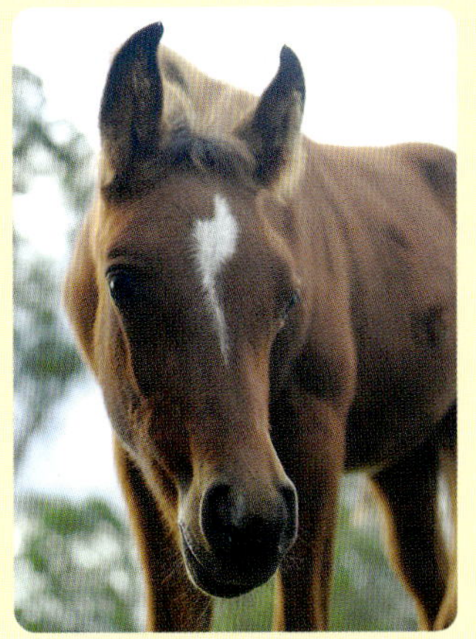

# 3 Principles of Posture

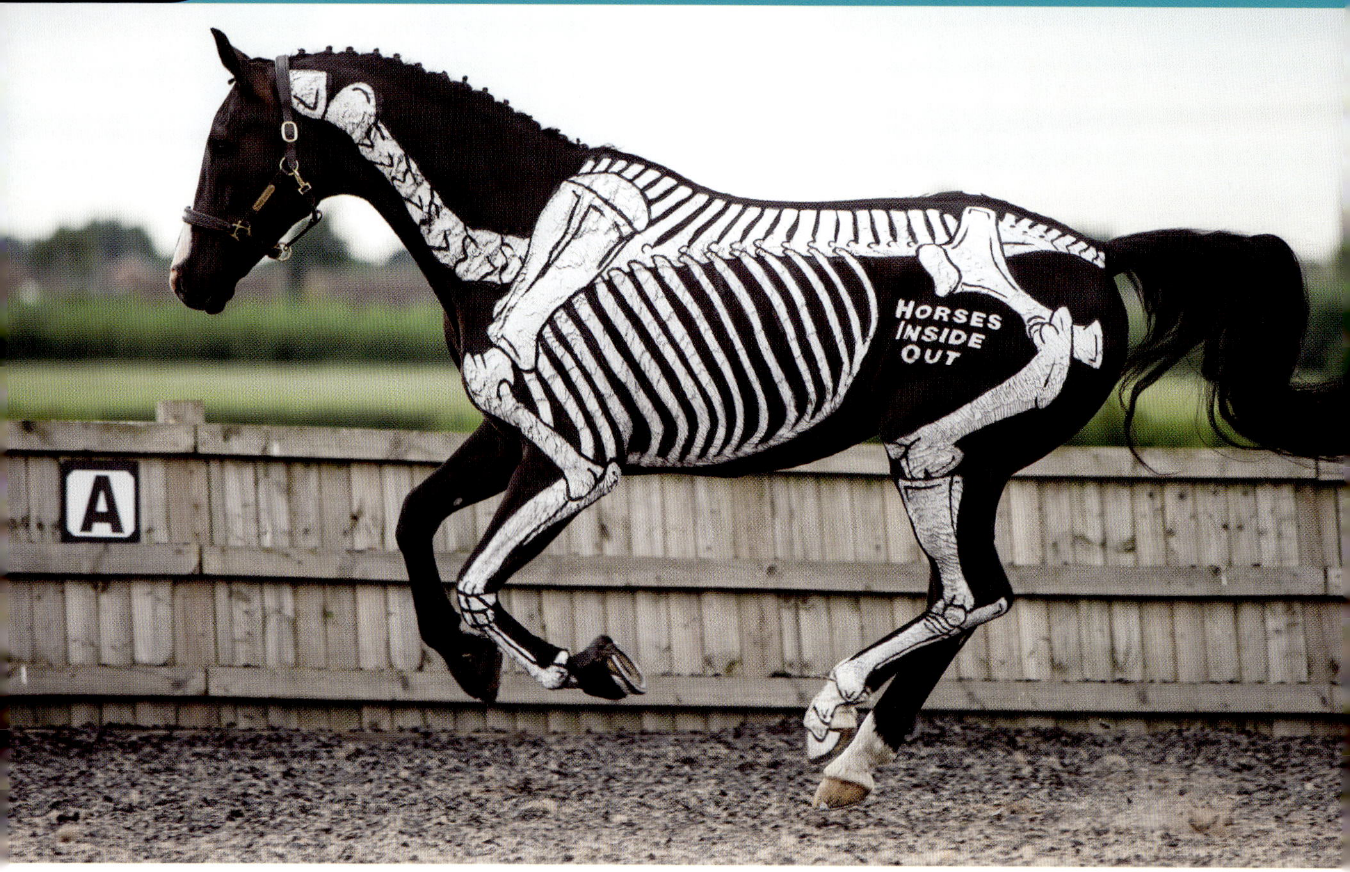

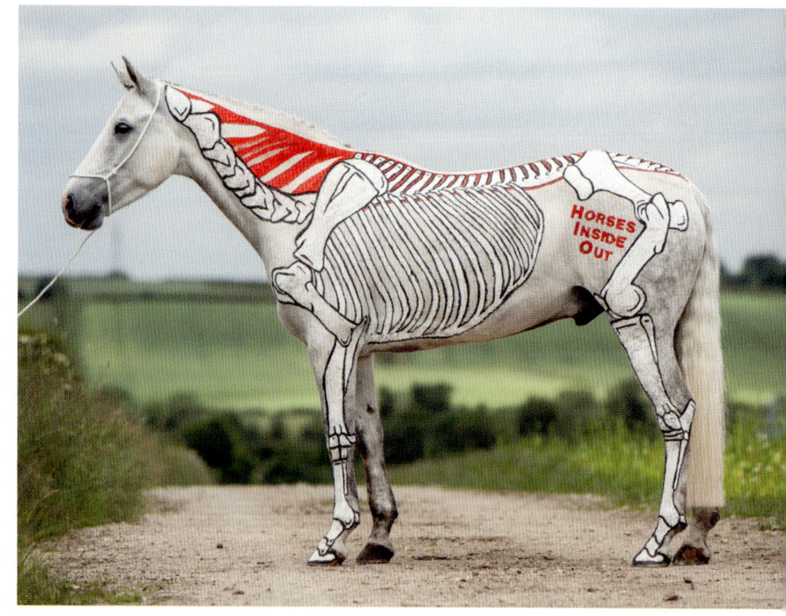

**ABOVE** *Maintaining good posture is an essential part of good horsemanship which will ensure comfort and well-being.*

Posture is the position in which the body is held. It is a dynamic relationship, maintained through a harmonious muscular and skeletal balance where each joint is correctly aligned and each muscle is working efficiently and correctly. In the moving horse, posture is concerned with self-carriage and optimum balance. Without good balance the horse cannot carry himself comfortably, gracefully and efficiently.

**RIGHT** *When standing square the weight should be evenly distributed around the centre of mass both from front to back and side to side.*

# What's so Important about Posture?

Good posture is vital for every ridden horse. It can be influenced by training and affects functional health. Maintaining it is an essential part of good horsemanship. It is a contributory factor in ensuring comfort and well-being, allows the horse to move with ease, efficiency and energy, puts a 'spring in his step' and extends his working life. Without good posture it is not possible to be truly physically fit and allow the horse to reach his full potential.

## Posture versus conformation

Conformation cannot be changed. It is determined by the skeletal structure, the characteristics of breed, genetics and how the horse is put together. If he is born with a long back, a sloping shoulder or short pasterns this will remain so. Conformation may sometimes *appear* to change; for example if the horse develops more muscle his back or topline may look different but the underlying anatomical structure will always remain the same.

Each discipline has different postural requirements but irrespective of breed, conformation or type, good posture makes the best of the horse's conformation. It is our responsibility to think of ourselves as personal trainers to our horses. This includes looking after every aspect of their well-being in general and their posture in particular.

## Benefits of good posture

Good posture suggests good health. Aesthetically it looks pleasing and anatomically it's important for the efficient functioning of the body. It:

- Keeps bones and joints correctly aligned to enable the correct functioning of the musculoskeletal system during all weight-bearing activities
- Minimises abnormal wear of joint surfaces that can result in premature degeneration
- Decreases stress on ligaments, tendons and fascia
- Prevents the back becoming fixed in an over-extended position
- Ensures muscles are used efficiently and effectively
- Reduces strain and overuse
- Allows optimum functioning of the internal organs
- Allows nervous system to work at optimal efficiency.

## Poor posture

Poor posture can be defined as any alignment that deviates from the ideal. Assuming a stressed position for a brief moment is not in itself a problem. The danger arises from cumulative effects which, if maintained over long periods, can have a detrimental effect on soft tissue. This can lead to biomechanically inefficient movement where even the most basic movements become tiring and uncomfortable. It can potentially affect demeanour and behaviour, lead to unsatisfactory training sessions, and result in frustration on the part of the rider.

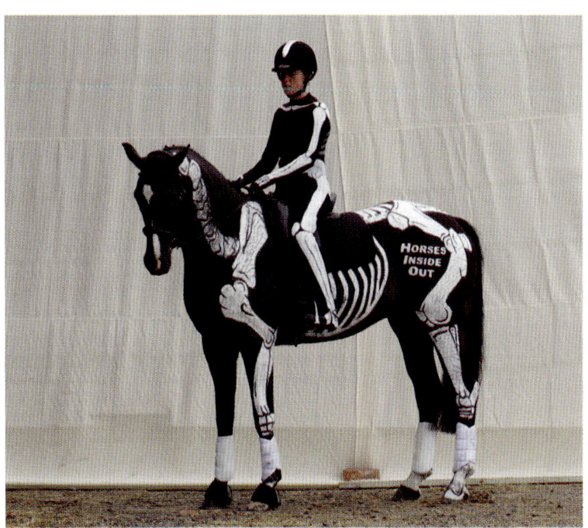


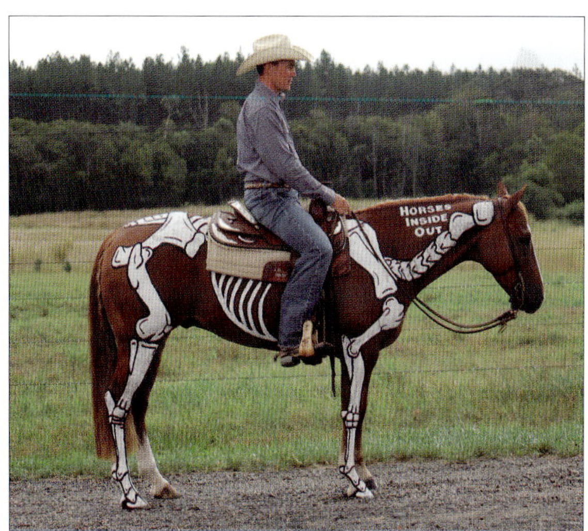


*Each discipline has different postural requirements.*

Factors that can contribute to poor posture are:

- Obesity
- Poor hoof balance
- Dental discomfort
- Poorly balanced or unskilled riders
- Carrying too heavy a rider for too long
- Lack of fitness
- Working in an inappropriate outline for the age and stage
- Psychological tension, negative tension and resistance
- Immobility where horses are stabled for long periods with lack of space in which to move
- Constantly eating out of a high hay rack
- Pain.

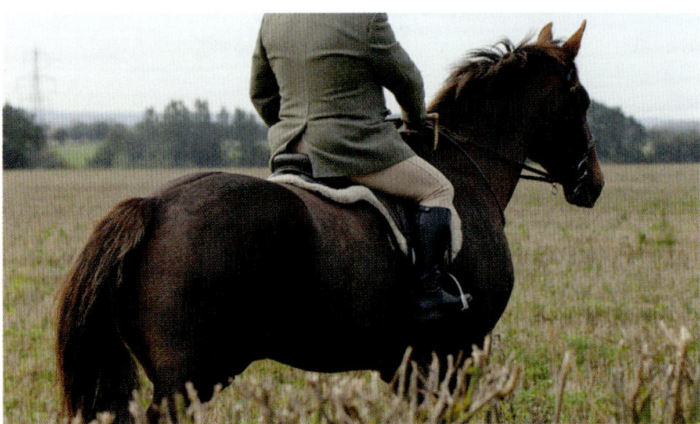

*As soon as a rider sits on the horse's back, the increase in gravitational force causes the back to extend. This horse is coping with both the weight of the rider from above and over-condition from below. In this case it is vital that the rider does everything in her power to support the spine.*

## Spinal Curves

One important indicator of posture is spinal curves. These are natural curves within the horse's spine. When referring to the curves, we are referring to the level of vertebral bodies and not the topline which can be influenced by the musculature.

1. The cervical vertebrae create an 'S' shape allowing the neck to protract and retract rather like a telescope. This enables the positioning of the head and neck to influence posture. At the top of the neck the cervical vertebrae curve upwards (dorsally concave). From mid-neck the curve changes direction with a dorsally convex curve. The thoracolumbar section of the spine should be straight or slightly curved upwards (dorsally concave).

2. When the upper curve rounds (flexes) and the lower curve hollows (extends) this shortens the neck.

3. When the neck elongates the upper and lower cervical curves flatten out.

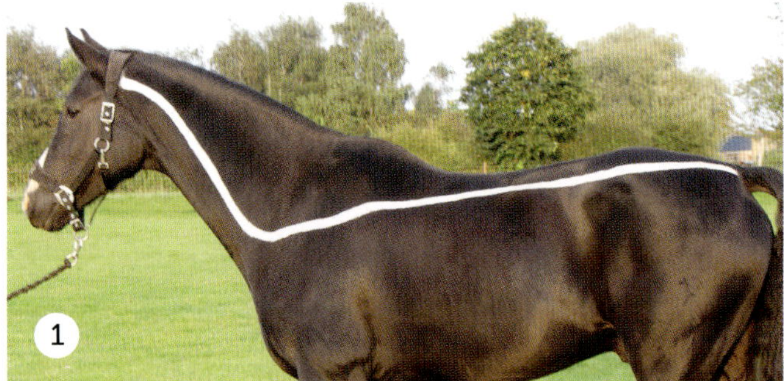

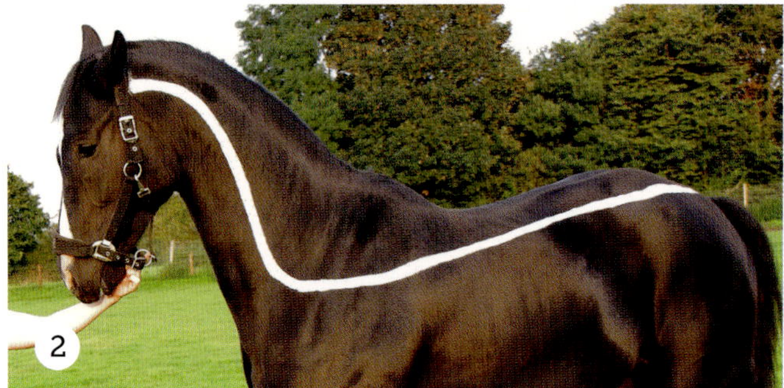

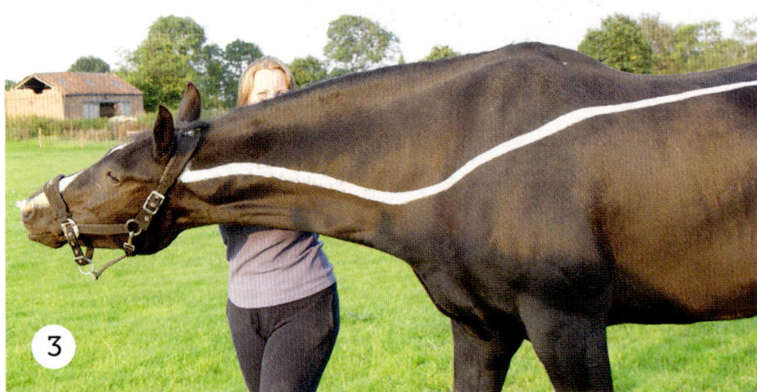

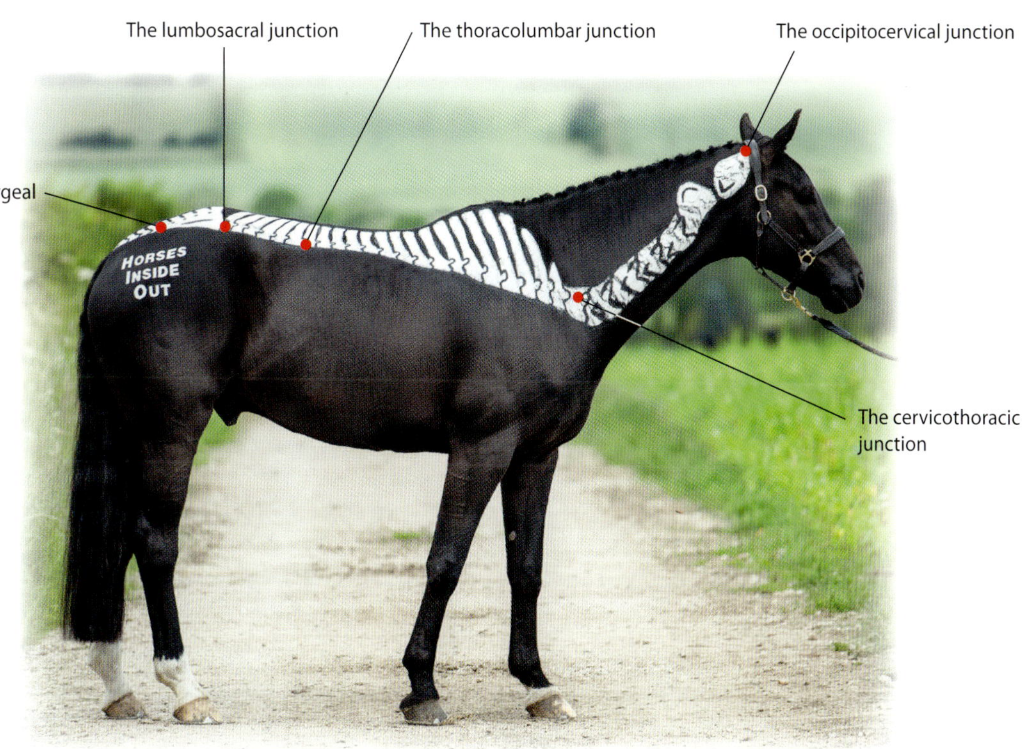



*This horse is illustrating basic good posture with well-positioned spinal curves.*

## Spinal junctions are key for posture

A spinal junction is the joint between the different sections of the spine. Their efficient functioning is fundamental to good posture. At each junction there is a change in the mechanics, anatomical configuration and amount of movement of the vertebrae.

Spinal curves are influenced by:

- Gravity
- Muscle development, fitness and tone
- The weight of the rider
- The weight of the digestive system
- Age.

The four mechanisms used by the horse to maintain good posture (see page 36) are also applicable to maintaining the optimum position of the spinal curves.

One of the most common poor postural positions is extension through the thoraco lumbar region. This detrimental posture, which is so well illustrated in this picture (see right), is coupled with a more extended curve through the base of neck (protraction through the cervicothoracic junction) and a more extended lumbosacral junction. This position will be uncomfortable for the horse, put strain through the joints of the spine and hindlimbs and add weight to the forelimb. These effects will be exacerbated in the immature horse where the growth plates of the spine are not yet fully fused.

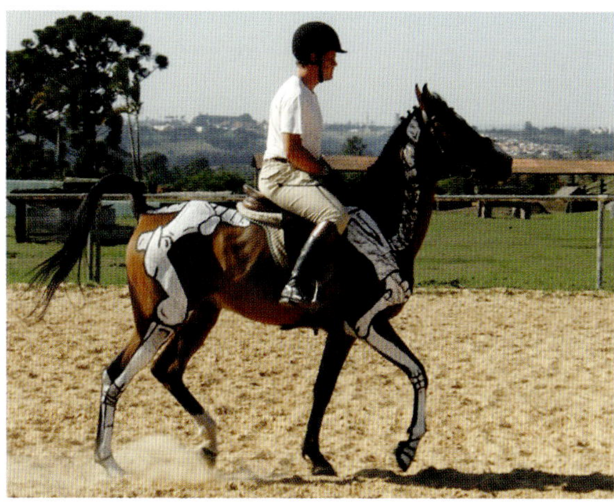

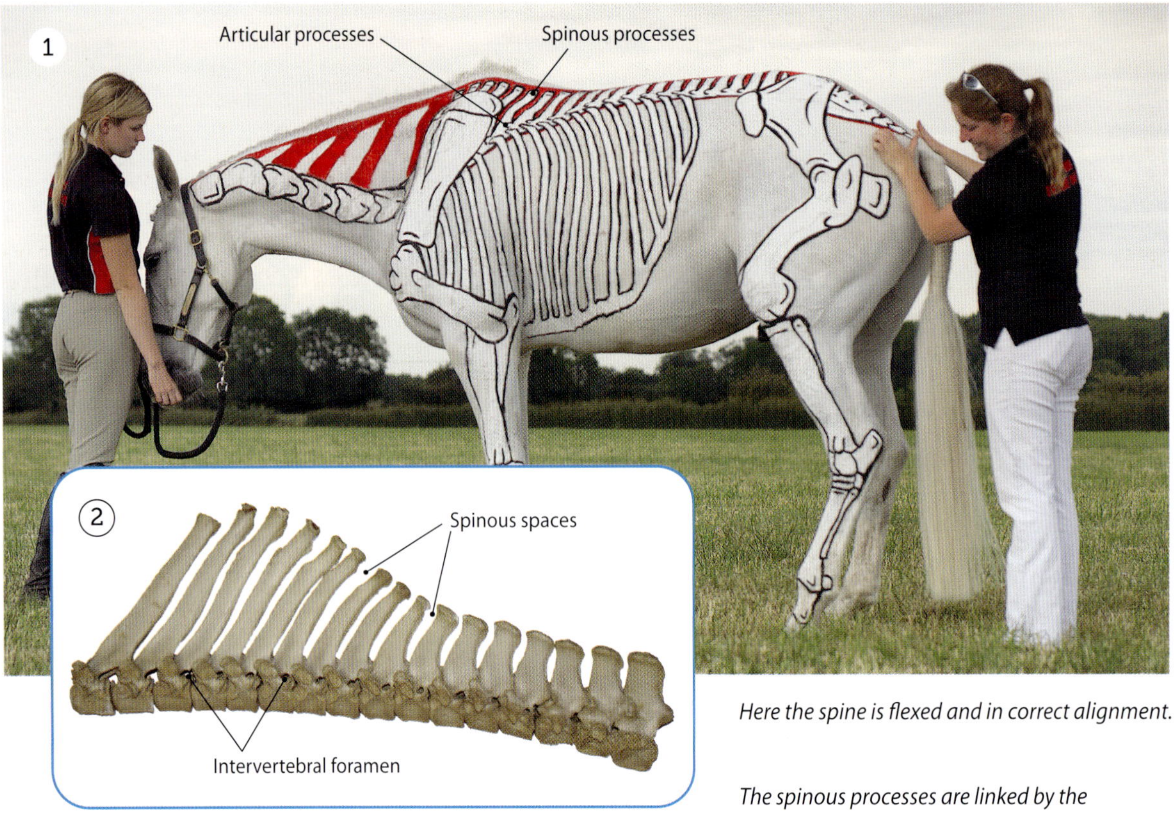

*Here the spine is flexed and in correct alignment.*

*The spinous processes are linked by the intraspinous ligament between them and the supraspinous ligament along the tops. In a normal fully flexed thoracolumbar spine (picture 1 and 2), the spaces between the spinous processes range approximately from 1mm to 7mm. When the spine is held in an extended position, the spaces reduce, increasing pressure on the intraspinous ligaments and causing the spinous processes themselves to support weight (picture 3 and 4). Over time this scenario may lead to kissing spines.*

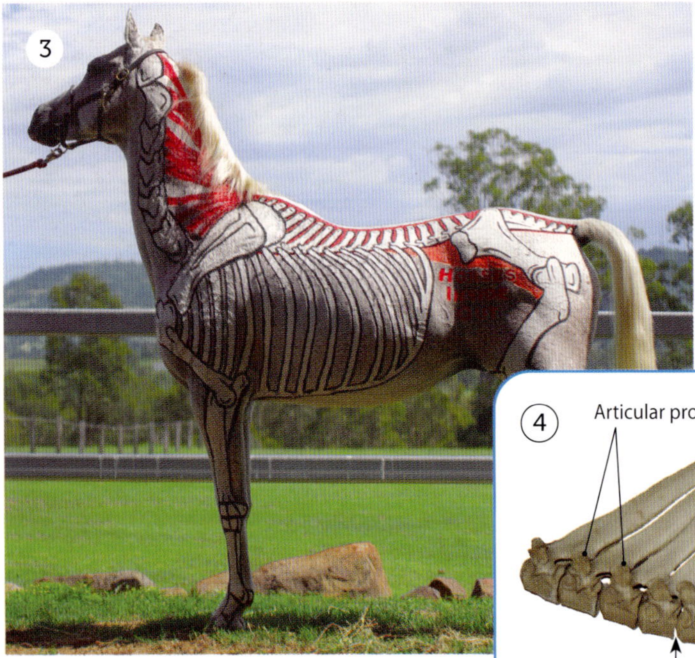

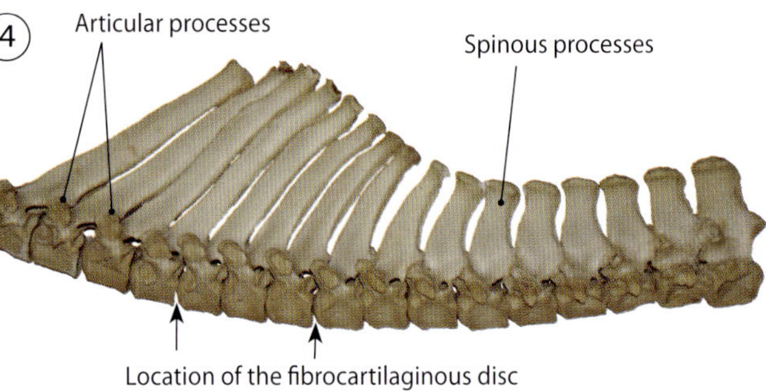


*Here the spinous processes are brought together as a result of poor extension and posture.*

# Some Examples of Posture from Different Angles

## Posture viewed from above

When the horse is standing square the spine should be straight, potentially making it easier to work evenly on both reins. Any curves in the spine indicate a spiral compensation pattern and alterations in muscle length on the right or left side. The dorsal stripe and position of the ribs on this horse indicates a slight curve to the right, suggesting he may find it easier to work on the right rein.

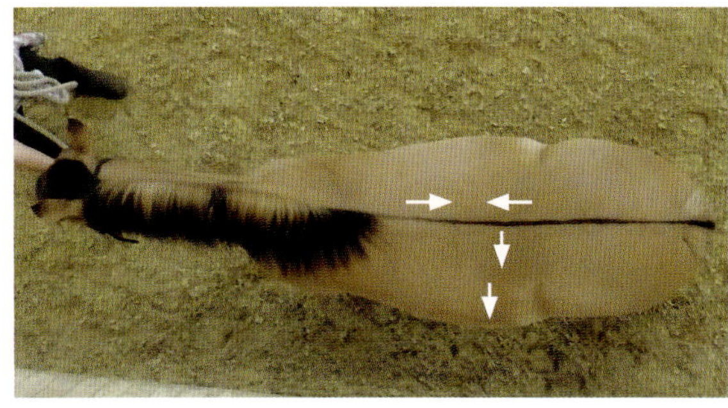

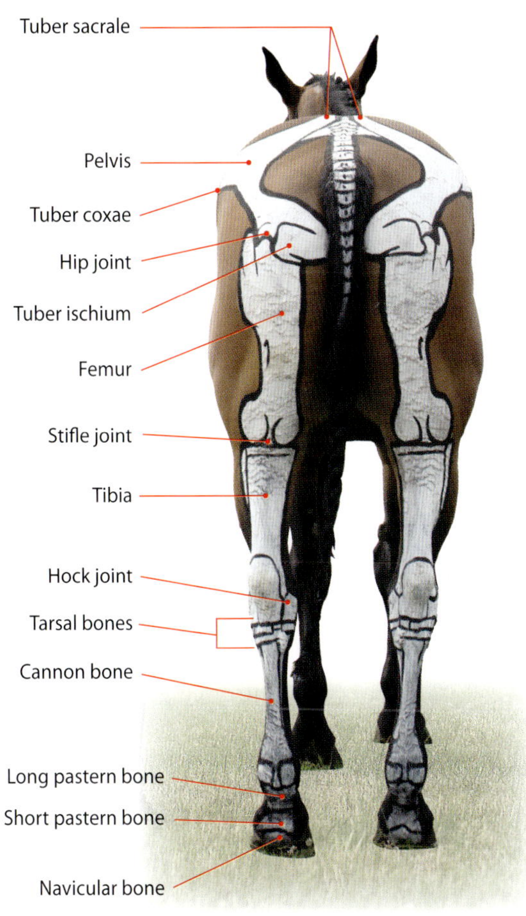


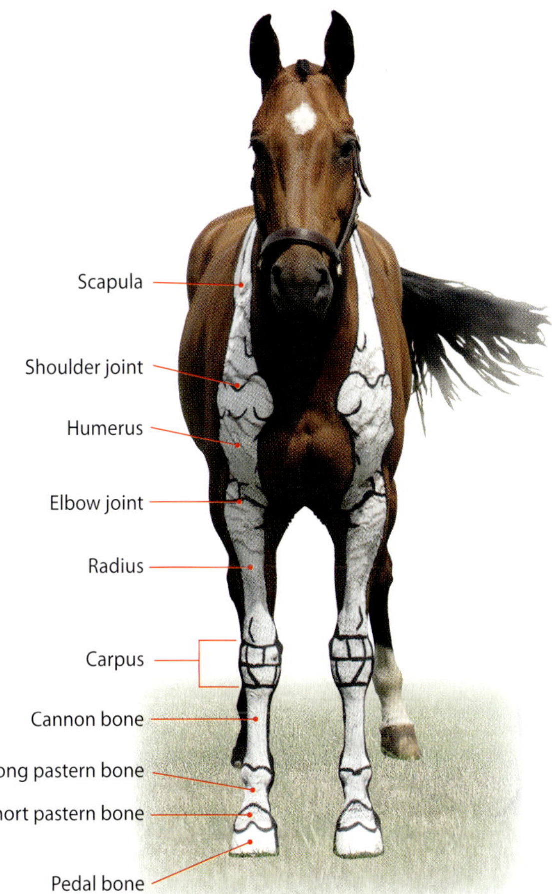


## Posture viewed from behind

When the horse is standing square, the weight should be evenly distributed and all the postural markers should be parallel and symmetrical. A horse with an asymmetrical spinal and hindlimb posture is more likely to show a difference in protraction and asymmetry in the flight arcs of his hind feet.

## Posture viewed from in front

This horse is displaying good posture. shoulder elbow and carpus bones are all in line. There is even distribution of weight and near symmetrical development of the pectoral muscles and forelimb joints.

# Effects of Poor Posture

## Skeleton and bones

Poor posture can lead to mis-alignment of the spine, subject muscles and joints to unnecessary stress, damage the supporting connective tissue and cause long-term pain.

Unnatural or uneven concussive forces as a result of poor posture can also precipitate bony or arthritic changes and can turn cartilage to bone. This can be laid down in the form of side bone, spurs or splints. Horses that tend to work on the forehand will have increased forces through the forelimb, making bony changes more likely and leading to a reduction in range of movement. See right, above and below.

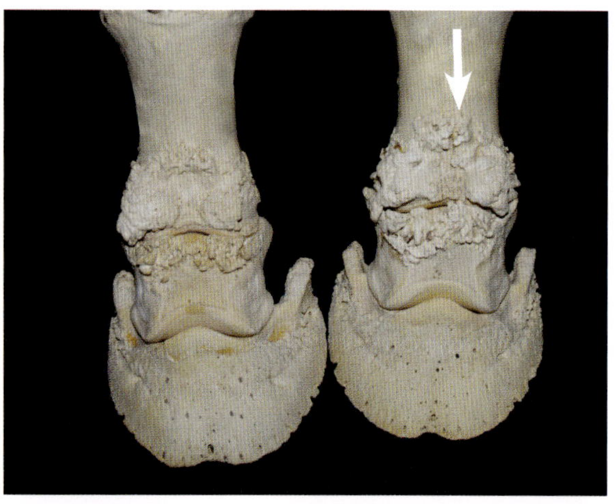

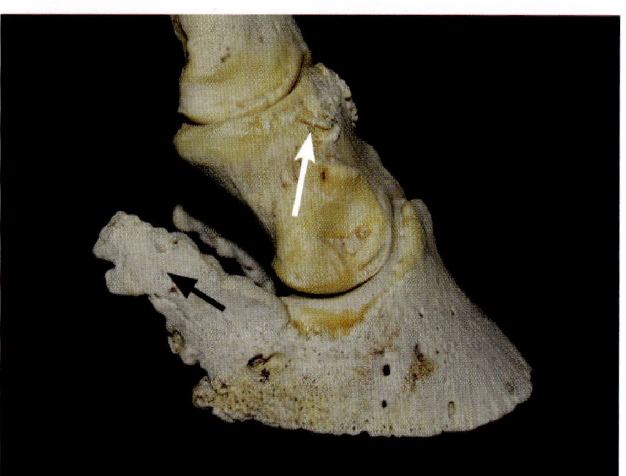

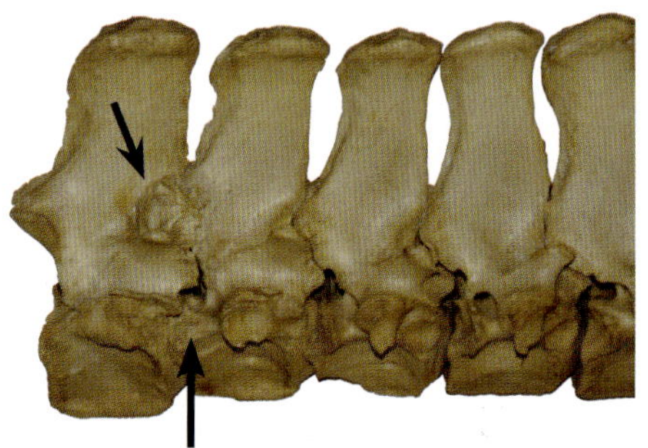

*In this photograph extra bone has developed around the vertebral bodies and facet joints.*

## WHAT ARE KISSING SPINES?

**K**issing spines or spinal impingement, is a common cause of back pain. It is often posture-related and most commonly occurs in the caudal thoracic section of the spine – the area on which we sit. As the spinous processes come closer together the intraspinous ligament is compressed and extra bone is laid down, causing them to fuse or even overlap. Onset is insidious, presenting as deterioration in performance or a progressive unwillingness to work. In some cases 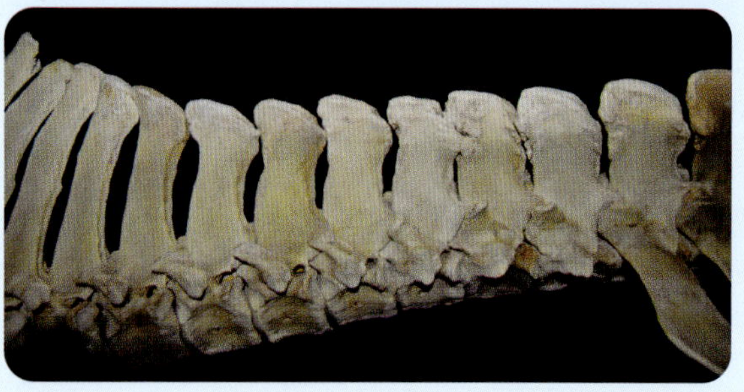 the condition is congenital but generally it is seen more in athletic, dressage, event and competition horses. This is possibly as a result of the greater physical demands placed on them. It may go unnoticed in horses used for hacking and low-level work. If kissing spines is suspected this can be verified by X-ray. Depending on the severity, treatment may range from training exercises, to drug therapy or, as a last resort, surgery.

## The effect of poor posture on muscles

Soft tissue damage is the most common cause of back pain in horses. Poor posture can alter muscle length and tone. This makes some muscles short and tight and others long and weak. Clear neural pathways develop so that the overused muscles are habitually recruited and the underused muscles weakened. This can lead to muscle overdevelopment (hypertrophy), muscle loss (atrophy), altered joint kinematics, faulty movement patterns and a cycle of poor posture and muscular imbalance.

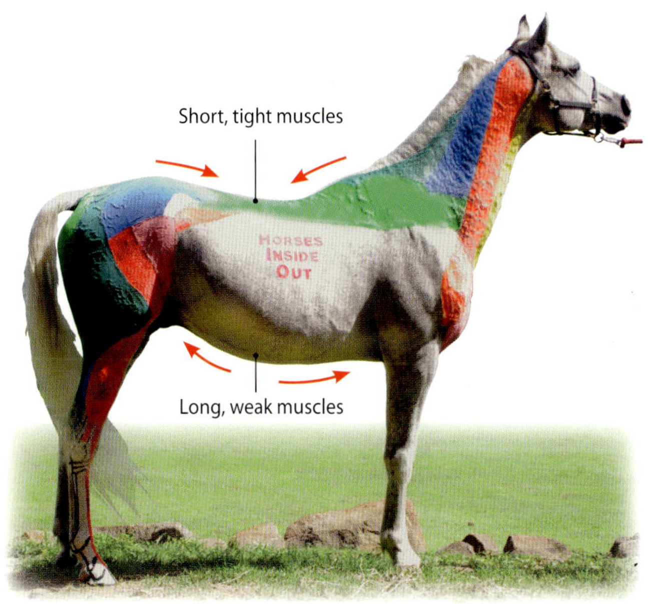


*RIGHT In this horse the longissimus dorsi, the main back extensor muscle, is short, tight and stiff; the abdominal muscles have lengthened, weakened and atrophied and the back is poorly supported.*

## The effect of poor posture on fascia

Because of its continuous nature, the fact that the fibres are laid down along the lines of tension and the manner in which it surrounds and permeates the muscles, fascia is influenced by and plays an important role in body positioning and posture. If a muscle is tight the fascia becomes restricted. This interconnectivity can affect the positioning of the muscle chains and even the joints. Once the fascia becomes restricted it can limit range of movement, flexibility and can hold the body in altered postural positions which will, in some cases, become ingrained as the norm.

*RIGHT An experienced therapist will be able to assess and identify which muscles are long and weak, which are short and tight, perform appropriate myofascial release and soft tissue therapy and suggest a relevant, manageable programme of stretching, suppling and ridden exercises.*

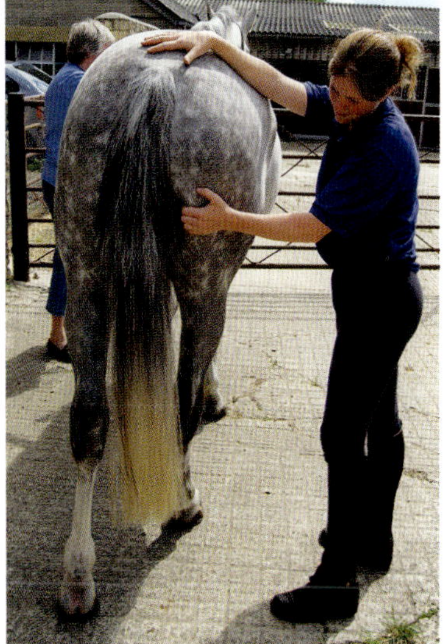

*BELOW Tension within muscles can affect blood circulation.*

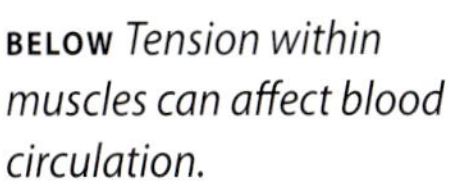

## The effect of poor posture on circulation

Tension within muscles can result in reduced blood circulation. This can affect metabolism, the supply of oxygen, the efficient delivery of energy derived from food groups as well as the removal of waste products such as broken cells, toxins and lactic acid. Lack of blood supply can increase the risk of muscle fatigue, microtrauma within the muscle fibres and contribute to delayed onset muscle soreness and the overuse syndrome.

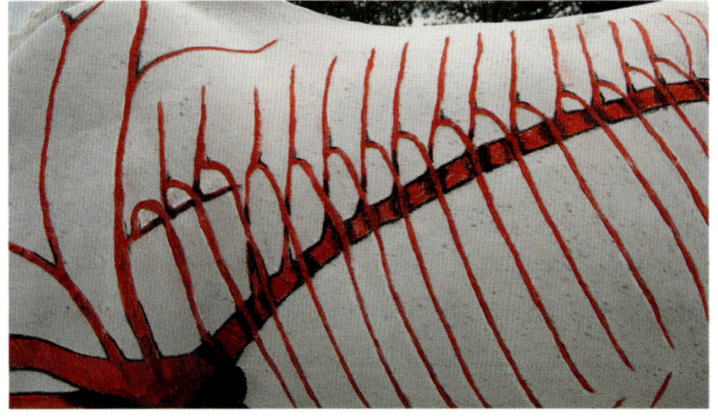

## The effect of poor posture on spinal nerves

The nervous system is the complex central computer which controls actions, voluntary and involuntary reactions, reflexes, the senses, feeling, response to the environment, behaviour and movement.

## The effect of poor posture on general health

In some cases, poor posture can cause constriction and affect the efficient functioning of the internal organs and digestive system. It can also upset the delicate balance of enzymes, nutrients, toxins and level of hydration within tissues at a cellular level.

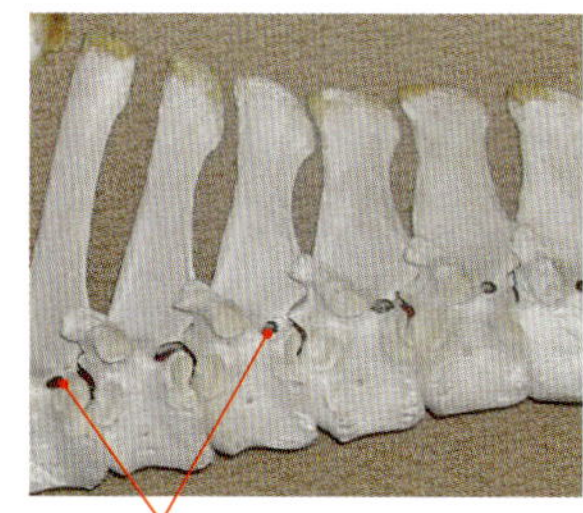
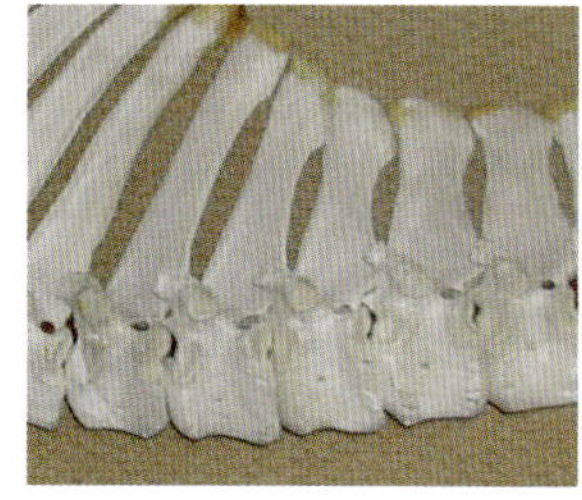

Intervertebral foramen

The spinal cord and nerves which relay information between the brain and the rest of the body are housed within the spine. Between each vertebra is a small hole, the intervertebral foramen, through which the spinal nerves pass. If the spine is over-extended, the diameter of the intervertebral foramen become restricted and it is possible for the spinal nerves to become pinched.

# Supporting Posture

There are four main mechanisms that maintain posture and support the weight of the rider. Understanding them will enable the rider to train more effectively.

1. Positioning of the head and neck

2. Positioning of the hind legs

3. Positioning of the thorax

4. Contribution of the flexor chain of muscles.

# 1. Positioning of the head and neck

The positioning of the head and neck is dependent on conformation, the biomechanical function of the spinal ligament system, muscle strength and condition. Understanding the mechanics of the spinal ligaments is useful for riders and trainers.

### The spinal ligament system

The spinal ligaments that have the greatest influence on posture and the positioning of the back are the nuchal, supraspinous and dorsal sacroiliac ligaments.

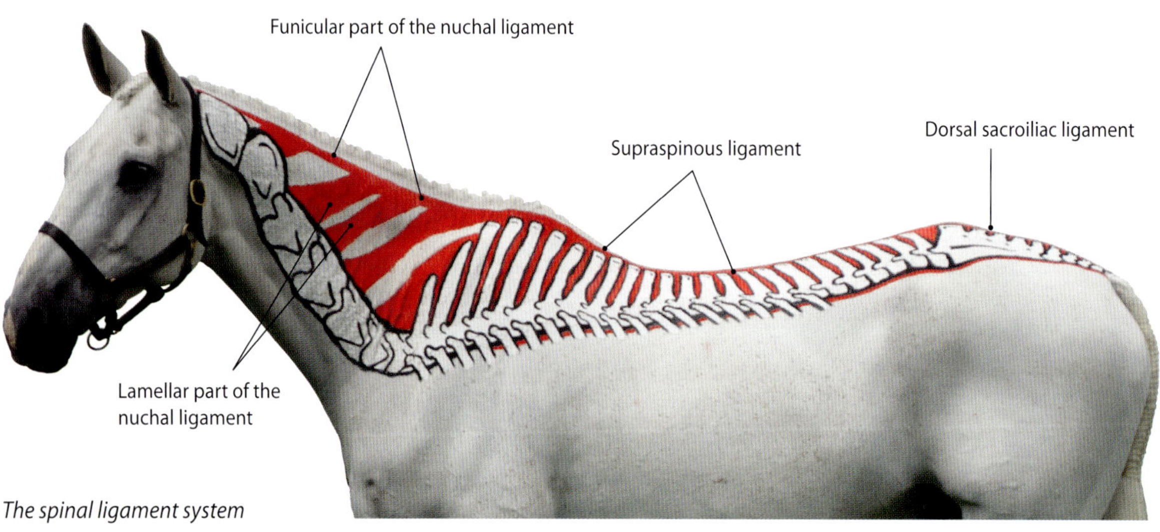


*The spinal ligament system*

Consisting of two parts, the strong, elastic nuchal ligament (NL) minimises muscular effort and is one of the most important structures in the horse's body. The funicular part runs from the occipital bone at the poll, underneath the fatty nuchal crest and attaches onto the spinous processes of the withers. The lamellar part consists of fan-like sheets of ligamental connective tissue which originate in the withers and funicular part of the ligament and attach onto the cervical vertebrae. The supraspinous ligament (SL), a continuation of the NL, continues in a less elastic form linking the tops of the spinous processes of the withers, thoracic and lumbar vertebrae. The dorsal sacroiliac ligament (DSL), a continuation of the SL, attaches to the tops of the sacral vertebrae, tuber sacrale and caudal vertebrae.

## How the spinal ligaments work

The main function of the NL is to support the head and neck, assist the work of the upper neck muscles and support the back. In a long and low outline, grazing stance, or as the cervical vertebrae flex, the NL becomes taut. Using the spinous processes of the withers as a fulcrum, this pulls on the SL which then raises the back, provides strength and stability, supports the weight of the rider and contributes to good posture.

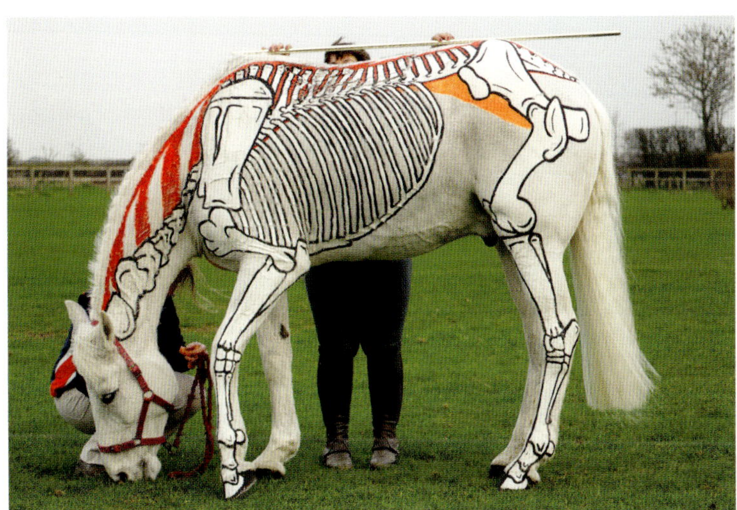

**LEFT** *When the head is down, tension in the NL and SL increases. This raises and supports the back.*

**LEFT, BELOW** *When the head is raised above the level of the withers, the NL and SL become slack, causing the back to hollow.*

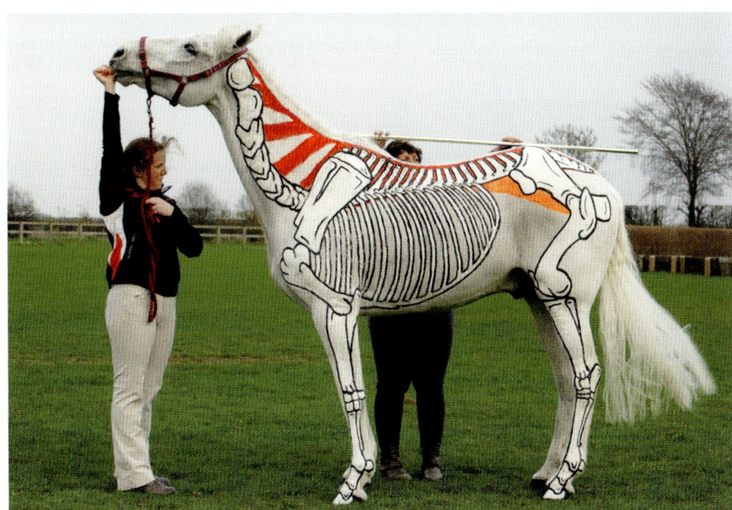

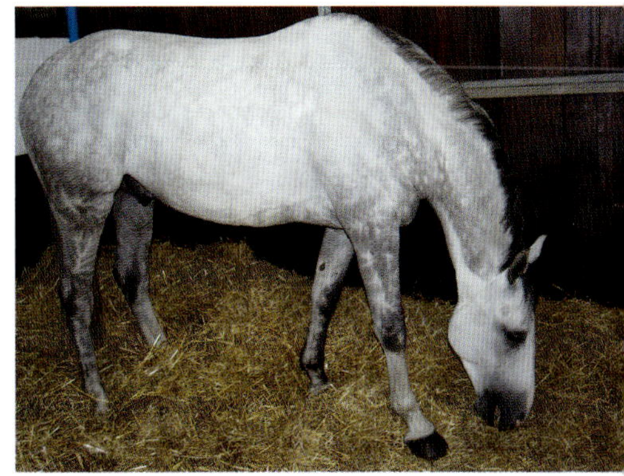

**ABOVE** *For good back posture, digestive and respiratory health and to maintain a low blood pressure horses should always be fed from the floor.*

## 2. Positioning of the hind legs

The further the hind legs come under the body, the more able they are to support back posture. The positioning of the hindlimbs is dependent on the configuration of the joints, muscles and ligaments.

### The sacroiliac joint

The sacroiliac joint is the junction between the pelvis, the highest bone in the hindlimb, and the spine. Here, the wing of the illium attaches to the large transverse process of the first sacral vertebra. This combined synovial and ligamentary joint has very little fluid, only a limited amount of movement, and is held in place by very strong ventral, dorsal and sacroiliac ligaments.

### The lumbosacral junction (LSJ)

The angles of the spinous processes change at the lumbosacral junction. This can be felt as a gap between the spinous processes.

This is the point at which the last lumbar vertebra and first sacral vertebra meet. It is a hinge joint which, after the neck and tail, forms the most flexible part of the spine. Flexion here allows the horse to round his back and tilt his pelvis during canter and gallop, when jumping, during dressage and in the sliding Western halt.

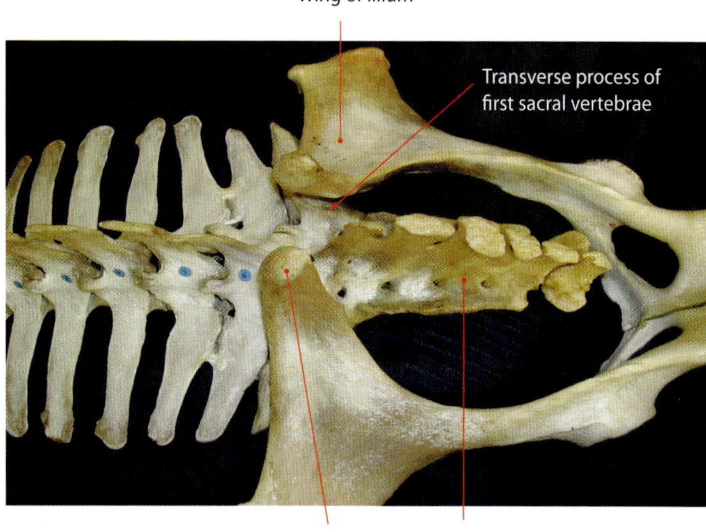


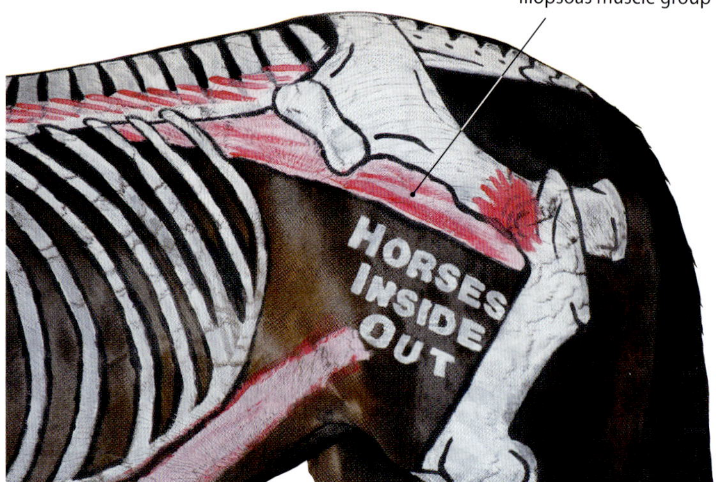


*The iliopsoas muscles are important flexors of the LSJ and hip joint.*

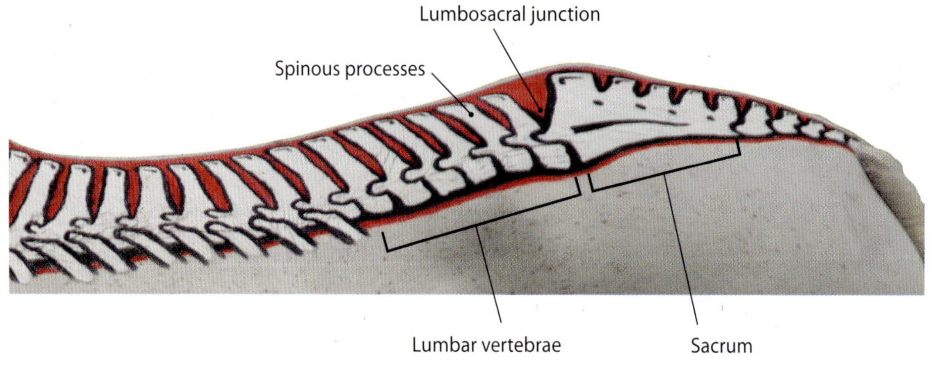

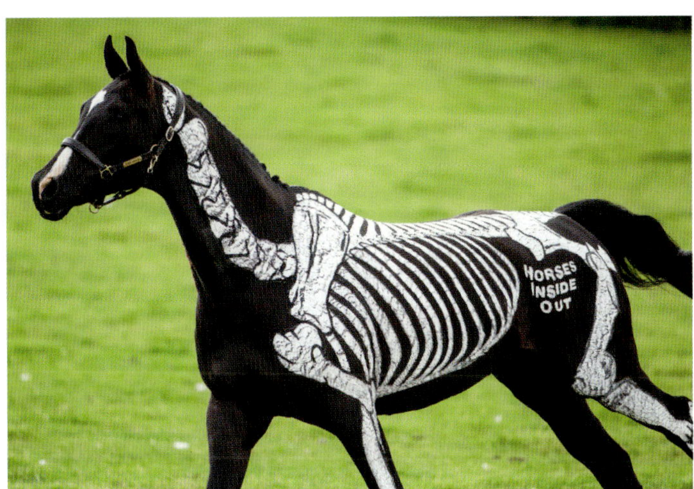

Extension of the LSJ allows the horse to extend his back, tilt the pelvis and thrust the hind legs out behind. This can be seen in gallop, canter, when jumping or bucking. There is no sideways flexion or rotation at the LSJ.

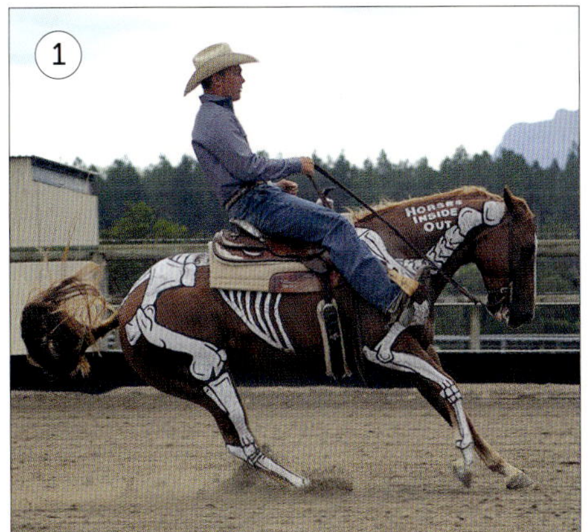

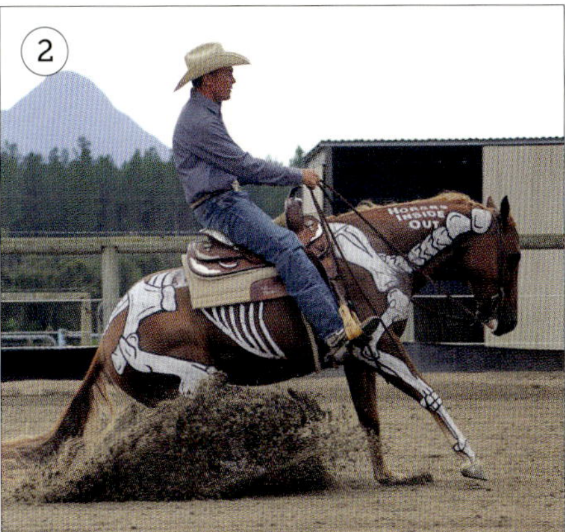

Although the pelvis can be seen to tilt, movement here is as a result of flexion at the LSJ rather than movement between the pelvis and the spine.

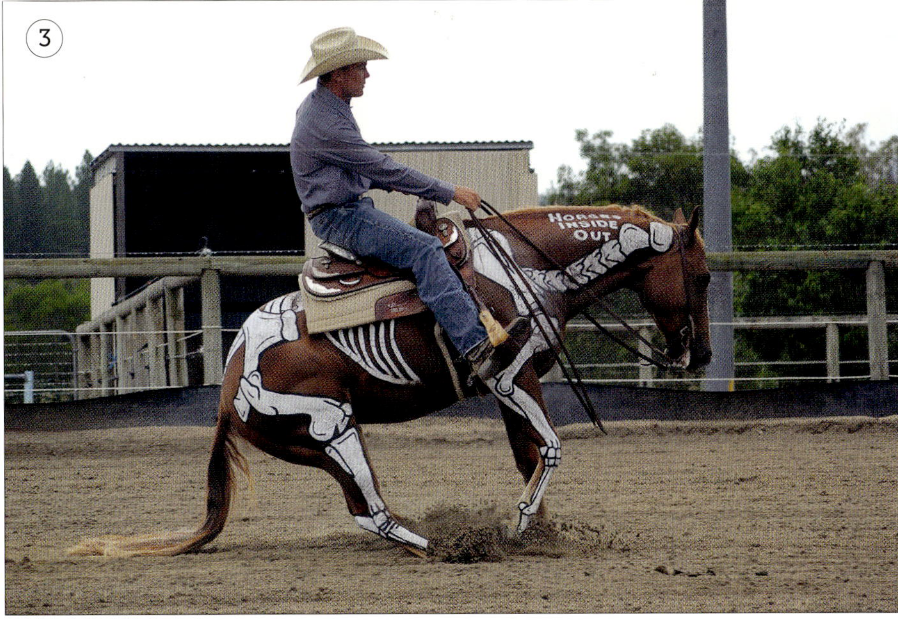

## Spinal ligament mechanism

As a continuation of the supraspinous ligament (SL), the dorsal sacroiliac ligament (DSL) stabilises the lumbar and sacral vertebrae. In a similar action to that of the NL pulling into the SL when the head is down, moving the sacrum affects the positioning of the lumbar region.

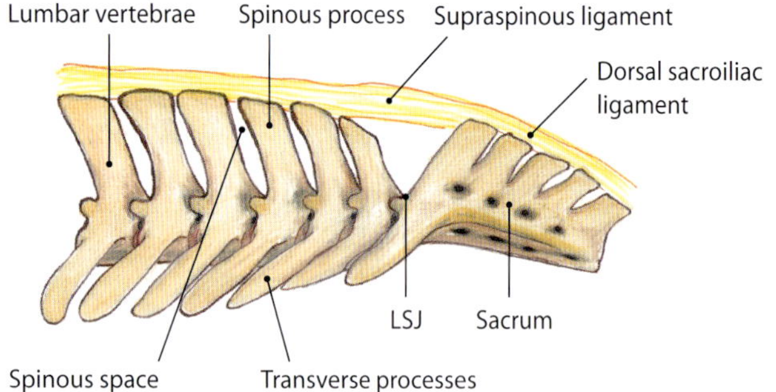


Picture 1: neutral LSJ position

*When the LSJ is flexed and the caudal end of the sacrum is down (Picture 2) traction from the DSL into the SL will open the spinous processes and raise the back in the caudal thoracic and lumbar region. When the LSJ is extended and the caudal end of the sacrum is up (Picture 3) the DSL and SL will be slack and unable to support the lumbar spine.*

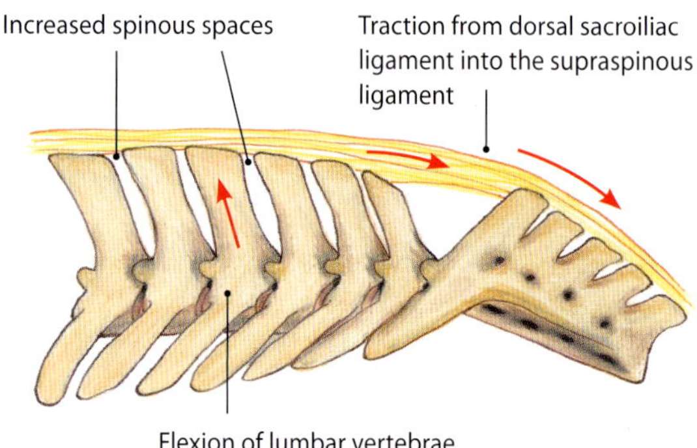


Picture 2: flexed LSJ position

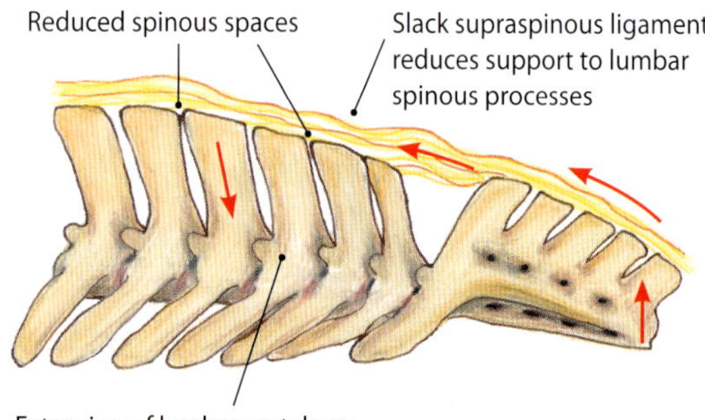


Picture 3: extended LSJ position

## The hip

The hip is a ball and socket joint where the head of the femur inserts into the pelvis. It controls the amount of protraction and retraction available to the hindlimb, allows the limb to be taken away from the body (abduction) and allows the horse to cross his hind legs (adduction). Its range of movement is restricted by the strong ligaments which attach it to the pelvis and by the fact it is buried deep under the gluteal muscles.

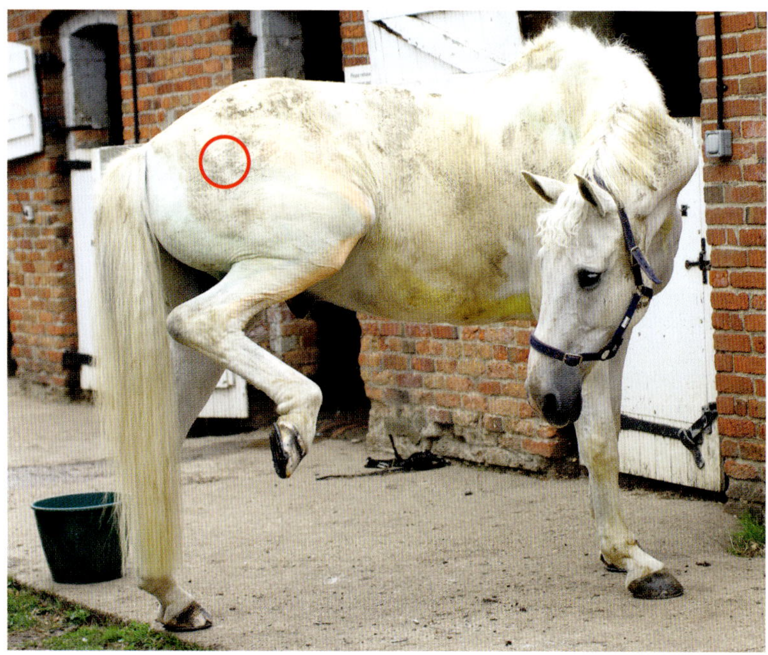

**RIGHT** *A demontration of hip rotation.*

## The stifle

The stifle, a compound joint of the femur, tibia and patella is equivalent to the human knee. It is the largest and most complex joint in the horse. The patella is connected to the tibia by three ligaments. Cartilaginous pads ('menisci') and specialised fluid contained in a thin capsule that surrounds the joint help with shock absorption and lubrication.

## The hock

Located between the tibia and cannon bone the hock is one of the most hard-working, complex and flexible joints in the body. Made up of multiple joints and individual bones all held in place by numerous ligaments and joint capsules it works as a hinge joint, moving by flexion and extension through one plane only. The upper joint between the tibia and talus is highly mobile while the lower tarsal joints are comparatively immobile. The hock is subject to significant concussive, weight-bearing, shock-absorbing, loading and rotational forces which make it the most common site for stress-related injuries in the hindlimb.

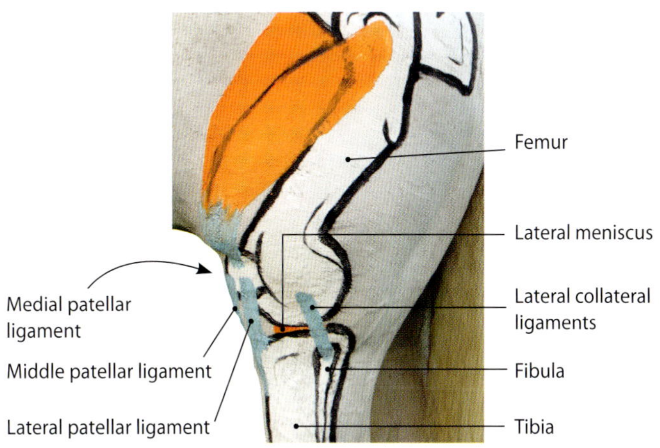


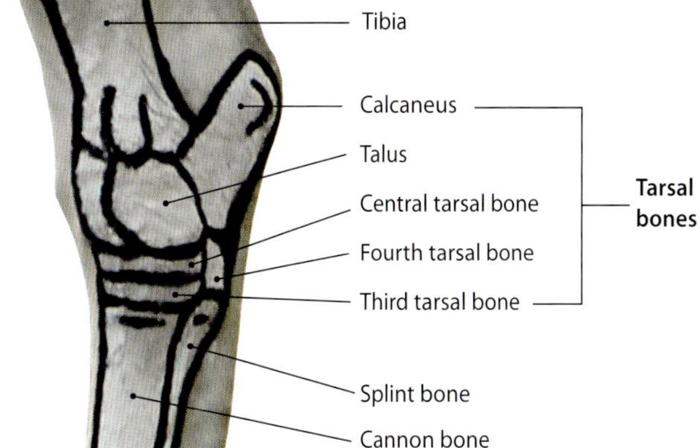


## THE LOCKING MECHANISM OF THE STIFLE

The patella is locked by the horse hooking the medial patellar ligament over a ridge on the inside of the femur. Once locked, little or no muscular effort is required to maintain position; more weight falling on the limb simply tightens the stifle. To 'unlock' the stifle, the quadriceps femoris and the glutofemoris muscles contract to pull the patella laterally and unhook the patellar ligaments. This allows the patella to once again run freely within its groove on the femur.

In some horses, this ligament gets caught or completely locked as the leg goes from extension to flexion. A locked stifle can present as a slight click or jolt, stilted movement when the horse first walks on from halt or, in extreme cases, a situation where the horse cannot walk forwards. Generally backing the horse up for a stride will unlock the stifle. Young horses may display a mild and inconsistent locking stifle as a result of weakness or tiredness in the quadriceps femoris and gluteofemoris muscles. These horses may benefit from a strengthening programme including backing up, hill, pole and water work. If the problem persists, there is a range of veterinary treatments available.

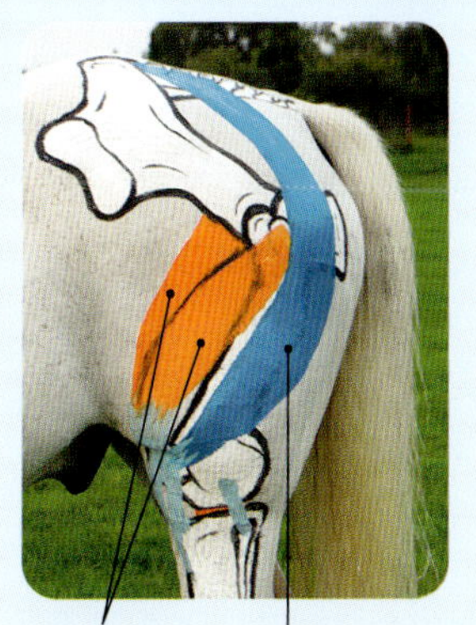

## The reciprocal system

Flexion or extension in the hock is a reflection of flexion or extension in the stifle and vice versa. This is because the high proportion of inelastic connective tissue within the peroneus tertius and the superficial digital flexor muscles causes them to function as ligaments rather than muscles. As the superficial digital flexor muscles have tendon attachments into the short pastern bones, flexion in the hock will also affect fetlock movement.

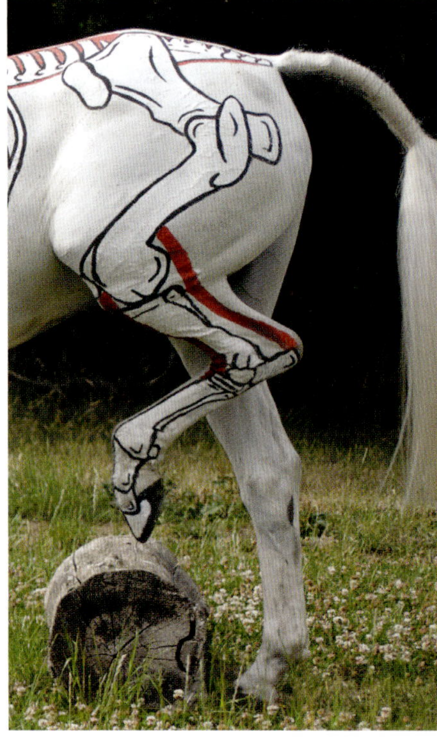
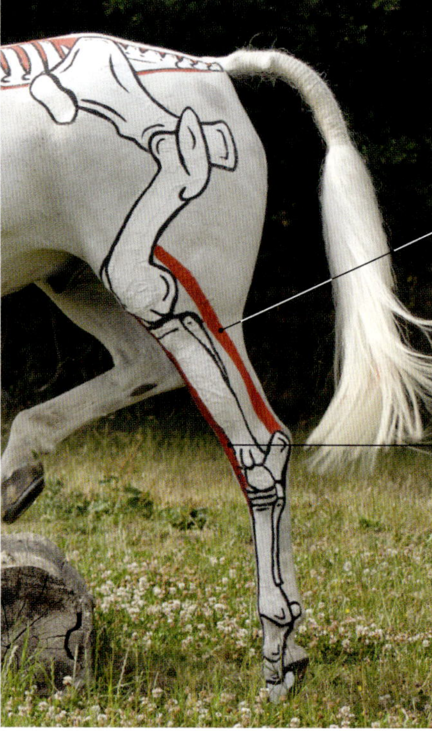



*Flexion or extension in the hock is a reflection of flexion or extension in the stifle and vice versa.*

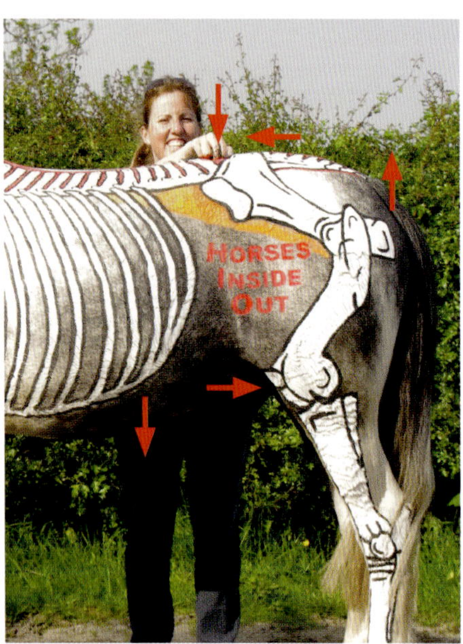


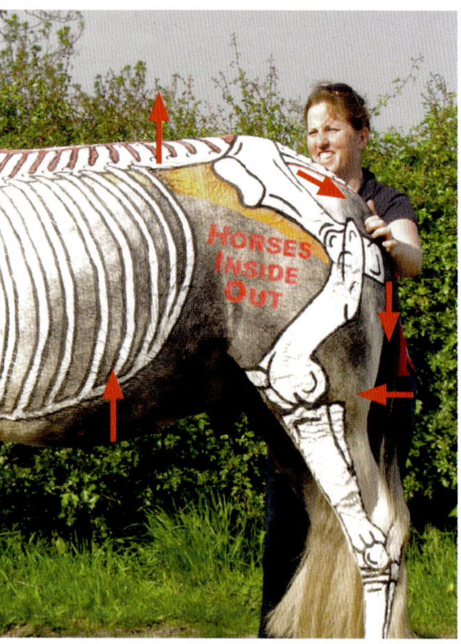


*When the LSJ extends, the back hollows and the stifle moves backwards. This is as a result of the function of the stay apparatus. In practical terms, it explains why a horse cannot work over the back if the hindlimbs are trailing. Conversely, when the back rounds, the stifle comes forwards allowing the hind legs to come well under the body to support the back.*

## Stay apparatus of the hindlimb

The stay apparatus is a series of muscles and ligaments which 'lock' the hindlimb joints in position. This allows the horse to stand with minimum muscular effort, rest one hindlimb whilst the weight is taken by the other and thus sleep standing up. It also has an important influence on joint movement and posture.

The stay apparatus has four main elements. They are the:

1. Muscles of the hindquarters
2. Locking mechanism of the stifle
3. Reciprocal system
4. Tendons and ligaments of the distal limb.

The lines in this painting represent how the muscles, tendons and ligaments of the stay apparatus are linked.

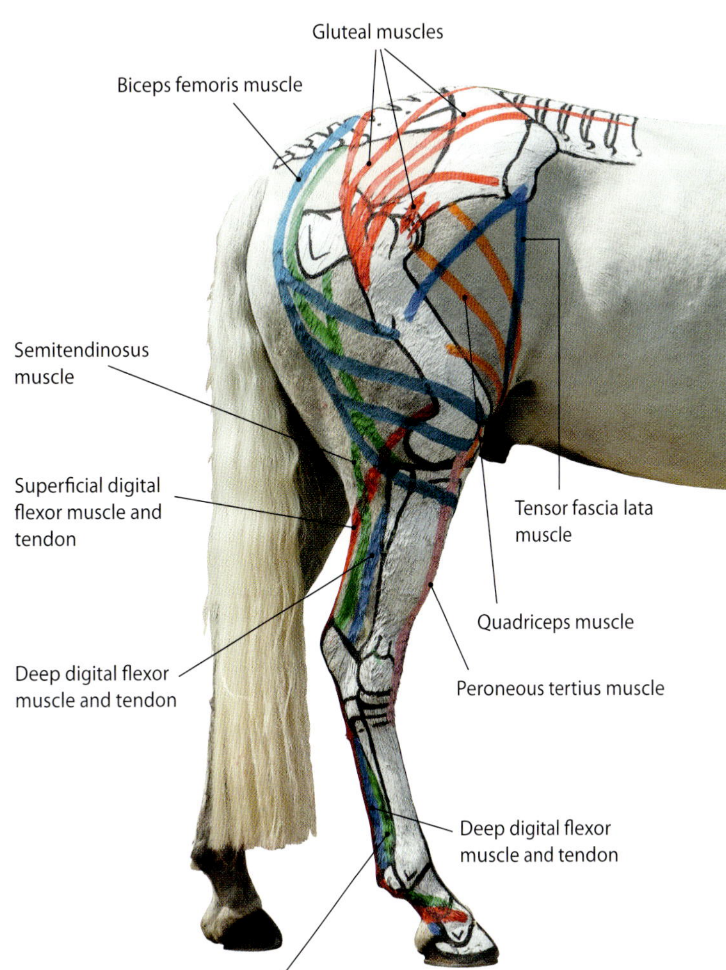


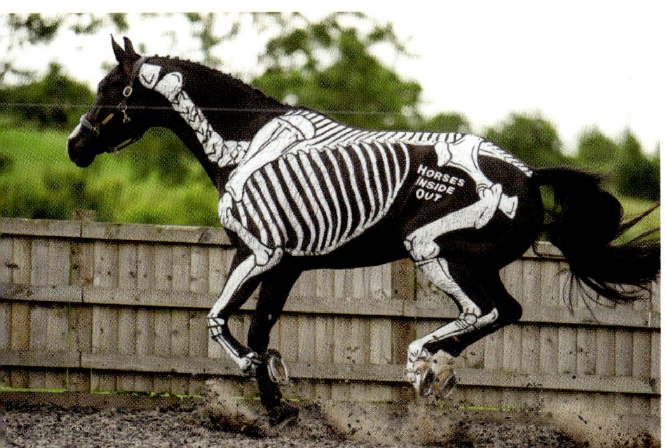


This horse is demonstrating how flexion of the lumbosacral junction is reflected in the hip, stifle and hock joints. Biomechanically it is not possible for one joint to work in isolation.

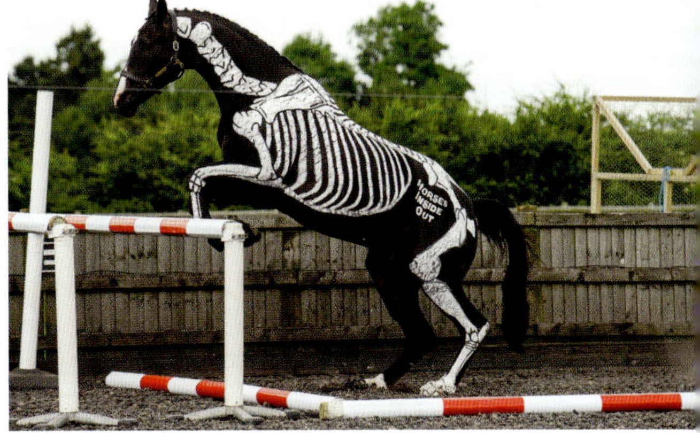


This horse is demonstrating how the mechanics of the stay apparatus cause the hindlimb joints to compress in unison to produce potential energy and then upward thrust.

## 3. Positioning of the thorax

As the horse has no collarbone, the thoracic sling connects the forelimb to the thorax and supports its weight between the front limbs. With correct training and conditioning, the thoracic sling muscles become shorter, stronger and more toned, holding the thorax in a higher position and contributing to improved posture.

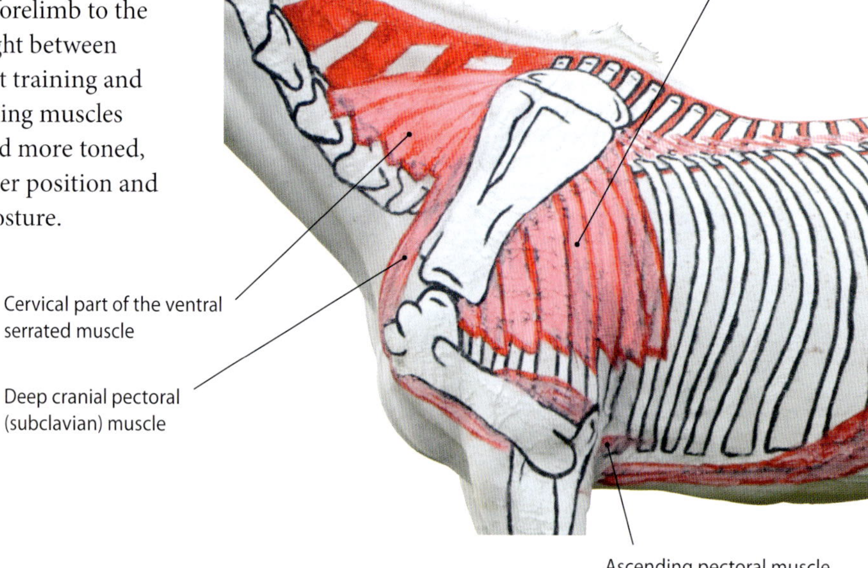


## Muscles that influence the base of the neck

In addition to the thoracic sling, muscles on the underside of the cervicothoracic junction support good posture.

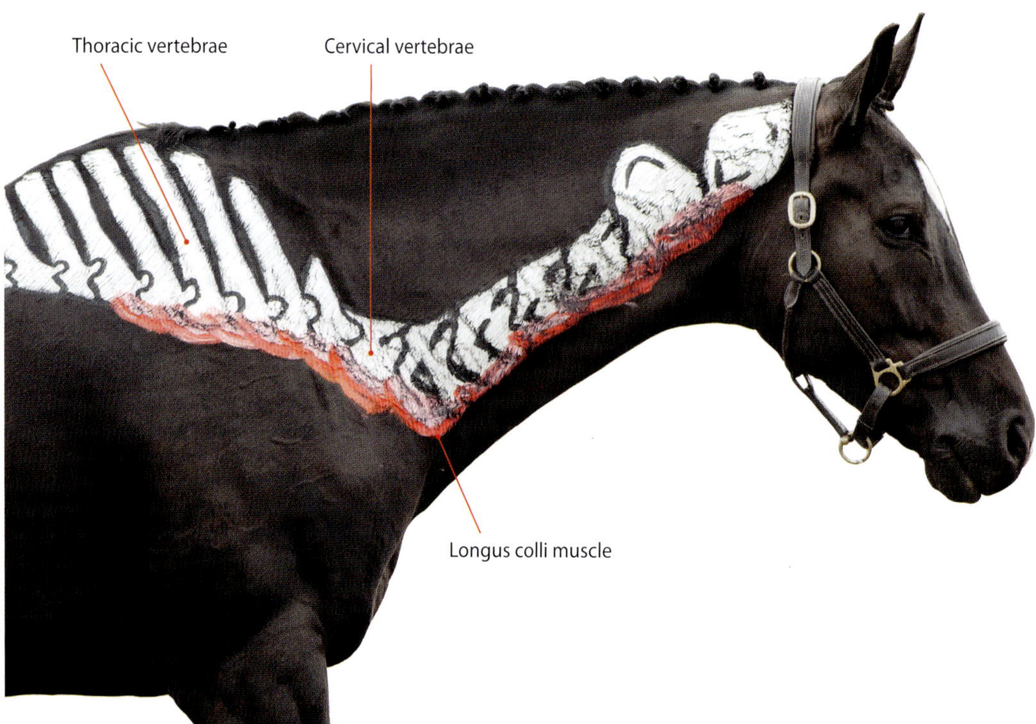

## 4. Contribution of the flexor chain of muscles

The spinal flexor and extensor muscle chains need to be in equilibrium in order to allow ideal posture and movement. Performing Pilates exercises is an ideal way of balancing these chains.

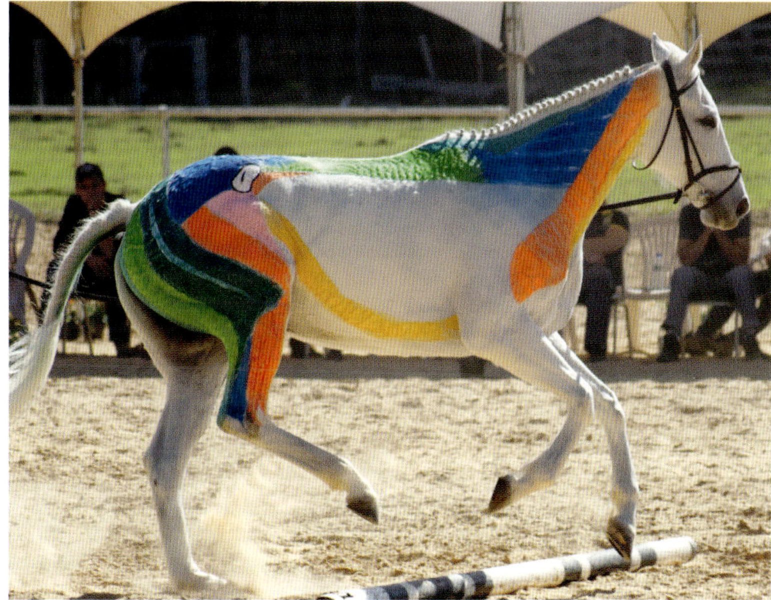

Four sheets of muscle cross the abdomen supporting its contents and lifting and flexing the back. Working in opposition to the back extensor muscles the abdominals need to be well toned to provide a strong back and core.

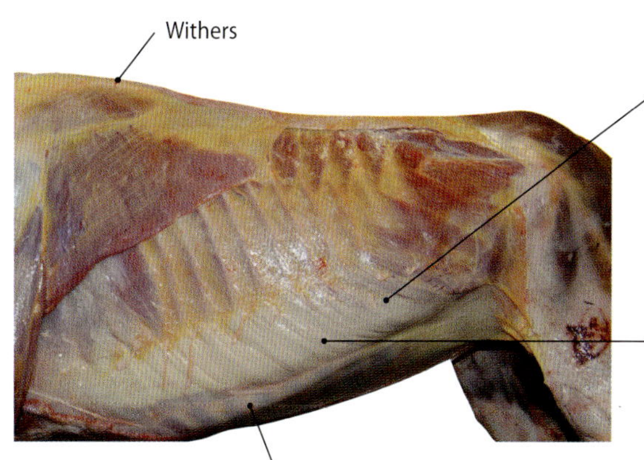


## SUMMARY

- Good posture can be influenced by training and is vital for every ridden horse.
- Long-term poor posture where some muscles are overused and overdeveloped and some are underused and atrophied will adversely affect the muscular, skeletal, fascial and neuromuscular systems.
- To maintain muscle tone, promote good posture and ensure spinal curves are correctly configured it is important that the horse always moves and is ridden with purpose.
- The four main mechanisms that influence posture are:
  1. Positioning of the head and neck
  2. Positioning of the hind legs
  3. Positioning of the thorax
  4. Development and tone of the flexor and extensor chain of muscles.

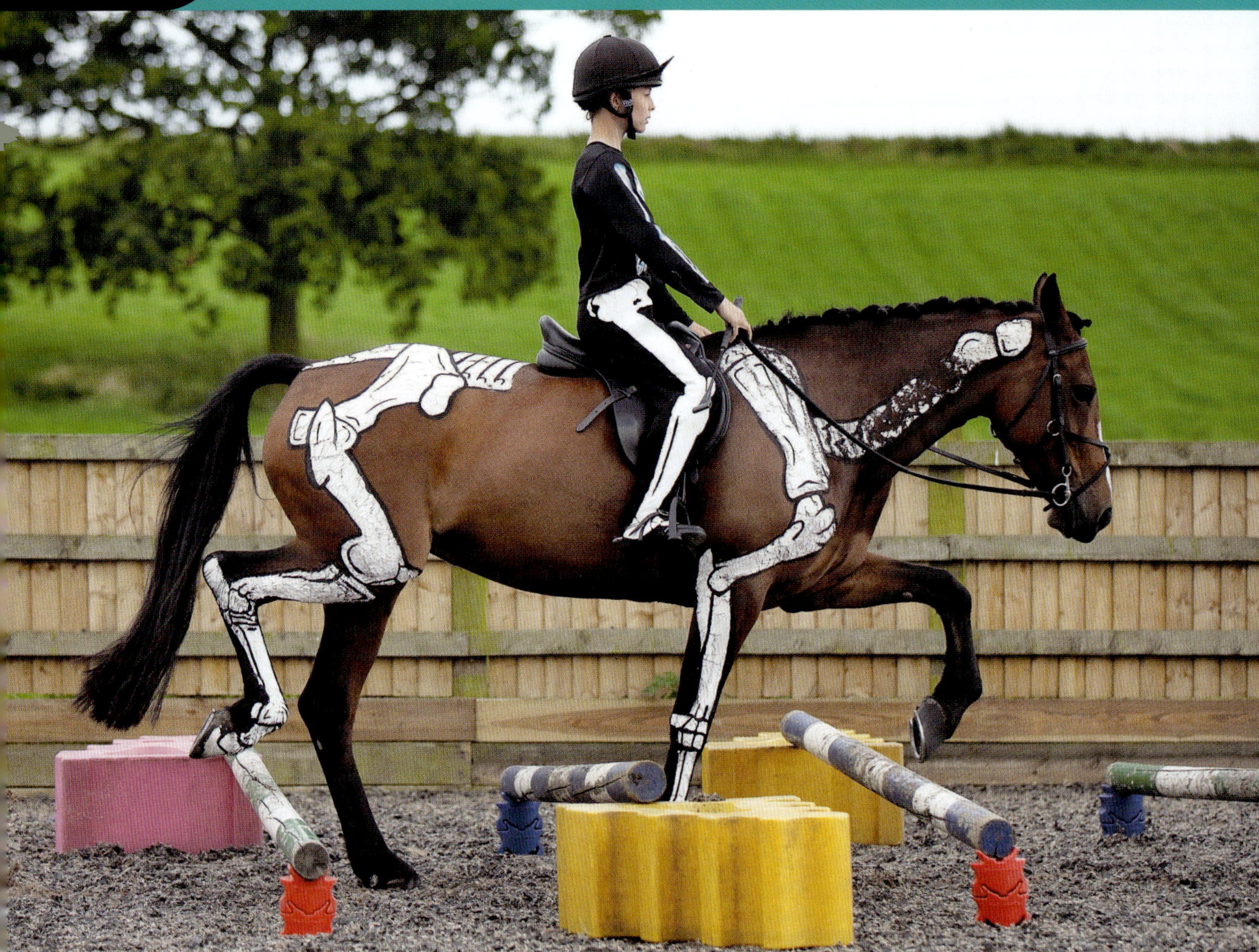

## Training the Systems

Before performing at any stage, horses need to be suitably physically fit. Fitness is having the ability to perform the desired activity with ease. This involves training the systems appropriately for soundness, performance and to avoid overload and injury. All systems respond best to a gradual increase of type, volume and intensity of workload and fitness training. It is especially important that young or previously untrained horses are allowed to build physical strength slowly through a well-planned basic training programme, before making discipline-specific demands.

**USEFUL RESTING STATISTICS FOR A HEALTHY HORSE**

Temperature: 37.2–38.3 °C (99–101°F)

Pulse/heart: 35–42 beats per minute

Respiration rate: 10–18 breaths per minute (bpm)

## Cardiovascular fitness

The horse has an enormous capacity to increase his cardiac output, which is the main response to exercise. During maximal exercise the heart rate can rise to 240 bpm. As the heart rate rises, more blood is pumped to the muscles for energy. At rest a fit horse's heart will push 1 litre of blood into the aorta with each heartbeat. During exercise this can increase to 1.7 litres per heartbeat. Blood pressure will increase as more blood is pumped around the body. This will result in greater aerobic efficiency, making it easier for the horse to work harder for longer.

Factors that raise the heart rate include: exercise, steepness of terrain, transitions, excitement, stress, stereotypical behaviour, fear, pain, infections, injuries or colic. Conversely, improved fitness, relaxation and contentment will lower the heart rate.

Using a heart rate monitor during an exercise session can be an interesting awareness exercise and a useful indicator of cardiac fitness as well as general health.

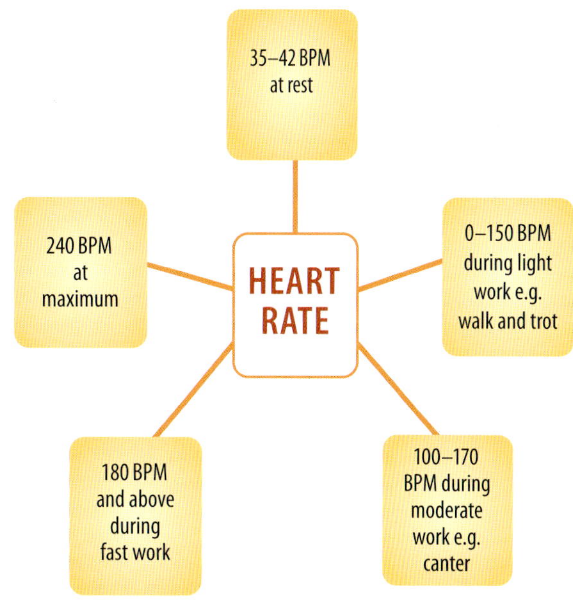


*This diagram illustrates normal expectations for heart rate in beats per minute according to the activity.*

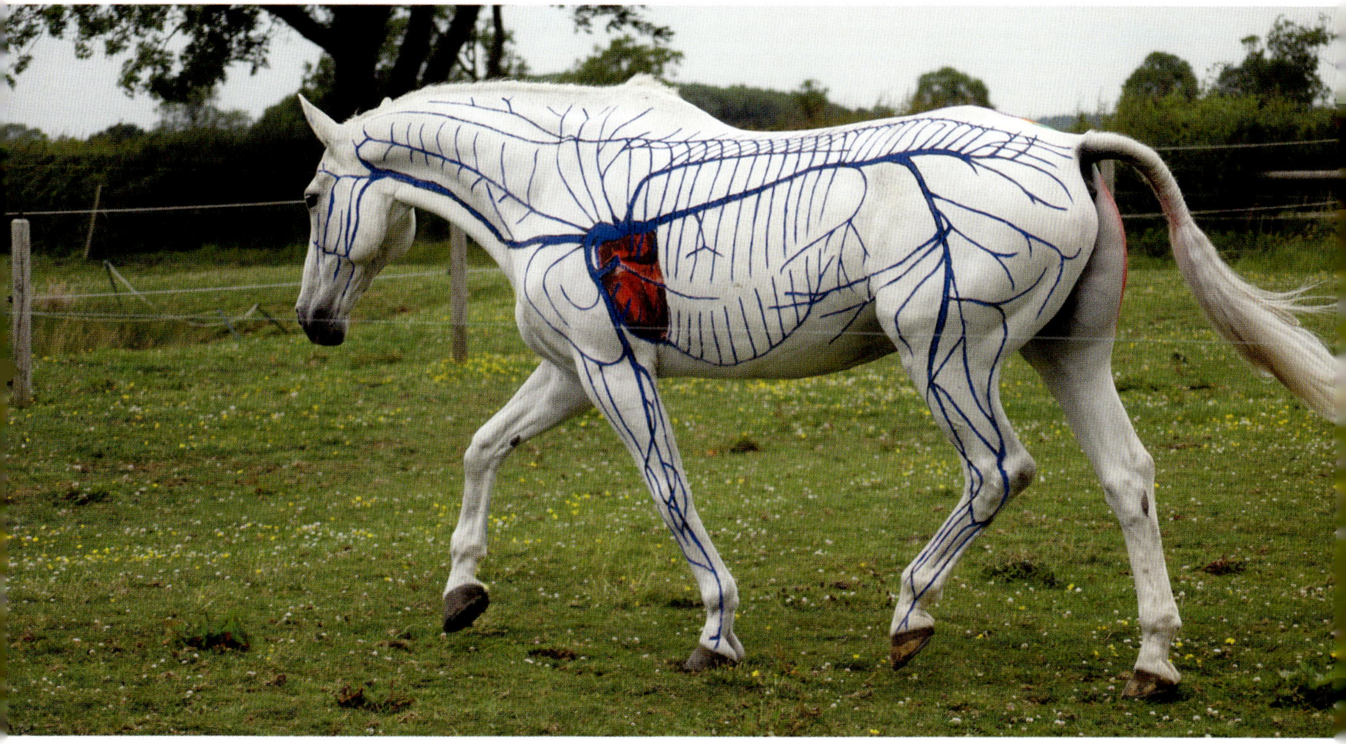

*This painting illustrates the major veins which return blood from the muscles to the heart during exercise.*

## Respiratory fitness

The main function of the respiratory system is to bring oxygen, vital for muscular function, energy, performance and fitness, into the lungs, circulate it to the rest of the body via the blood then exchange it for carbon dioxide. Efficient lung function is essential for optimum performance. At gallop, breathing is coupled with stride in a 1:1 ratio. Maximum respiration rate therefore is determined by the number of strides. Limiting factors to respiratory efficiency include the volume of the lungs, the diameter of the airway from the nostrils through the windpipe, outline and gait. Respiratory fitness cannot be improved in the same way or to the same degree as cardiovascular fitness.

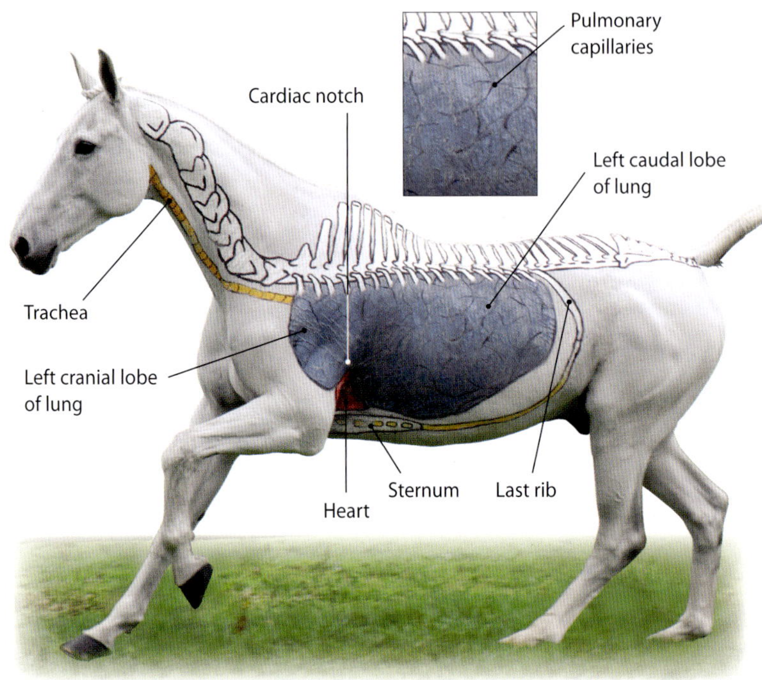


*The main function of the respiratory system is to bring oxygen into the lungs.*

**1. Long Slow Distance Work (LSD)** is the basic requirement for all conditioning programmes. For a previously fit horse coming back from three months at grass it can take a minimum of six weeks to reach the desired level of fitness. LSD can be performed as a ridden activity, on the lunge, in long-reins or on a horse walker.

### There are three main types of exercise that condition the cardiovascular system.

**2. Interval Training (IT)** improves aerobic capacity by alternating bursts of faster work with short rests. The aim is to raise the heart rate to around 180 bpm, walk until the heart rate drops to about 100 bpm then repeat the exercise. As fitness increases recovery times reduce.

**3. Sprint Training (ST)** improves anaerobic capacity through high-speed conditioning. It is used mainly with race and event horses, although all can benefit from occasional sprint training appropriate to their age, stage and fitness. To ensure muscular recovery times it is important only to perform fast work every fifth day.

## Musculoskeletal fitness

### Strengthening and conditioning bone

Strong bone, supported by good nutrition and exercise, is essential if the horse is to perform successfully and remain sound.

*Bone remodelling*

Healthy bone, which continually increases in density and strength, is strong, but not brittle. Triggered by a need for calcium and in an ongoing response to mechanical stresses on the bone tissue, it is constantly being remodelled in a process known as Wolff's Law. Maximum bone density is generally not achieved until the horse is 6 years old, by which time many horses are already being ridden and competed. Horses need to work on a variety of surfaces to elicit good bone strength. Those who are only worked on soft surfaces or that spend a lot of time stabled or inactive will be more prone to sore bones and concussion problems when exposed to a harder surface than those who have very short bursts of daily training, such as a brief period of working trot or canter over a slightly firmer surface. Grassland in summer for example will elicit a greater bone response than sand.

Bone requires a low level of concussion to stimulate conditioning and strengthening. Walking horses on the road can be incorporated with LSD work and is a good way, particularly with young and unfit horses, of achieving the correct balance of enough G-Force for bone conditioning without causing too much concussion. This exercise is also an effective way of stimulating and hardening the tendons.

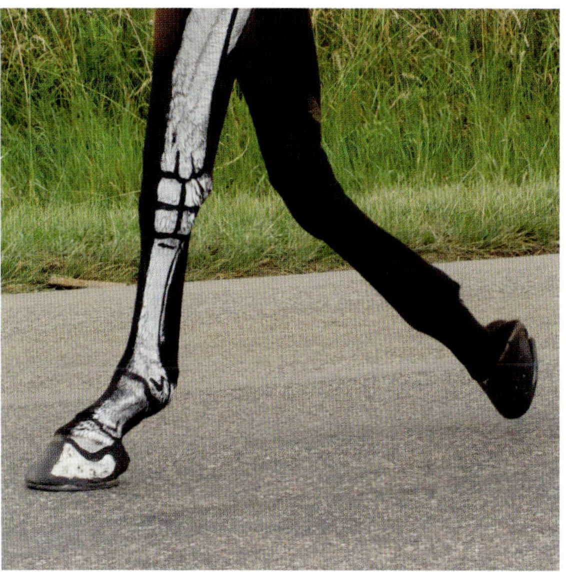

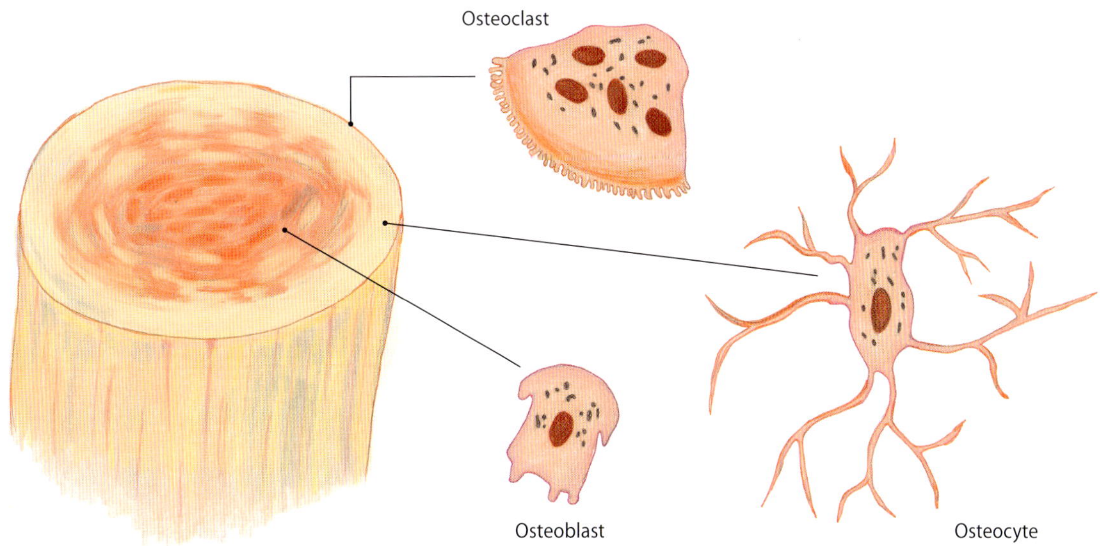


*The three bone remodelling cell types.*

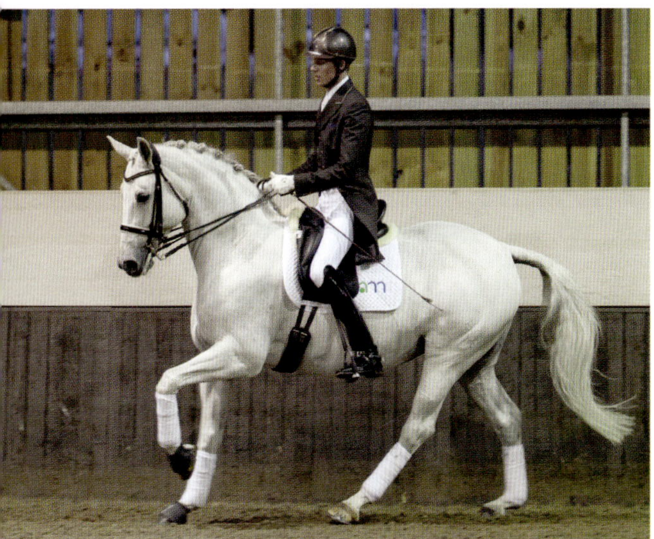

**ABOVE** *Exercise that stretches and strengthens muscle will also condition connective tissue. A well conditioned, strong, supple horse is more likely to have stable joints and the muscular strength and tone to facilitate good posture, power, endurance, expression, balance and accuracy. He will also be better prepared to cope with varying terrain and any turn of speed or direction required. Conversely, short, tight muscles will restrict movement and contribute to poor performance and injury.*

## Strengthening muscle

A strong, supple muscular system goes hand in hand with a well-conditioned cardiovascular system as the increase in oxygen allows the muscles to work more efficiently. To increase the quality of muscle fibres, which are improved through performing repeated contractions, it is necessary to increase the intensity, duration and frequency of the exercise. This requires a regular, structured, strengthening exercise programme dependent on age, breed, fitness and condition. Muscle adapts, gets larger, stronger and is rebuilt slowly. Asking too much in the form of speed, distance or carrying weight for long periods before the horse is physically able results in stiff, fatigued, sore or damaged muscles which delays the strengthening programme and is counterproductive. After intense training sessions, to avoid strain, fatigue and to allow the muscles time to recover, only perform focused, intense strength training sessions two or three times per week.

## Stretching

Stretching is an important part of ridden work. Whether undertaking stretching as part of a warm up, cool down or stand alone activity it is a major contributing factor to achieving muscular fitness and has enormous benefits for both horse and rider. It:

* Keeps muscles supple and comfortable, enhances body awareness and proprioception, improves coordination, optimises athletic ability and reduces stiffness
* Elongates the muscle fibres, ensuring optimum range of movement
* Lessens tension on joints, tendons, muscles and ligaments
* Improves the circulation of blood and lymphatic fluids, allowing more oxygen and nutrients to enrich the muscles
* Contributes to the efficient removal of toxic by-products of metabolism; an important factor in preventing fatigue and reducing recovery time
* Contributes to mental and physical relaxation.

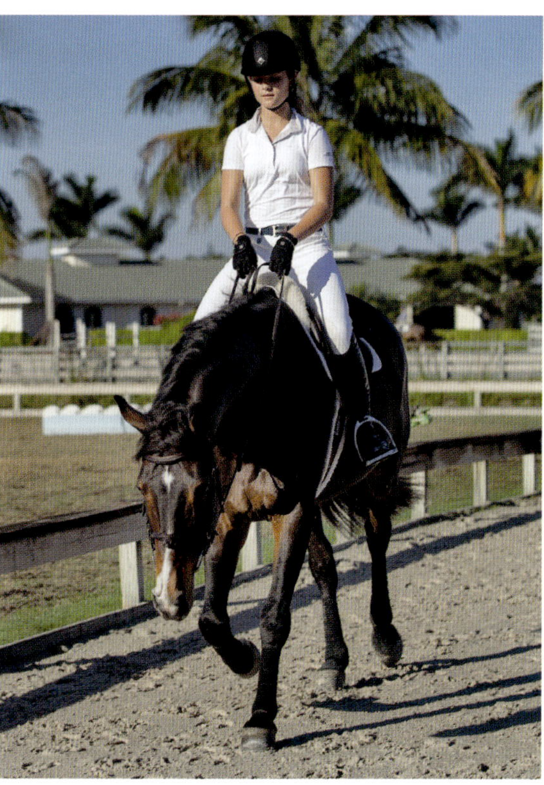

*Stretching is an important part of ridden work.*

## Types of Stretching

There are two main types of stretching – see photos and captions below.

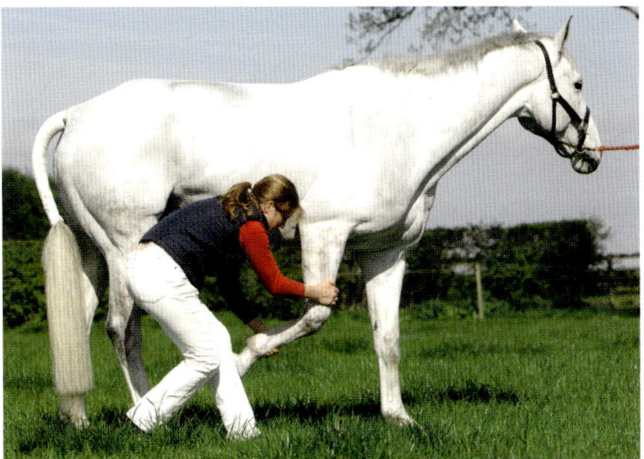

**Passive stretches** *are performed by a handler. To achieve these the horse needs to be warm, relaxed and confident. Cold connective tissue, which has low blood saturation, can be more susceptible to injury.*

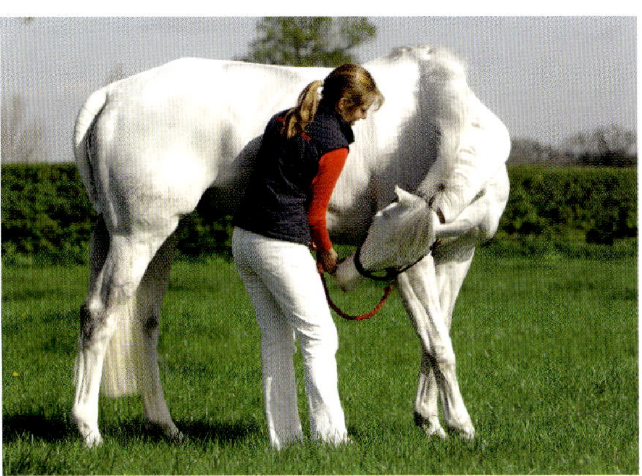

**Active Stretches** *require the horse to move the body parts to create the stretch himself. These can be performed during ridden or groundwork exercises, and also with the use of carrots.*

To perform passive stretches:

- Begin slowly. Once maximum stretch is reached hold it for 5–15 seconds to allow the fibres to relax before taking the stretch a little further
- Work a manageable programme into your daily routine
- Be patient. Benefits of stretching will only be seen if performed regularly and consistently.

## The stretch reflex

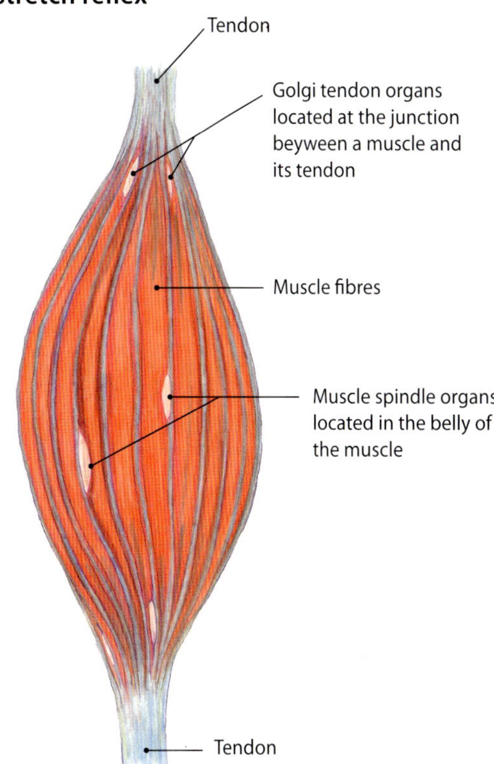


These are the two main types of stretch receptors which provide automatic regulation of skeletal length and prevent the muscle and connective tissue from overstretching. They are essential for coordinating muscle activity and operate by relaying information about the state of muscles to the central nervous system. Stretching a muscle too quickly stimulates the stretch receptors to contract. This reaction protects the musculoskeletal system from injury and explains why it is important to stretch gradually. Holding the stretch for as long as possible gives time for the stretch receptors to adjust and allows the muscle to lengthen.

Stretch receptors can also have a useful role in movement. When a muscle stretches quickly and powerfully, for example when landing from a fence, the receptors respond by causing a strong contraction of the muscle. In the case of the landing horse this helps him push up into the next stride. The more suddenly a muscle elongates, the stronger it contracts.

# Conditioning cartilage, tendons and ligaments

When galloping, landing from a large fence or when performing advanced dressage movements, the tendons of the lower leg are stretched to the limit as the limb absorbs many times the body weight (see right).

Tendon and ligament injury, for which lengthy recuperation is required, is often caused by repetitive strain associated with vigorous athletic pursuits. A progressive, planned conditioning and training regime can reduce the risk of these injuries. As with conditioning bone, tendons respond well to walking on a firm surface. If tendon or ligament injury does occur it is important to seek advice from a vet.

Cartilage, which increases in thickness and fluidity, and tendons and ligaments, which benefit from improved coordination and proprioception, take much longer than lungs or muscles to adapt to new activity or an increase in intensity and volume.

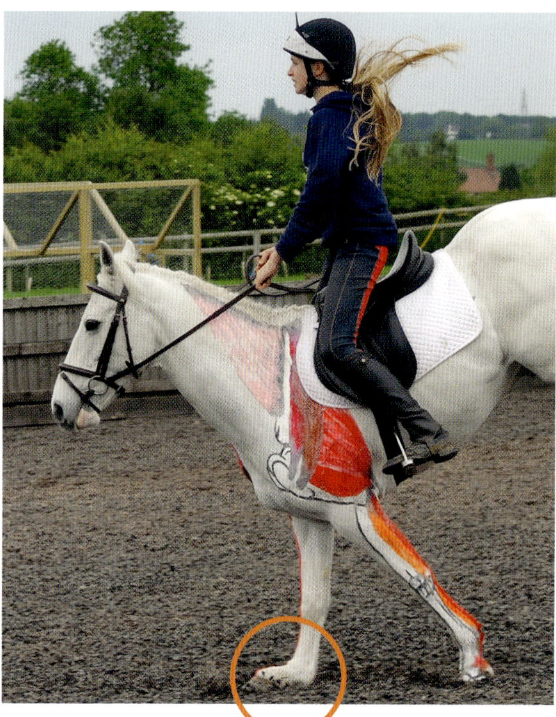

*Hyper extended fetlock.*

*The tendons and suspensory ligament of the lower limb.*

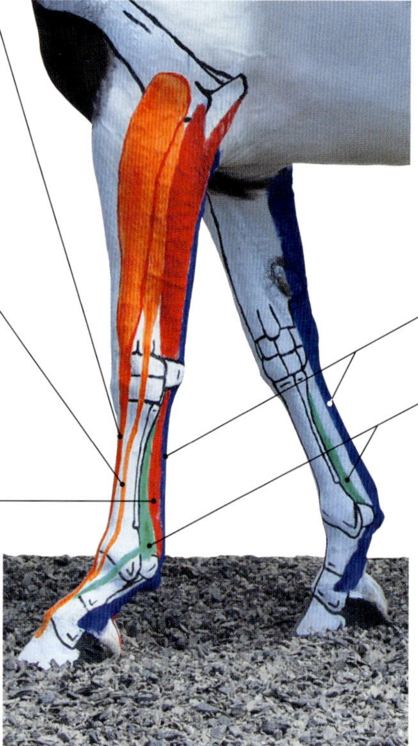

**Common digital extensor tendon (CDET)**
**Origin:** Common digital extensor muscle
**Insertion:** Front of the short pastern bone and the centre of the pedal bone
**Action:** Lifts the toe, extends the fetlock, pastern and coffin joints.

**Lateral digital extensor tendon (LDET)**
**Origin:** Lateral digital extensor muscle
**Insertion:** Outside of the long pastern bone
**Action:** Assists the CDET, lifts the toe and extends the fetlock, pastern and coffin joints.

**Deep digital flexor tendon (DDFT)**
**Origin:** Deep digital flexor muscle and check ligament
**Insertion:** Underside of the pedal bone
**Action:** Flexes the joints of the lower leg, particularly the coffin joint and supports them during weight-bearing.

**Superficial digital flexor tendon (SDFT)**
**Origin:** Superficial digital flexor muscle
**Insertion:** Medial and lateral side of the short pastern bone
**Action:** Flexes the joints of the lower leg, supports them during weight-bearing and limits fetlock hyperextension.

**Suspensory ligament**
**Origin:** Bottom row of carpal bones between splint bones. It branches into two above the fetlock to join with the sesamoid bones
**Insertion:** Blends with CDET at the level of the short pastern bone
**Action:** Supports and prevents over-extension of fetlock joint.

The main risk factors that contribute to overload and breakdown of tendons and ligaments are:

1. Repetitive movements
2. Cumulative stress from long-term training
3. Lack of conditioning
4. Uneven, deep or slippery terrain
5. Poor conformation such as long sloping pasterns, long toes or low heels
6. Insufficient warm up.

## Nerve conditioning, coordination and proprioception

Whatever the task, age or stage, a calm, relaxed atmosphere combined with patience, consistency and repetition is conducive to learning and provides an optimum environment for the function of the nervous system.

Proprioception is spatial awareness. Proprioceptors in the form of sensory and motor nerves are situated in muscles, tendons, ligaments and joints. These relay information about the musculoskeletal system to the central nervous system and allow the horse to unconsciously monitor the position of all his body parts in relation to each other and his surroundings. As increased body temperature speeds the interaction between nerve impulses and the receptors, body awareness is enhanced if the horse is calm and comfortable and warm. Proprioception and muscle coordination directly determine athletic ability and although some horses are more naturally balanced and athletic than others, both in hand and ridden exercises can improve these attributes. Lateral work, walking over and between poles, passive stretching, dressage movements, hill work and gymnastic jumping all encourage coordination and balance.

Proprioception is reduced if the horse is cold, fatigued or in pain, lacks exercise or is stressed or excited. In this state he is less aware of his body and more likely to be uncoordinated, perform badly, trip or knock down a pole when showjumping.

*Some imprinted responses are unhelpful. For example if a young horse is always led from the left, he will associate pressure on the nose with turning his head to the left. This can be an unwelcome response as he comes into training. Avoiding a bad habit is better than trying to break it!*

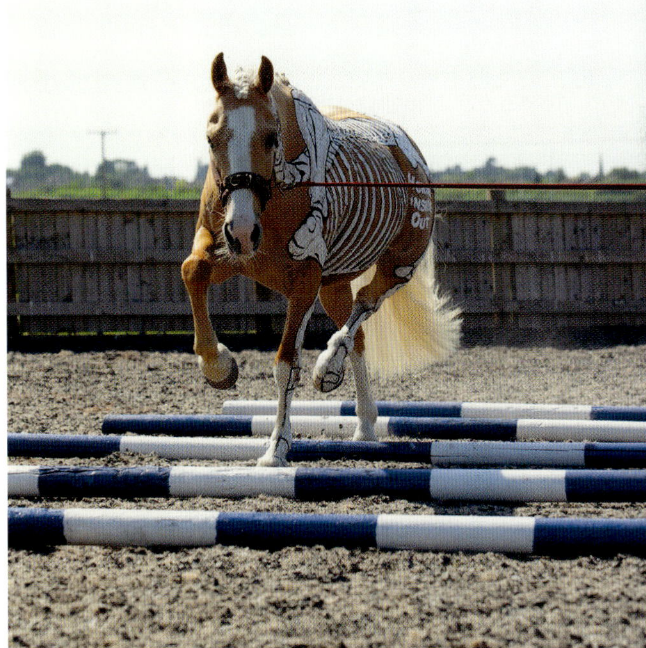

*Hoof/brain coordination relies on a number of factors including nerve conditioning, proprioception, coordination and speed of muscular contraction.*

# Warm Up

Before performing any exercise it is essential that the horse is prepared. Warming up and cooling down are very important parts of any physical activity whether for horse or human. The warm up should:

- Increase blood flow to muscles and vital organs
- Improve mechanical efficiency, power, pulse and respiration rate
- Awaken the core
- Allow for greater utilisation of fatty acids in early work so that less lactic acid is produced in subsequent exercise
- Stretch the muscles, ligaments and tendons
- Take the joints through a full range of movement
- Increase flexibility and range of movement
- Focus the mind.

Warming up appropriately cannot be guaranteed to prevent injury but certainly reduces the risk. There is no hard and fast rule but, as a general guide, the horse needs 15–20 minutes to warm up. Older horses, who are more susceptible to injury, or who have suffered injury in the past, might need longer

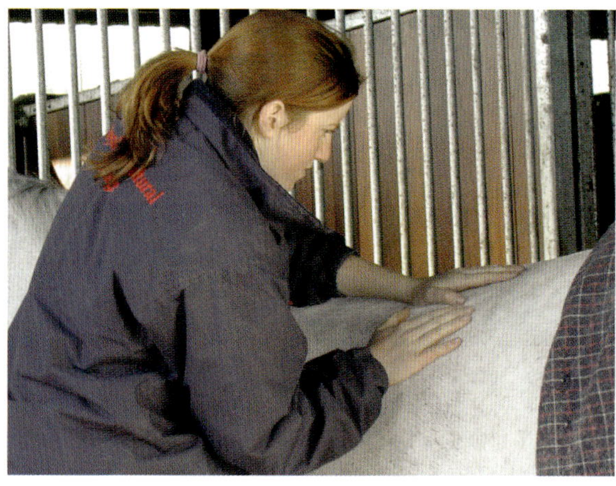

*Warm up can begin with a good groom, massage and passive stretches.*

or a different workout than horses that are younger or have been injury free.

## Ridden warm up

Ridden warm up should begin with a purposeful, forward free walk on a long rein. This enables the spinal ligament system to raise the back, support the weight of the rider, allow the back to swing and elongate the topline and back muscles.

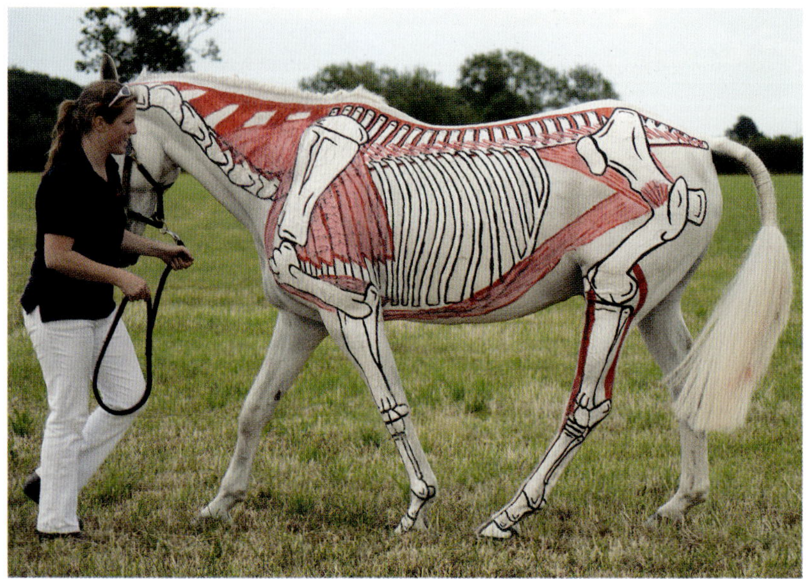

*Essential groundwork: Circling the horse to the left and right and backing up a minimum of ten steps with the head lowered is advantageous before mounting. This encourages the back to lift, supple and stretch.*

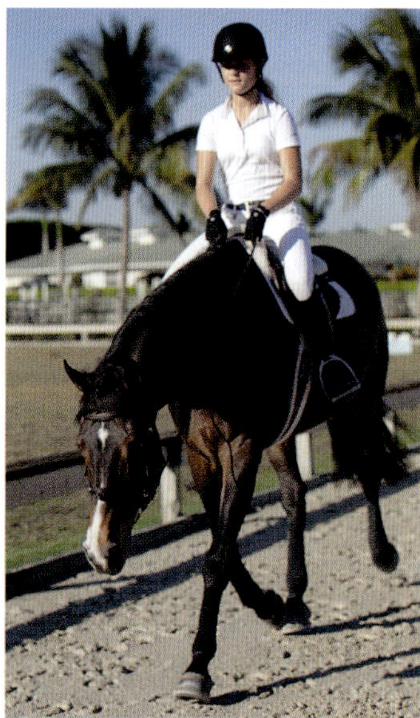

*Stretching over the back is an important part of warming up.*

A short hack in walk followed by riding large schooling figures, such as circles of varying sizes, serpentines and figures of eight engages attention and prepares muscles for work. Be methodical and include changes of rein and lateral work such as leg-yield, shoulder-in and travers, which are good movements to stretch joints, encourage the hind legs to step under and across the body, generally loosen and supple the horse and recruit the core. Following the walk work and still on a long rein, progressing to an even, active trot then canter whilst continuing the schooling figures and introducing transitions lifts the back, benefits musculoskeletal suppleness, begins to open the airways and increases the respiration rate and circulation.

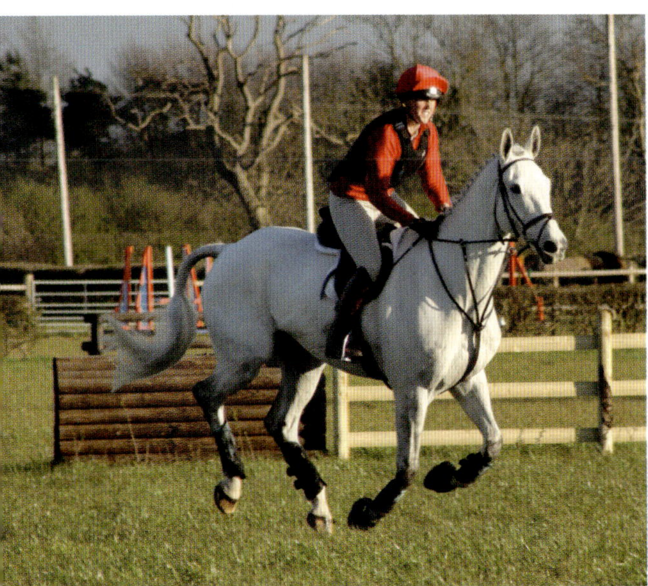

*As the horse rocks from the fore to hindlimbs and brings both hind legs through together, warming up in canter with the rider in the two-point position alleviates stiffness, is kinder on the back and is beneficial for horses with any kind of back problem. Cantering in a long and low outline will also elongate and strengthen the topline muscles in preparation for picking up a contact later in the session.*

## Cool down

Cooling down at the end of a session is as important for the health of the musculoskeletal system as the warm up. Stretching down in a long and low outline helps to relax and elongate the muscles and gives the circulatory system the opportunity to remove toxins, draw lactic acid from the soft tissues, reduce the likelihood of inflammation and allow the heart and respiration rates to return to normal. It is also a positive, calming and relaxing experience for both horse and rider.

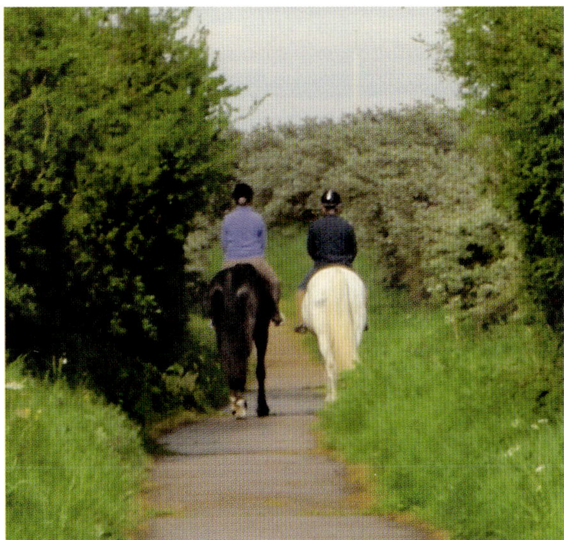

*A ten-minute hack is an excellent cool down activity.*

## Training Principles

For a well-coordinated, forward-going, agile, athletic horse, there are three main aspects to his training we need to consider. They are rhythm, balance and suppleness, without which it is difficult to achieve a good contact, impulsion, straightness and collection.

### Rhythm

Rhythm refers to the pattern and regularity of the steps, which should cover equal distances and be of equal duration. It is not concerned with speed.

A consistent rhythm will:

- Improve core stability and balance
- Facilitate relaxed movement within the gaits
- Enable the horse to extend and collect with ease
- Strengthen muscle, bone and connective tissue
- Establish correct neural pathways
- Reduce the risk of injury, as movement is predictable rather than erratic.

## Balance

Balance refers to the ability to maintain a laterally
(side to side) and longitudinally (from fore to hind)
balanced posture with an air of graceful efficiency,
effortlessness and ease regardless of activity. Lateral
balance is improved with equal bending in both
directions which, in turn, will allow the rider to keep
the horse straight. Longitudinal balance is improved
by working on transitions both within and between
the gaits.

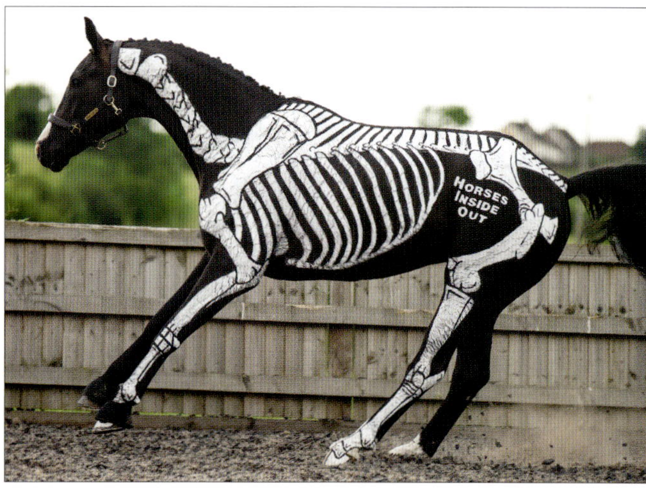


RIGHT *When running free, the horse continually uses his
head and neck to balance and counteract momentum. His
challenge is to move and remain in balance when we as
riders require him to keep his head still!*

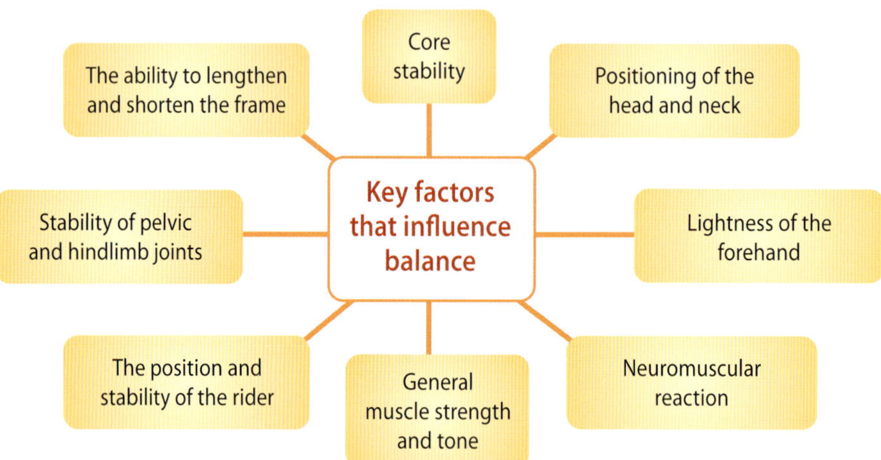


### CENTRE OF MASS

The centre of gravity around
which the mass of the horse is
equally distributed, is located in
the centre of the body, slightly
behind the heart and about two-
thirds of the way down the body
below the withers. This point is
transient and dependent on the
position of the head and neck,
the position of the hind legs,
conformation, posture and a
combination of speed and degree
of collection.

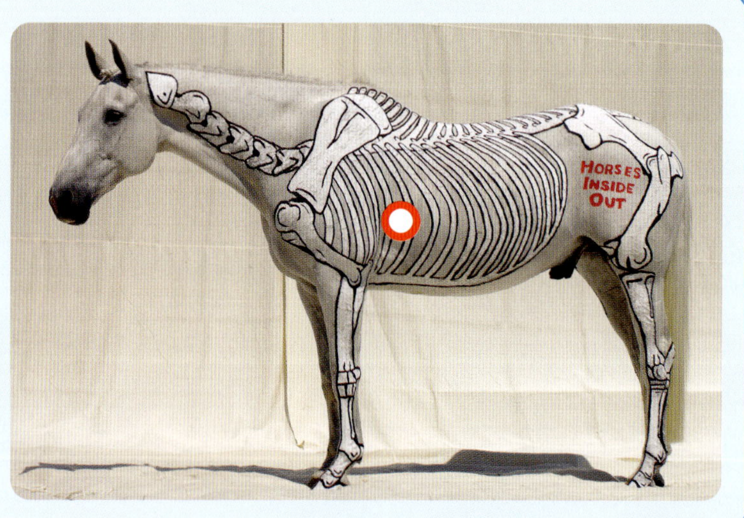

## The core muscles

Good core strength is essential for balance. The core muscles enable the horse to recruit the musculature of the trunk effectively and thus influence the position and stability of the spine, pelvis and limbs during dynamic movements. It enhances coordination, performance and control, is important for maintaining self-carriage, carrying the weight of the rider, performing highly engaged dressage movements, jumping and working at speed. Weak core muscles can lead to fatigue, loss of balance, poor performance and an increased risk of injury particularly in the back, neck and pelvis. Strengthening the core with regular, good quality exercise should be a particularly important training aim.

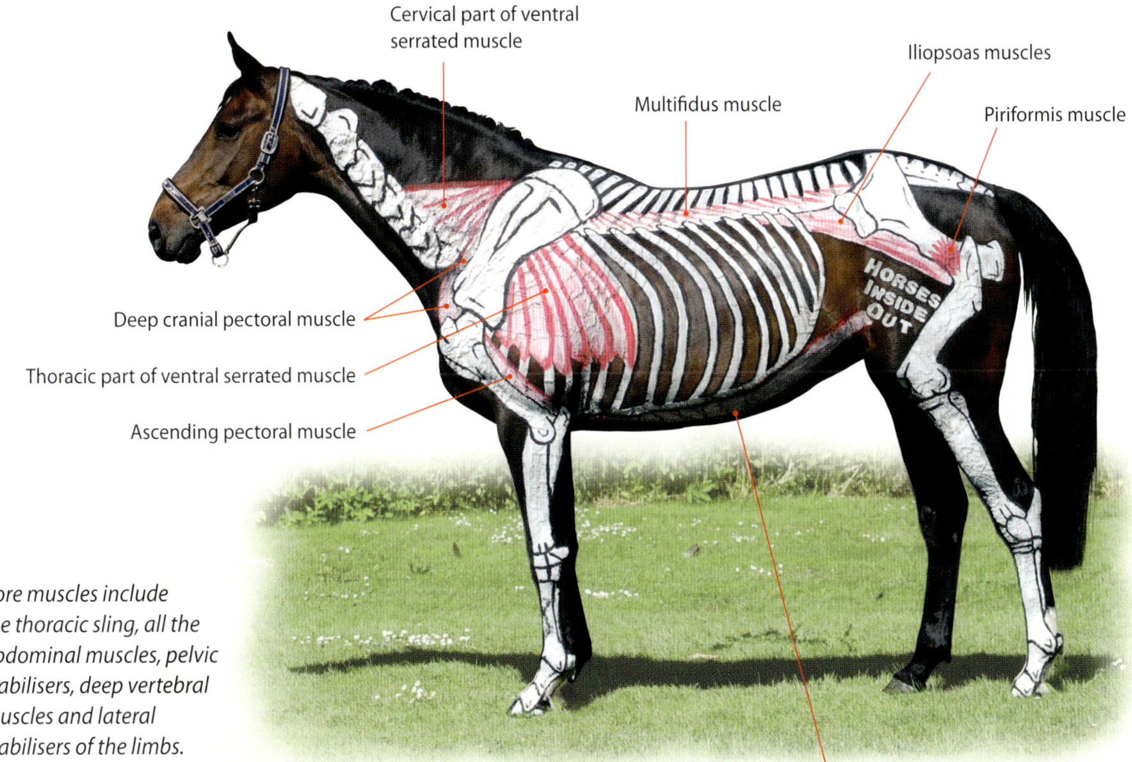


*Core muscles include the thoracic sling, all the abdominal muscles, pelvic stabilisers, deep vertebral muscles and lateral stabilisers of the limbs.*

*The multifidus muscle contributes to vertebral posture and stability by attaching the base of each individual spinous process to the bodies of neighbouring vertebrae. With a well-endowed nerve supply it is sensitive to any changes in segmental alignment. If back pain causes the multifidus to atrophy, its role will be assumed by the longissimus dorsi. As this is a movement rather than a stabilising muscle this will adversely affect performance.*

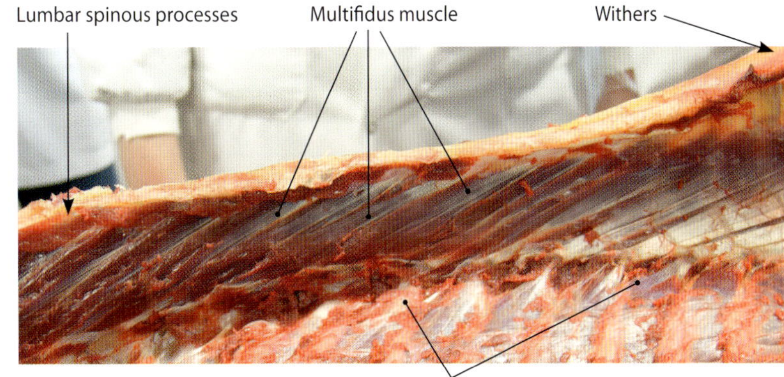

## Suppleness

Suppleness is sometimes referred to as looseness or relaxation. It requires the muscles to be sufficiently conditioned and free from tension to allow the horse to cope both mentally and physically with the work required of him. To be truly supple both laterally and longitudinally the horse must be able to:

- Demonstrate elasticity through the muscles
- Bend comfortably to the left and right
- Adjust his head position
- Stretch the head and neck forwards and downwards in all gaits
- Swing through the back
- Lengthen and shorten the stride without losing rhythm or balance
- Engage the hindquarters
- Move with rhythmic, flowing natural gaits
- Perform stretch exercises with ease.

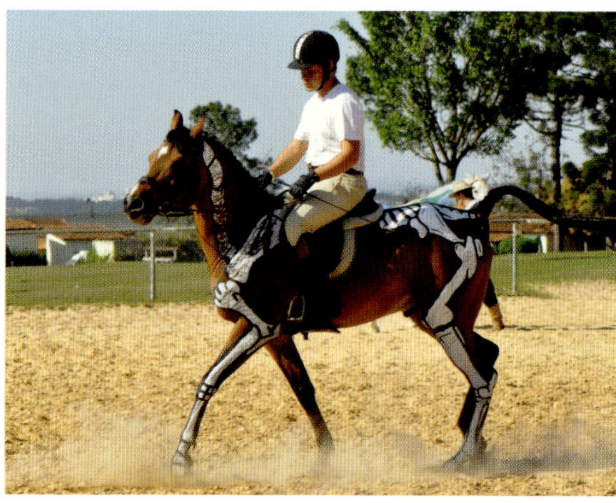

*An inflexible horse that carries tension, lack of muscle tone, or is stiff or rigid in any part of his body will hollow through the back, be uncomfortable to ride and be unable to use himself effectively. This will result in irregular gaits, falling 'in' or 'out' through the shoulder, a general unwillingness to work and an increased likelihood of muscle strain.*

### Balancing flexibility with stability

When choosing an exercise programme it is important to consider each horse's general stability and strength in relation to flexibility, suppleness and range of movement. A good sports therapist or coach will be able to advise. Once they have completed their assessment, they will suggest a correctly balanced programme of strengthening and flexibility exercises.

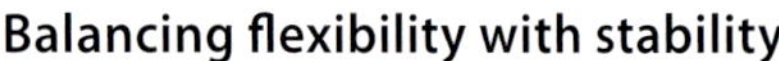

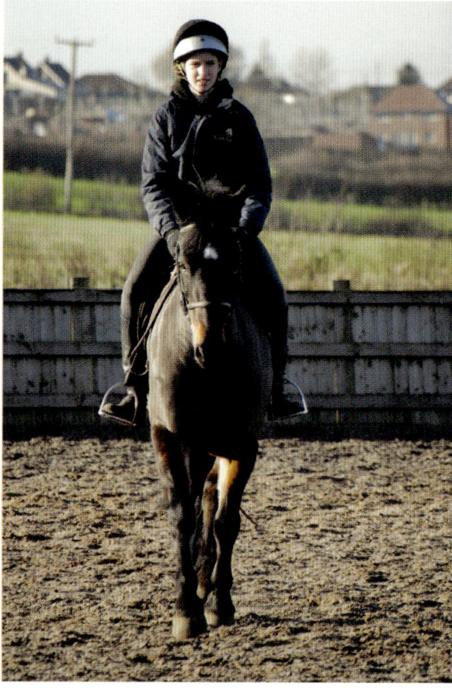

*A flexible supple young horse may struggle with balance and straightness. A well-balanced, stiffer, straight horse that neither falls in nor out may struggle with lateral suppleness and range of movement. The first horse (**LEFT**) will require a higher proportion of strengthening, balance and stability exercises, whilst the second (**RIGHT**) a higher proportion of stretching, suppling and flexibility exercises.*

Some suggestions for balancing flexibility with stability are:

- Work a manageable programme of in-hand stretching, strengthening and 'Pilates' type exercises into your daily routine
- Take the joints and muscles through a full range of movement on a regular basis
- Intersperse strengthening and fast work with flexibility sessions
- Perform ridden active stretches
- Vary the outline
- Perform lateral suppling exercises regularly
- Perform stretching, flexibility and strengthening exercises on the lunge
- Vary hacking surface and terrain
- Practise regular pole work and gymnastic jumping exercises.

## SUMMARY

- Horses need to be physically fit to work at their best.
- Long slow distance work is the basic requirement for conditioning all systems.
- Walking on hard ground is good for conditioning bone and hardening tendons.
- Warming up increases blood flow to muscles and vital organs, stretches the muscles, tendons and ligaments and prepares the body for exercise.
- Rhythm, balance and suppleness are prerequisites for contact, impulsion, straightness and collection.
- Regular stretching is beneficial for keeping muscles in optimum condition.
- It is important to balance stability with flexibility.

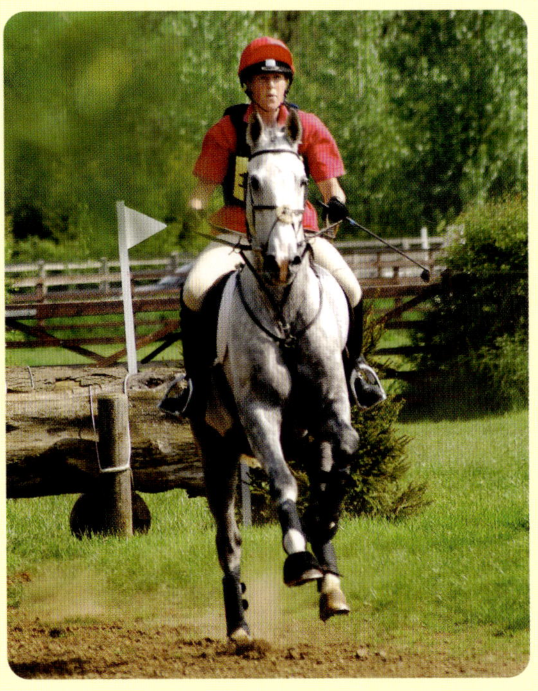

*As activity intensifies the horse breathes faster.*

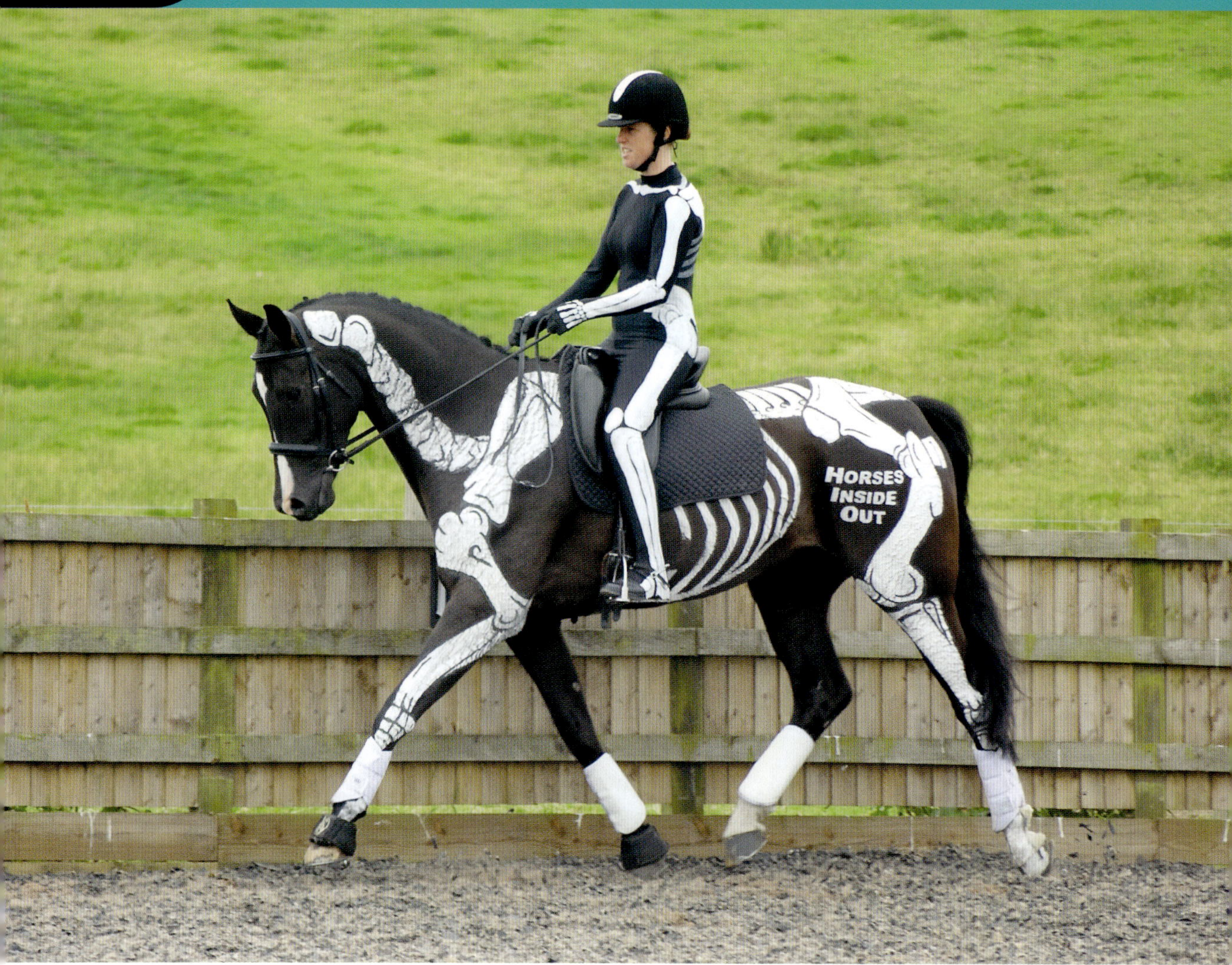


As soon as a weight is placed on the horse's back it will affect his posture, comfort, balance and confidence. Horses have evolved to carry weight – not the weight of a rider but that of the heavy hind gut suspended below the rigid spine. It is the rigidity of the spine which forms a bridge between the fore and hind ends which allows us to ride our horses. Making it easier for the horse to carry weight must be a primary aim. To do this it is important to ensure his back is raised and well supported with the rider sitting in a correct balanced position.

## Rider's Position and Posture

To enable the horse to move in balance whilst carrying weight, the rider must apply timely, precise, independent aids whilst continually assessing and maintaining a quiet balanced position following the movement. Because the horse's centre of mass is transient, the rider needs to constantly adjust his position to reflect this. This desirable quiet state of equilibrium can be more effectively achieved with the help of someone on the ground, mirrors and video.

# Reducing the Burden

This rider's balanced position will reduce the burden on the horse. With the leg directly below his centre of mass he has created a vertically correct 'ear – shoulder – hip – heel' line. If the horse were removed the rider would land on the ground in perfect balance.

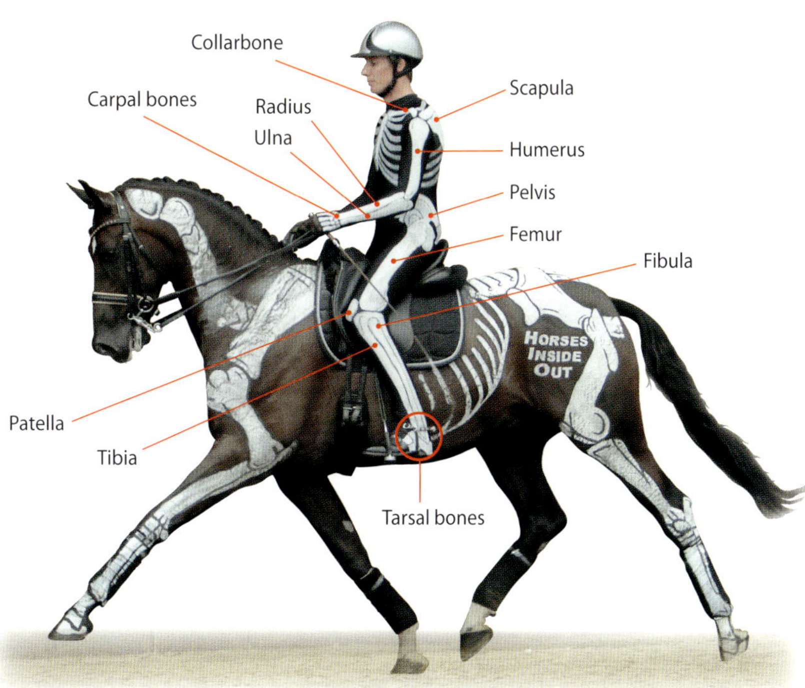


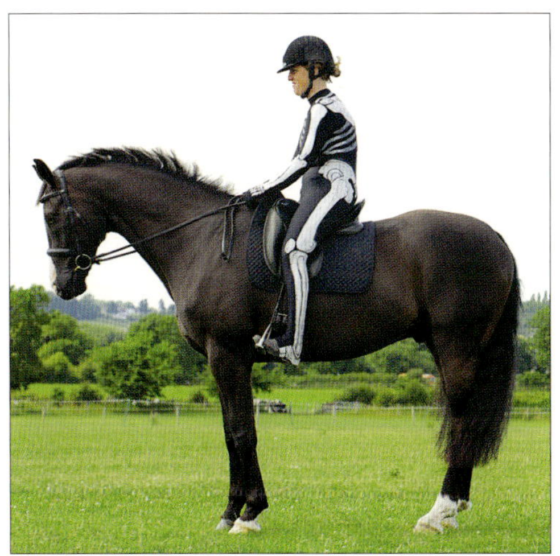

ABOVE *This rider is creating a greater burden for the horse to carry. The chest is collapsed and the spinal vertebrae, rather than being vertically stacked, are curved forwards. The 'ear – shoulder – hip – heel' are not aligned. This common poor postural position can be as a result of sitting slumped with the arms and head forwards when at a computer or driving. If the horse were removed the rider would be unable to maintain her balance on the ground.*

RIGHT *Position should be assessed from all angles. Here, the vertical axis of the rider's spine and the horizontal line of the hips are correctly aligned with those of the horse.*

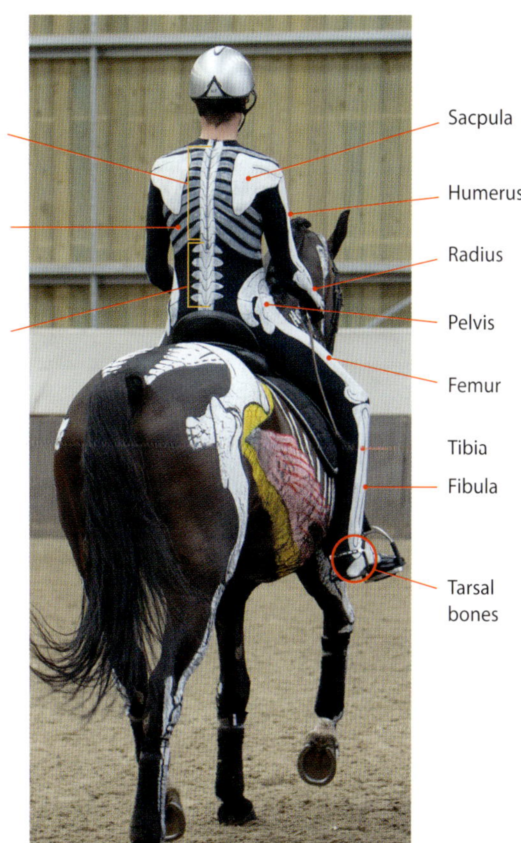

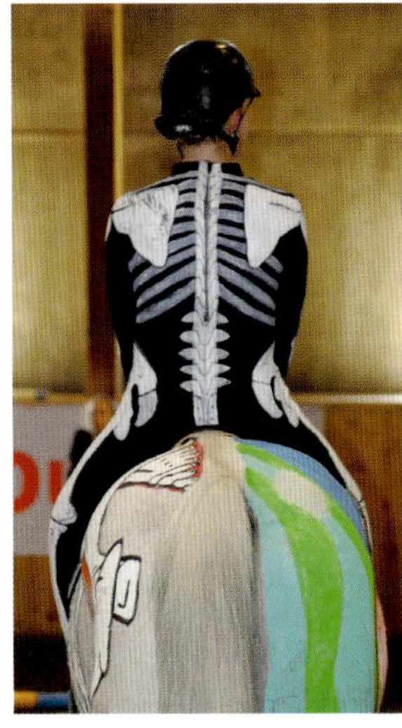

This rider's crookedness will affect the horse's straightness and balance.

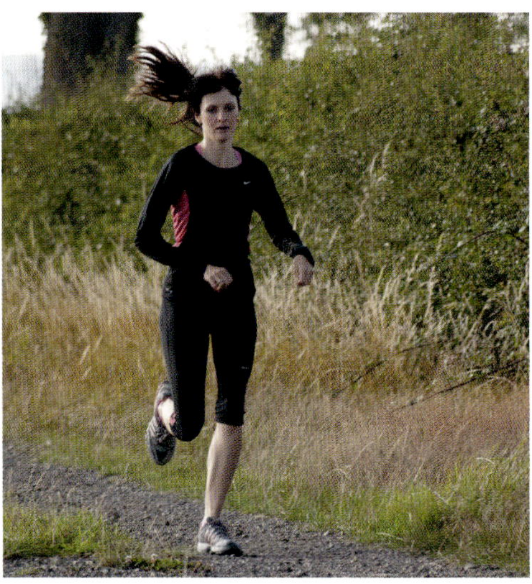

Although horses can carry 20% of their body weight, to reduce the burden it is important to perform exercises both on and off the horse and pay attention to personal fitness, weight, posture, reactions and balance.

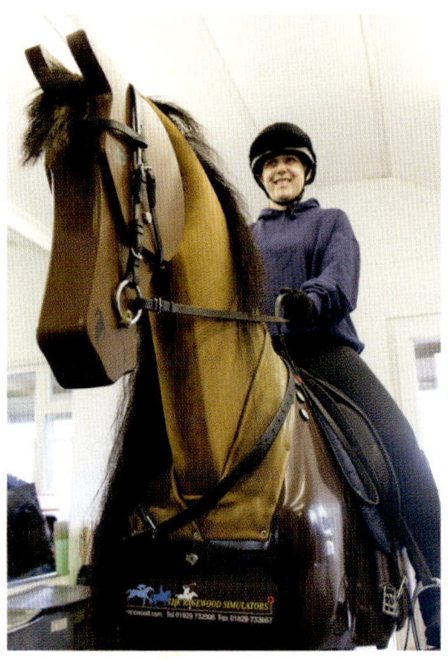

When starting to ride or to hone skills, practising on a mechanical horse before moving onto a live animal is advantageous. Perfect balance comes from practice and the ability to predict movement.

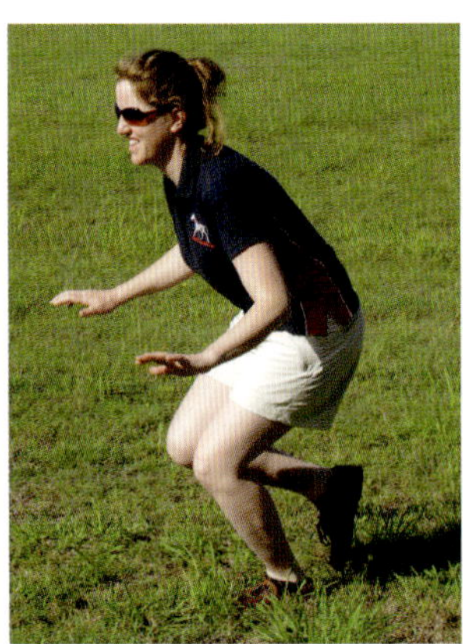

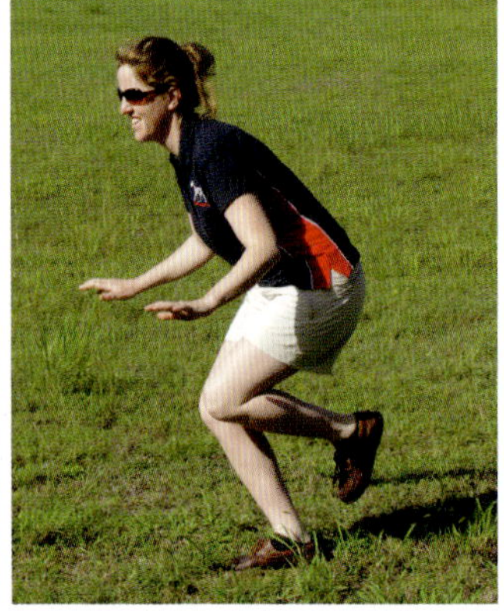

**LEFT** This is a good balance and strengthening exercise for riders.

**SEQUENCE BELOW** This is an excellent exercise for opening the chest, stretching the pectoral muscles and improving riding position. It can be performed both on and off the horse.

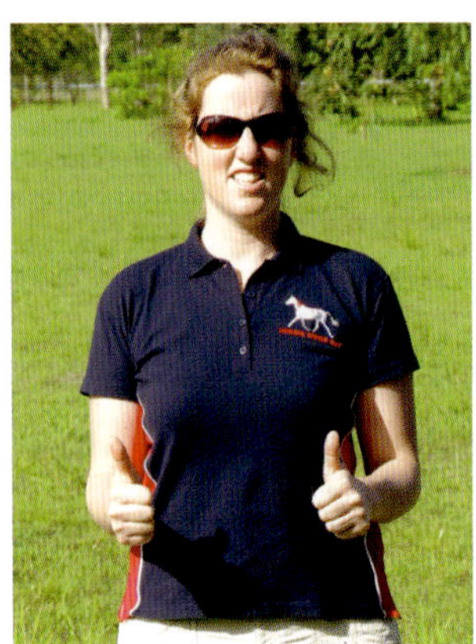

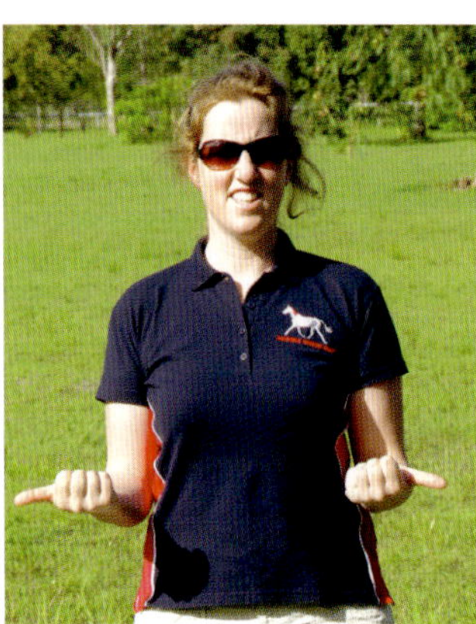

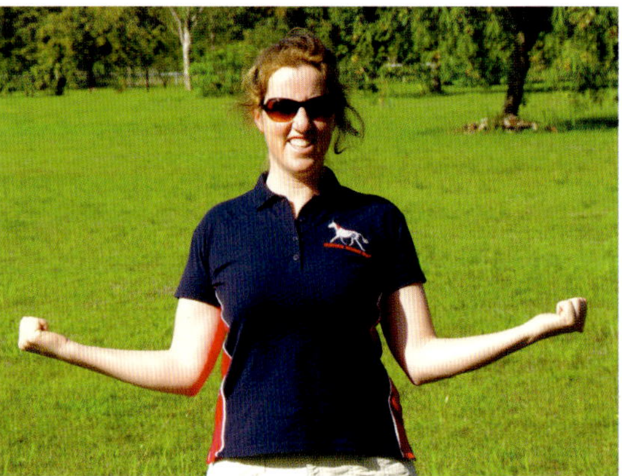

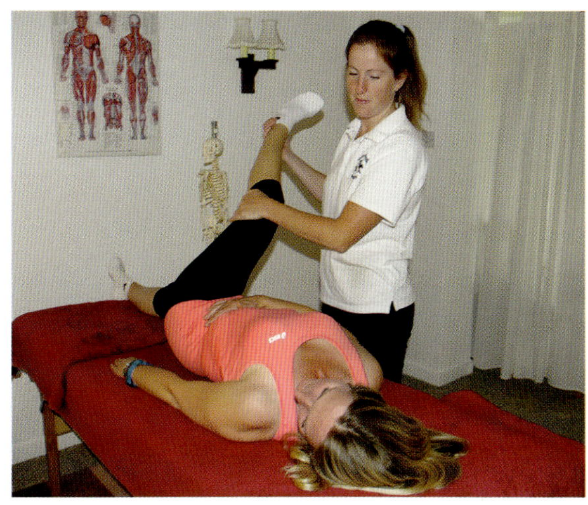

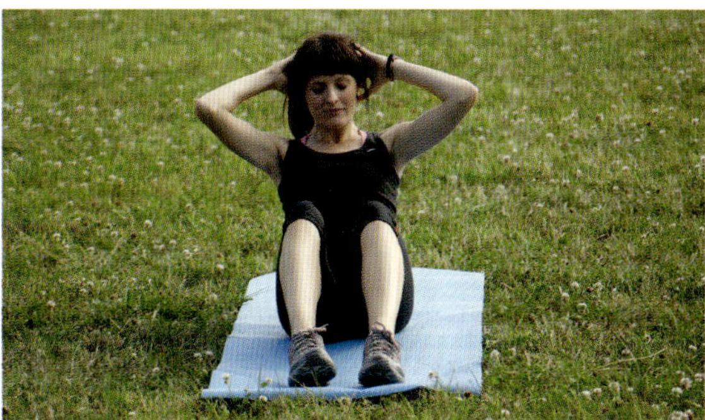

**ABOVE** *Pilates is a wonderful way to improve posture, balance and core strength.*

**LEFT** *Paying attention to our own musculoskeletal system is good for both flexibility and relaxation.*

# Influencing Structures

Sympathetic, intuitive riding requires a thorough understanding of the structures on which we sit and enables the aids to be applied in tune with the horse's rib movement and muscle contraction.

## Cutaneous muscle

The cutaneous muscle lies between the skin, the largest organ of the body, and the superficial muscles. It is thickest at the girth, tapering and merging with fascia at the edges. This muscle, which has the ability to shiver, envelops the trunk and legs down to the knee. To remove a fly from his neck or lower leg the horse must either shake his head or stamp his foot. To rid the body of a fly landing on the area covered by the panniculus carnosus the horse merely twitches his skin. As this muscle is highly innervated and sensitive, it is important to apply heel pressure lightly. An overtight girth, heavy kicking or overuse of spurs will potentially cause bruising, thickening or 'deadening' of the cutaneous and subcutaneous layers. The cutaneous muscle also acts as a shock absorber, a reservoir for fluids and for insulation.

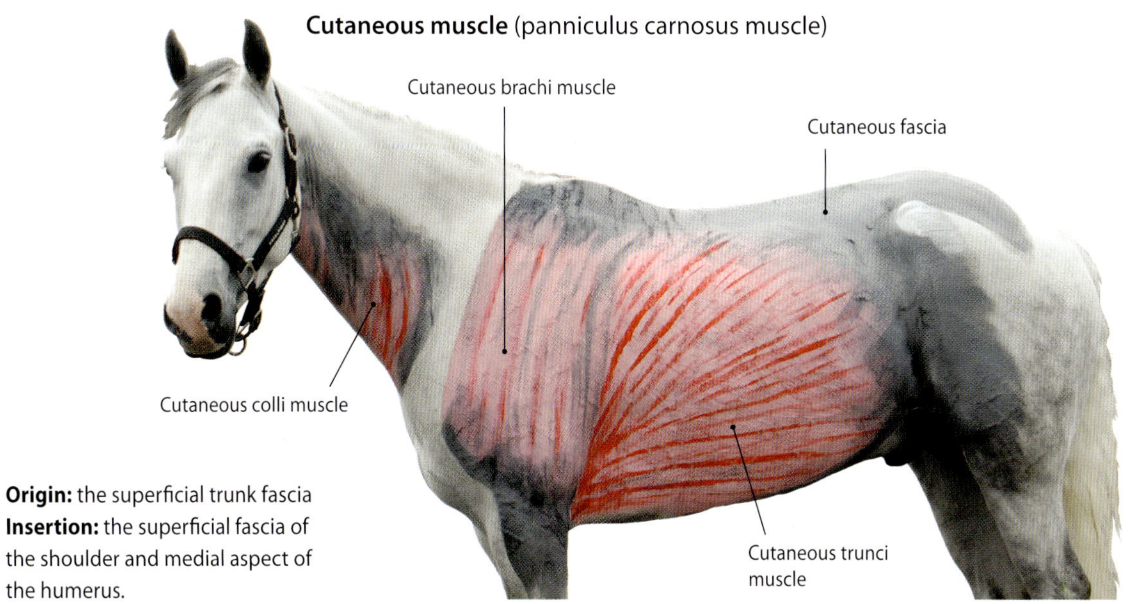


**Origin:** the superficial trunk fascia
**Insertion:** the superficial fascia of the shoulder and medial aspect of the humerus.

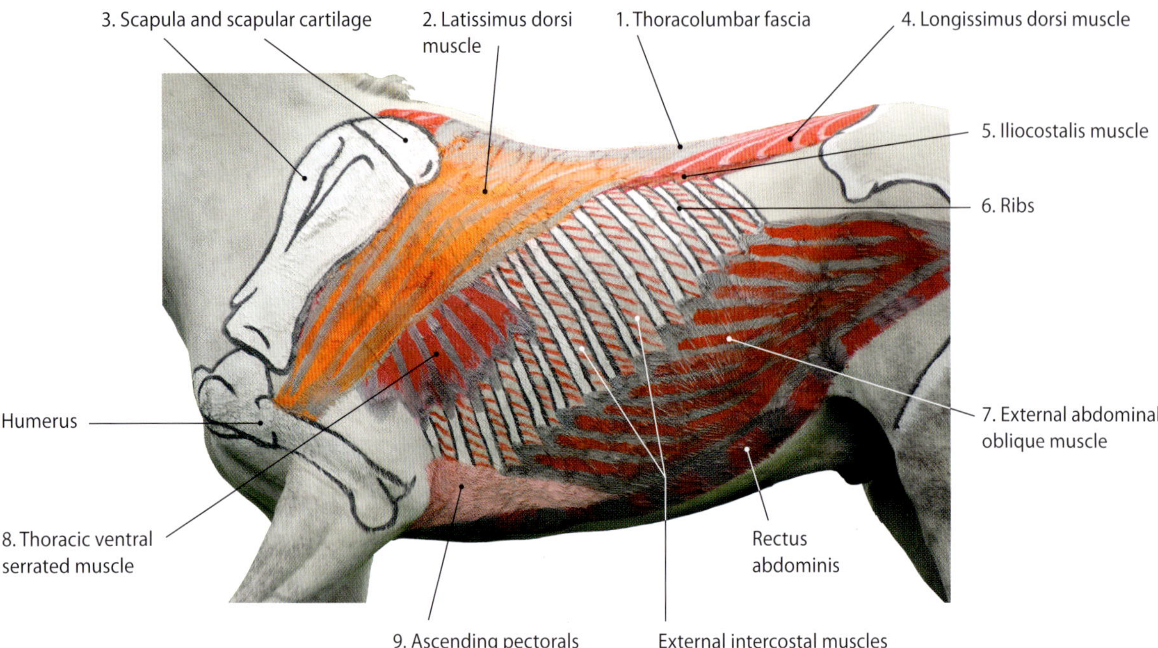


*The saddle, girth and rider's seat and legs are in direct contact with these muscles and anatomical structures.*

# 1. Thoracolumbar fascia

The thoracolumbar fascia which plays an important part in the support and transfer of forces for movement and which influences the muscles of the back, thorax, neck, tail, forelimbs and hindlimbs, many of which originate here, is situated directly underneath the saddle. It is important that it remains flexible, hydrated and does not become restricted by an unstable 'heavy' rider or a poorly fitting saddle.

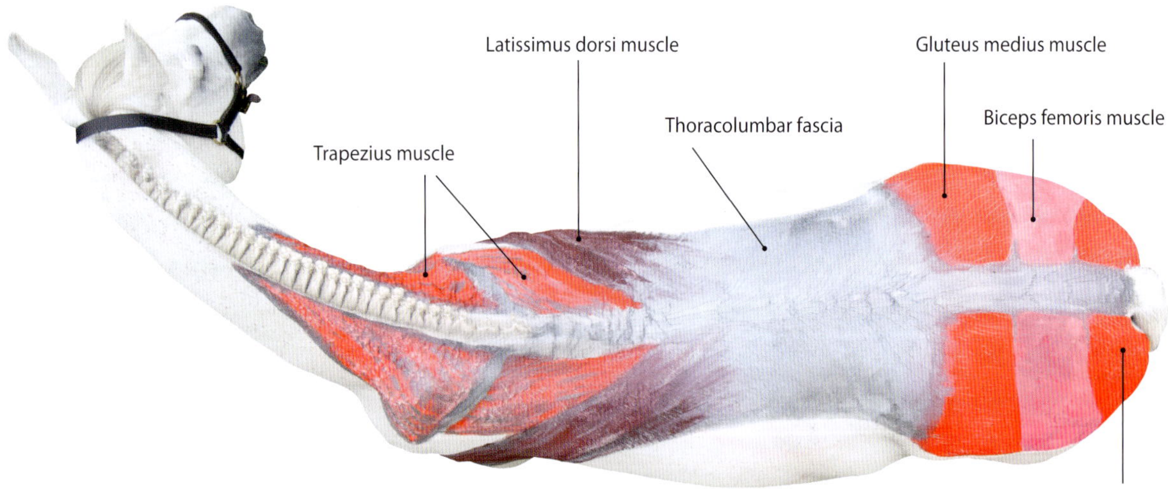

## 2. Latissimus dorsi muscle

Contraction of the latissimus dorsi, which originates in the thoracolumbar fascia, helps to flex the shoulder and pull the body forwards over the planted limb.

During protraction, the latissimus dorsi elongates to allow greater expression. Reducing stride length in a downward transition can be achieved by squeezing with the knee or thigh to encourage the latissimus dorsi to shorten. An overtight girth, a poorly fitting saddle which physically restricts the muscle, or a rider who continually grips with the knee can have a similar but negative effect and will inhibit maximum forelimb expression.

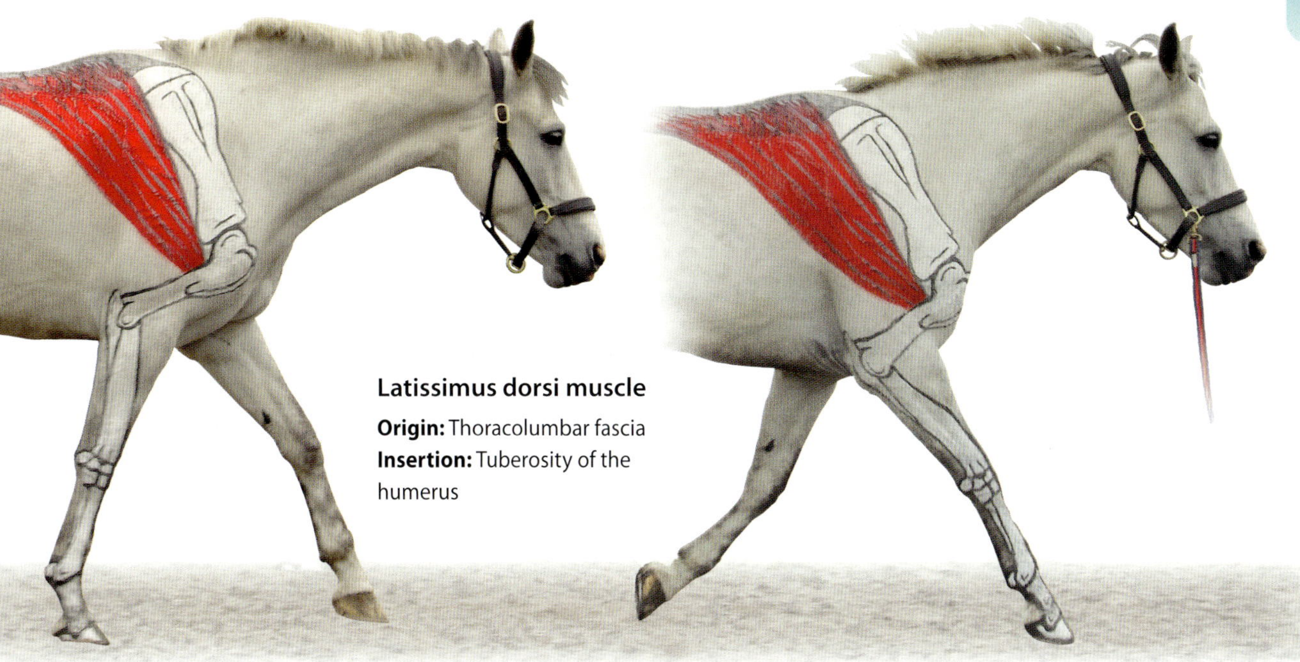

**Latissimus dorsi muscle**
**Origin:** Thoracolumbar fascia
**Insertion:** Tuberosity of the humerus

*Contraction of the latissimus dorsi.*

*Elongation of the latissimus dorsi.*

## 3. Scapula and scapular cartilage

Scapular cartilage is a semicircular extension of the scapula. It feels and acts like bone. As the forelimb moves through the stride cycle the top of the scapula moves elliptically. It is important the fit and positioning of the point of tree allows space for this movement.

If the saddle is too narrow or too far forward this may cause:

- Reduced forelimb protraction and expression
- An unwillingness to move forwards or downhill
- Discomfort landing from a jump, especially drops and downhill fences.

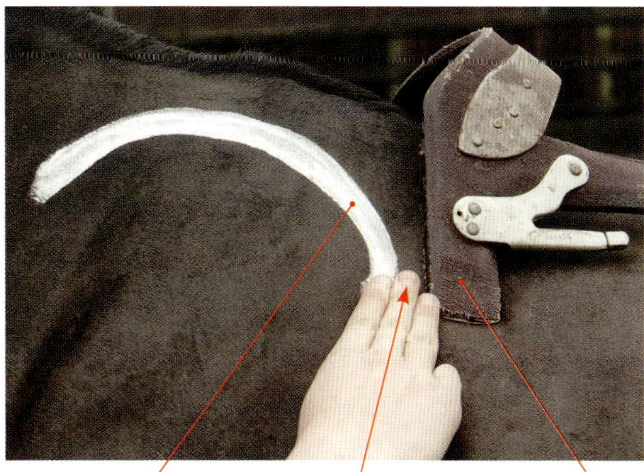

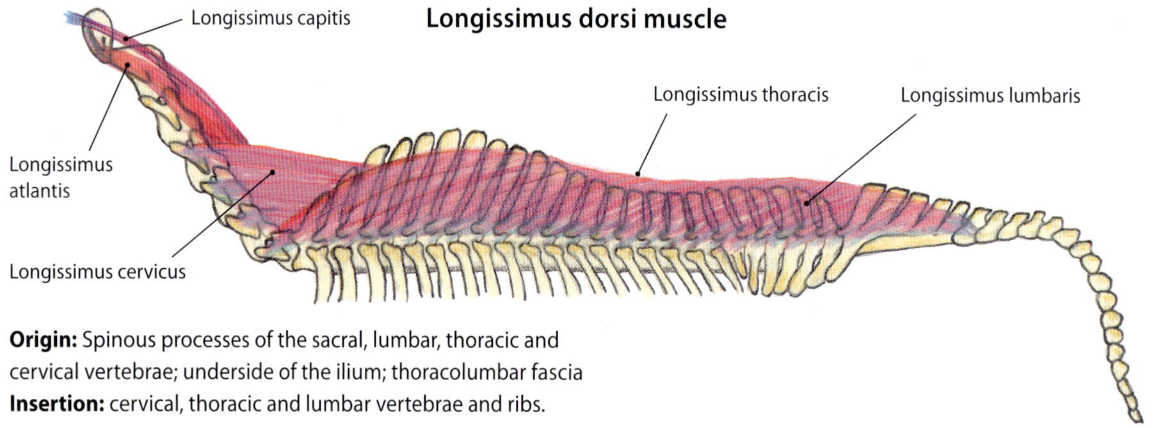



**Origin:** Spinous processes of the sacral, lumbar, thoracic and cervical vertebrae; underside of the ilium; thoracolumbar fascia
**Insertion:** cervical, thoracic and lumbar vertebrae and ribs.

## 4. Longissimus dorsi

Situated directly underneath the thoracolumbar fascia, the longissimus dorsi, the longest muscle in the body, creates the bulk of the soft tissue mass on which we sit. As a movement muscle, it is responsible for extension and hollowing of the back and contributes to forward propulsion by transferring energy created in the hindlimbs during the retraction phase of the stride forwards through the spine. As the horse bends, for example on a circle, the longissimus dorsi shortens on the inside and lengthens on the outside of the bend, stabilises the spine and prevents over flexion during the moment of suspension in trot.

Tension within the longissimus dorsi results in a hollow back usually accompanied by a high head carriage, unwillingness to stretch down, disengagement of hindlimbs and an inability to work correctly over the back when ridden. As a superficial muscle, although it is prone to soreness from poor posture, unsympathetic riding, incorrect saddle fit, asymmetry and hindlimb lameness its accessibility makes it easy to assess and positively influence with massage techniques.

## 5. Iliocostalis muscle

This muscle contributes to stabilising the thoracic spine and ribs. When it contracts the back will extend. When just one side contacts it contributes to lateral flexion in the back and rib movement. Tension within this muscle can result in altered rib positioning and potential discomfort.

**RIGHT** *There are a number of reflex points along the edge of the iliocostalis where it meets the angle of the ribs. Some half pads used under the saddle can create a ridge causing irritation, discomfort or continual stimulation of the reflex points.*

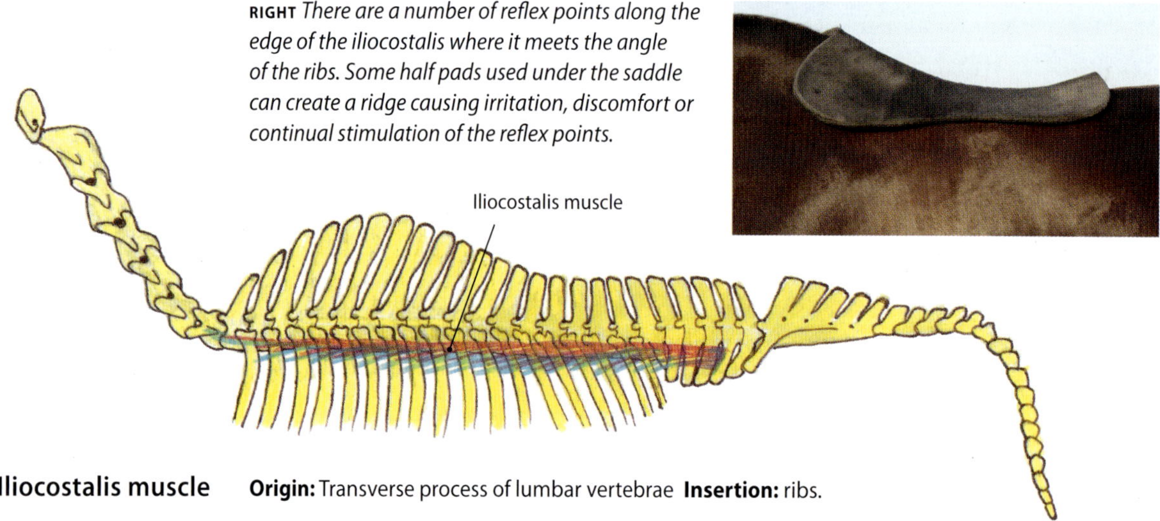



**Iliocostalis muscle**    **Origin:** Transverse process of lumbar vertebrae  **Insertion:** ribs.

## 6. Ribs

Each rib rotates around an axis which connects the head and tubercle of the rib to its two adjacent thoracic vertebrae. The ten false ribs which connect indirectly to the sternum via a fascial attachment have a degree of spring which as well as allowing the chest to expand as the horse breathes, contributes to bend.

As each hindlimb comes under the body in walk or trot, the barrel of the ribs swings to the opposite side. The longer the stride length, the greater the rib movement. Understanding and developing a 'feel' for both rib movement and the position of the hind leg allows leg aids to be applied alternately, accurately and effectively as the ribs swing towards each of the rider's leg in turn. Adjusting the amount of rider leg pressure applied can then influence stride length and positioning of the hind legs. This is particularly useful in lateral work. Applying heel pressure lightly is important to avoid damage and keep the muscles covering the ribs soft and supple.

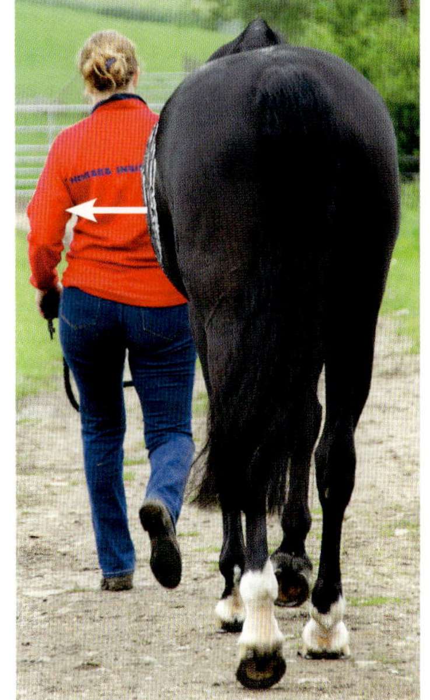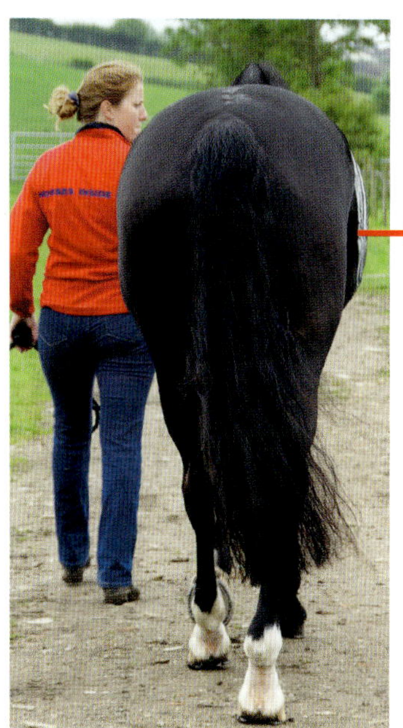

Mobilisation of the ribs achieved by gently and rhythmically pushing in the area indicated (see below) is useful for:

- Maintaining range of movement in the thoracic vertebral joints
- Maintaining suppleness in the longissimus dorsi, iliocostalis, diaphragm and abdominal muscles
- Improving lateral work
- Maximising the horse's ability to bend.

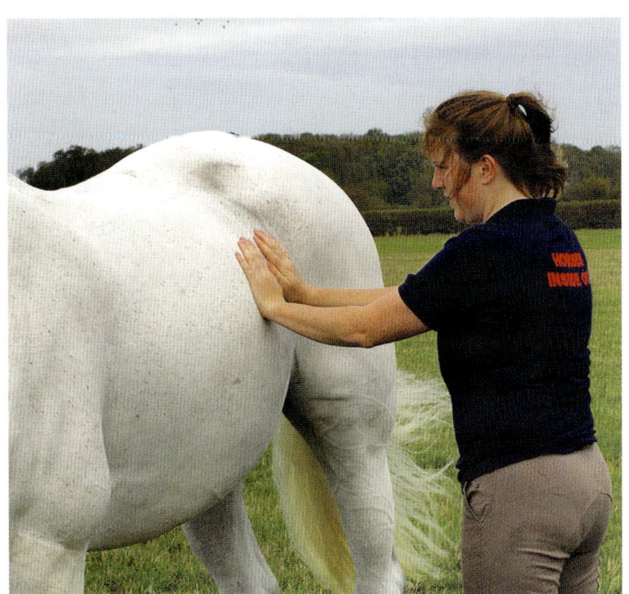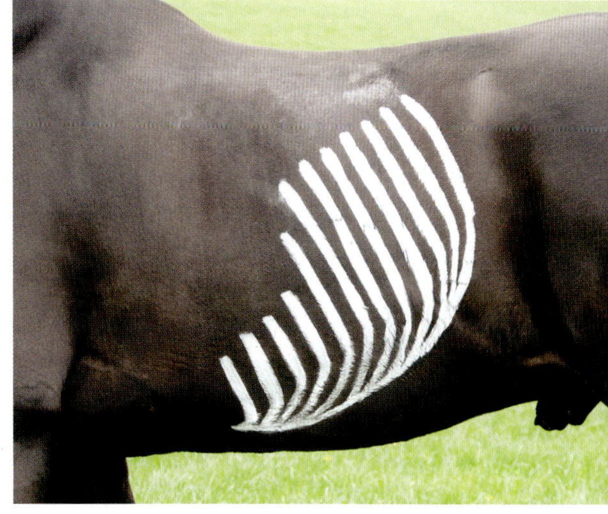

**LEFT AND ABOVE** *Mobilise the ribs by gently and rhythmically pushing in the area indicated.*

## 7. External abdominal oblique muscle

The primary role of the external abdominal oblique muscle is to support the weight of the abdomen and assist with defecation and expiration. It also contributes to back flexion, rib movement and hind leg protraction. When riding, our lower leg and heel lie directly on top of the external abdominal oblique muscle. As with the cutaneous muscle and ribs this muscle is particularly vulnerable to bruising.

**Origin:** Ribs –18 and thoracolumbar fascia
**Insertion:** Pelvic ligaments and fascial connection to the femur.

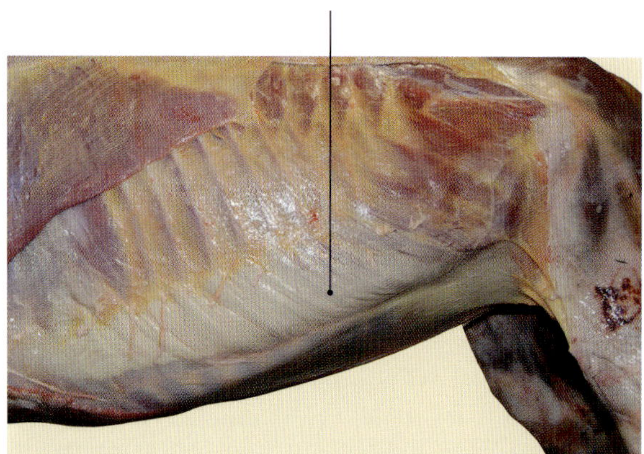



**RIGHT** *In this picture the right external abdominal oblique muscle is just starting to contract. Applying a right leg aid at this moment encourages the horse to snap the leg forward a little quicker.*

**BELOW LEFT** *Here the right external abdominal oblique muscle is shortened in full contraction. A right leg aid applied at this moment will encourage the hind leg to come higher and further under the body.*

**BELOW RIGHT** *Applying a right leg aid at this moment will not directly influence hindlimb protraction but will help flex the back.*

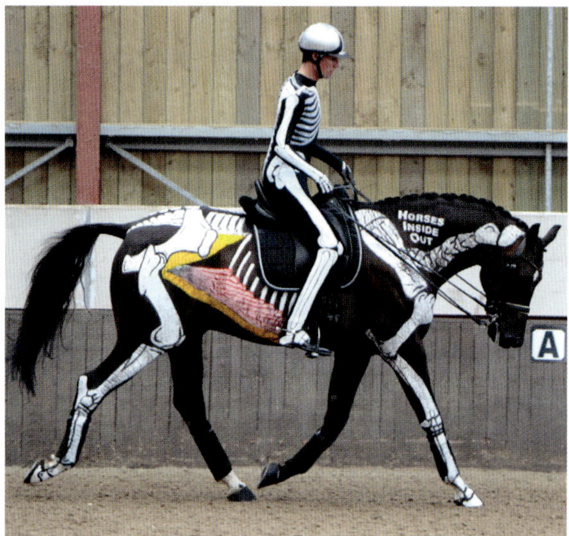



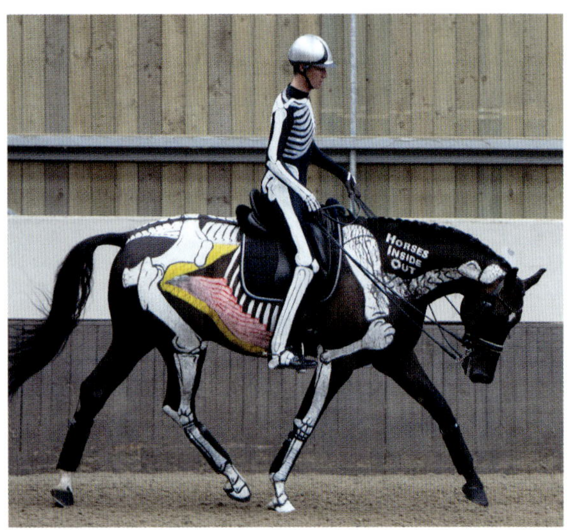



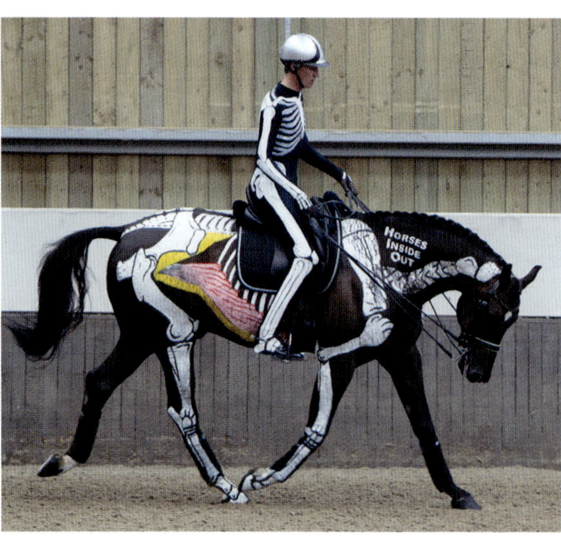

## 8. Thoracic ventral serrated muscle

The thoracic part of the ventral serrated muscle lies mainly beneath the flap of a saddle. It can therefore be influenced by pressure applied on it through the saddle by the inside of the rider's knee and upper calf.

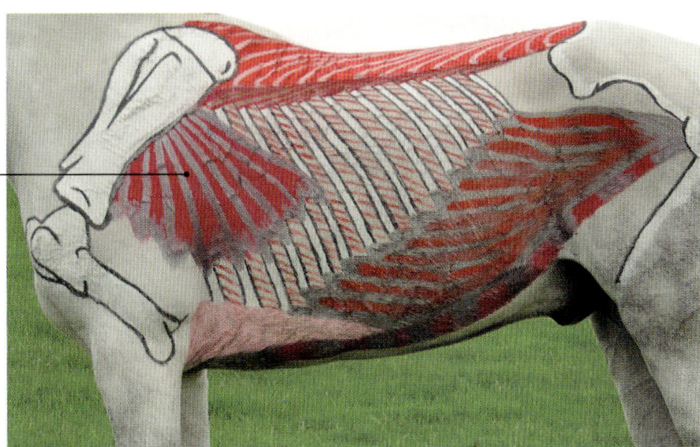



**Origin:** Ribs 1–8
**Insertion:** Underside of scapula and the scapular cartilage.

*As part of the thoracic sling, the thoracic part of the ventral serrated muscle helps to lift the thorax between the forelegs when the forelimb is planted. Applying leg aids further forward stimulates nerves and muscles of the thoracic sling which encourage the horse to come up through the shoulders.*

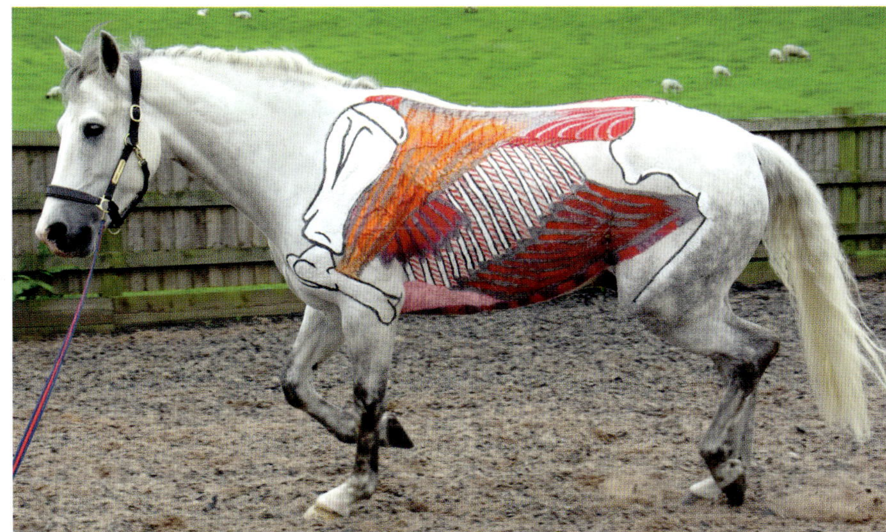

*During the swing phase the thoracic part of the ventral serrated muscle helps stabilise the scapula, facilitating crisper movement, expression and greater protraction of the forelimb.*

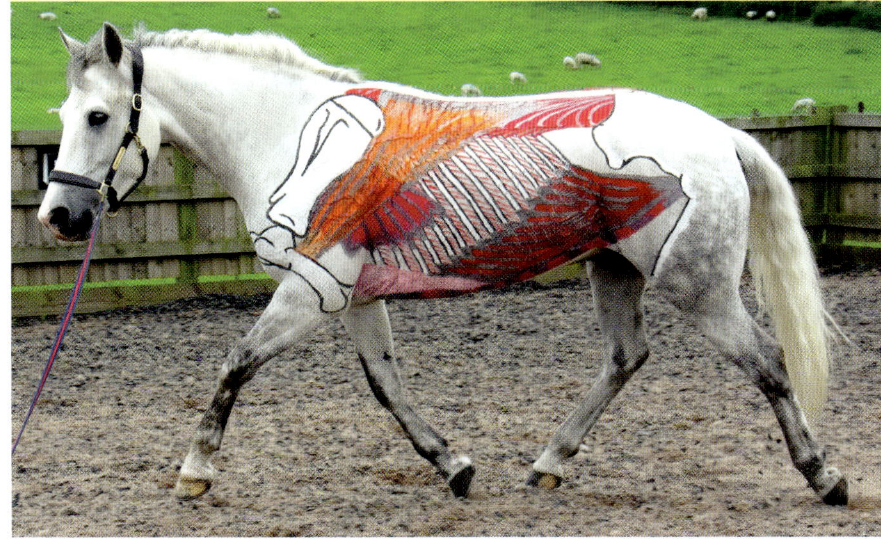

## 9. Ascending pectoral muscle

When the ascending pectoral muscle shortens it pulls the body forward over the planted limb. It also adducts the leg, supports the trunk and contributes to stabilising the shoulder joint.

The ascending pectoral cannot easily be affected by leg pressure but it can be directly influenced by the girth. An overtight girth will prevent the muscles from functioning correctly, reduce forelimb range of movement and be uncomfortable for the horse.

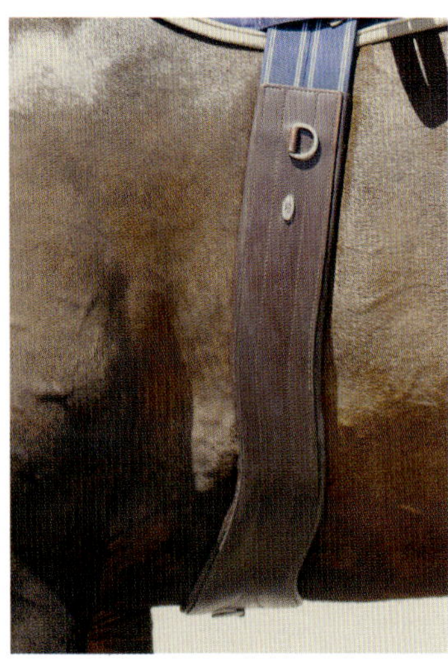

*This ergonomically designed girth fits well and allows space for movement of the forelimb.*

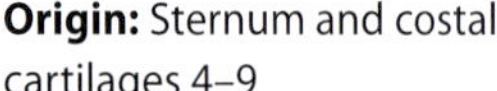

**Origin:** Sternum and costal cartilages 4–9
**Insertion:** Humerus and fascia of the forelimb.

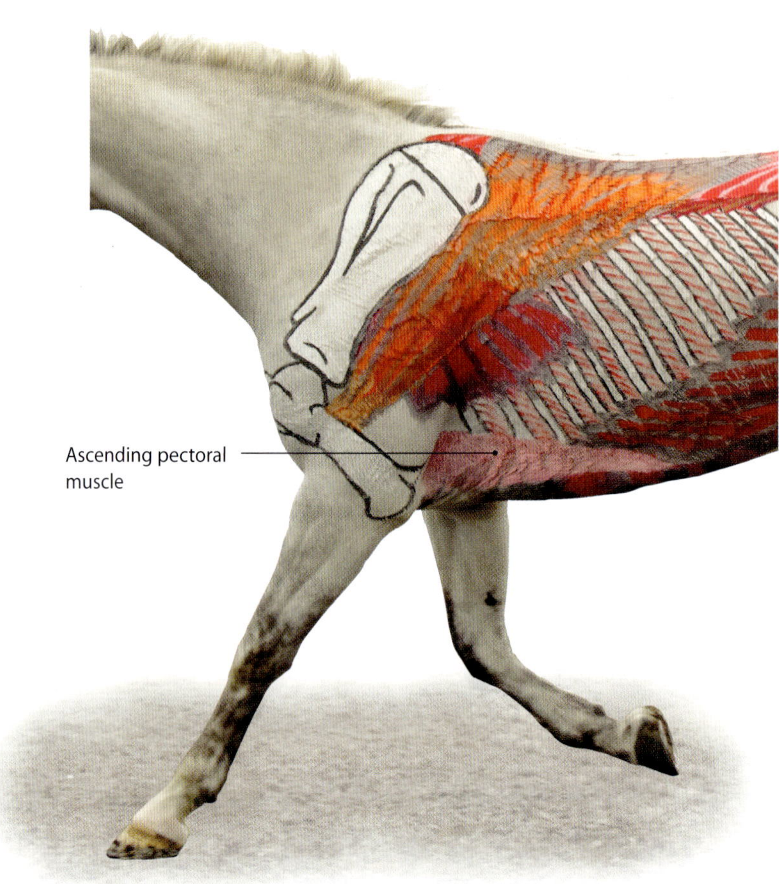

# The Head

As riders and handlers, we use the head more than any other part of the horse for influence and control. Incorrectly fitting tack, poll, nose and jaw pressure, injury and accidents can all lead to patterns of pain, imbalance, behavioural changes, movement compensation patterns and decreased overall harmony, contentment and performance.

## Outer head structures

The skull is made up of twenty-six connecting plates joined by fibrocellular joints known as sutures. These are designed to disperse energy from impact, such as when the horse lands from a jump, or in response to trauma. As the horse matures some of the sutures fuse. Understanding the external structures of the head is important for how we handle our horses and for bridle fit.

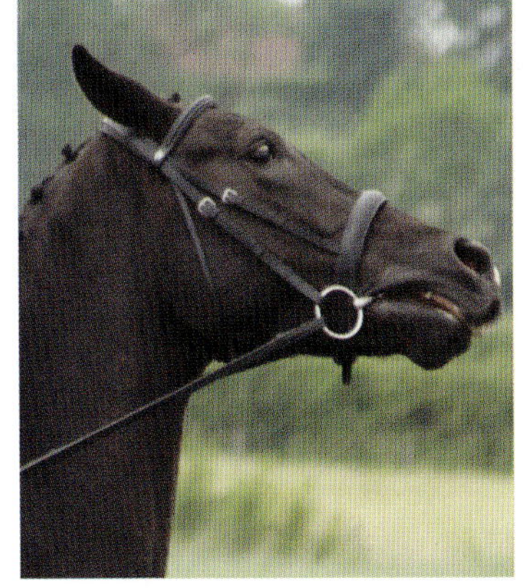
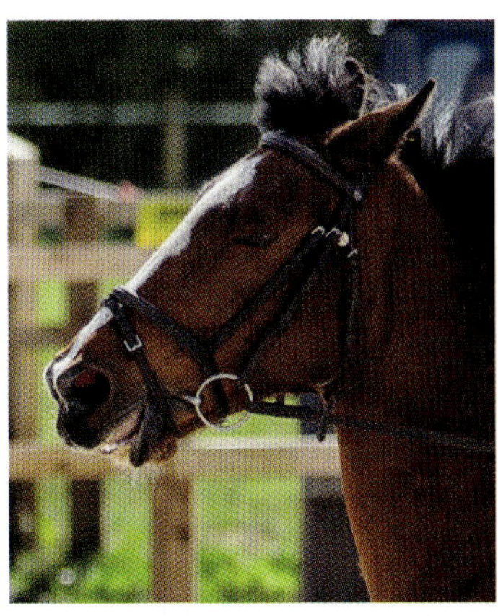

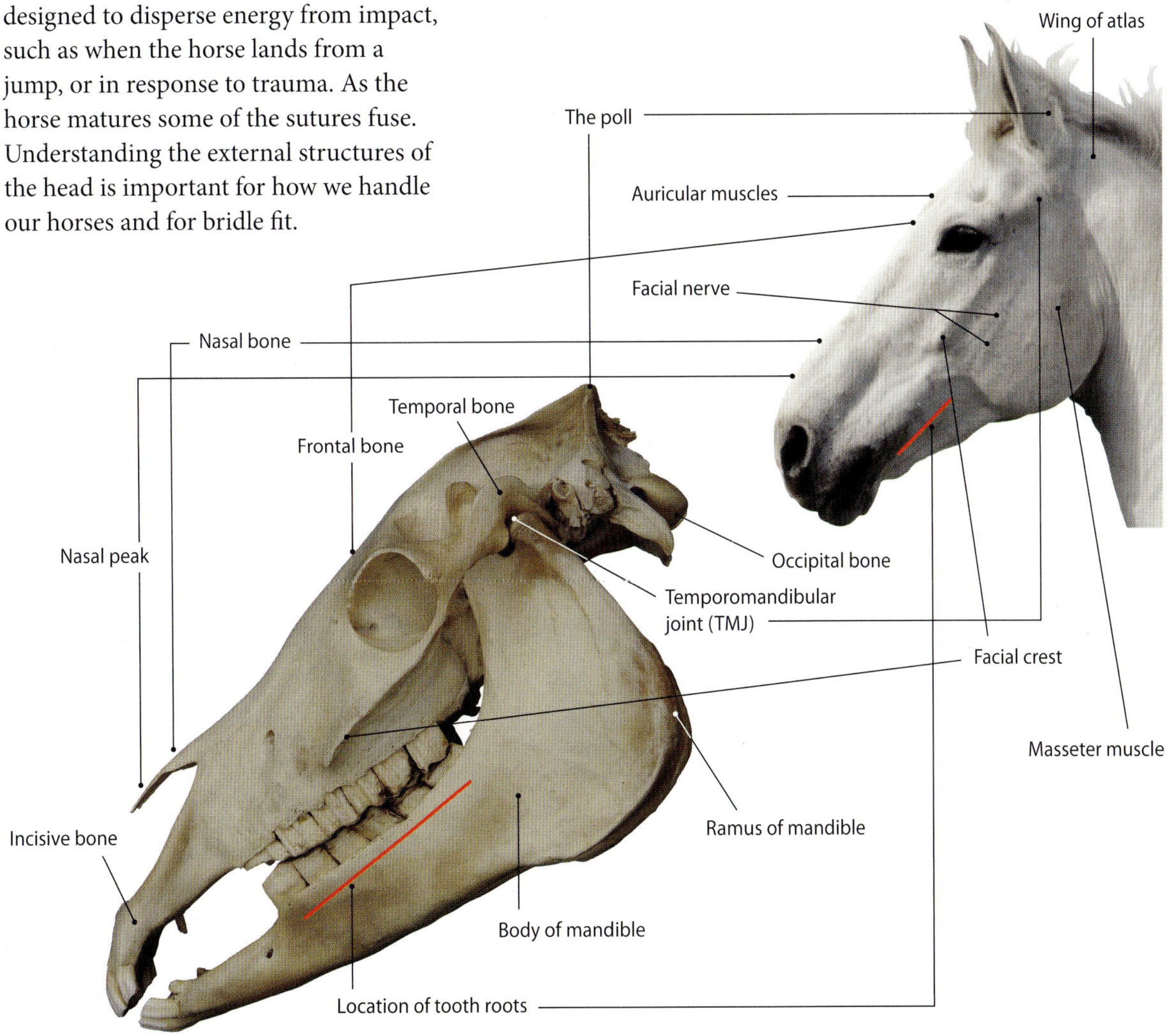

*Understanding the anatomy of the head will enable us to handle the horse more sensitively, appreciate the effect we have on delicate vulnerable structures and recognise the importance of still, quiet hands and a consistent, even, gentle contact when riding.*

## The poll area

Technically the poll or occipital bone is the highest point of the skull. Many riders and trainers however recognise and refer to the poll as the area just behind the ears between the skull and the first cervical vertebra, the atlas. Many muscles and tendons attach into the poll. The vitally important and influential nuchal ligament originates here. The poll is particularly sensitive to pressure. This is the area where the bridle, headpiece, or halter passes over the top of the head and comes into contact with the skull. By applying even slight pressure to the bridle or headcollar, a rider or handler can significantly influence the horse.

If a horse panics and pulls back hard against a tie ring, hits his head on a solid bar above a stable door, has too tightly fitting a headpiece, or is repeatedly 'jerked' by a leadrope when being led, this can cause swelling and discomfort at the poll. If this happens it is important to assess the amount of damage and act accordingly. If the poll is bruised a cold compress, gentle stretching and massage may help. If there is bruising it may be advisable to allow the structures to recover before applying pressure. If the horse seems disorientated or undergoes behaviuoral changes it is essential to call the vet.

## The nose

A horse uses his nose for communication, by emitting a variety of whickers, snorts and neighs as well as mutual grooming.

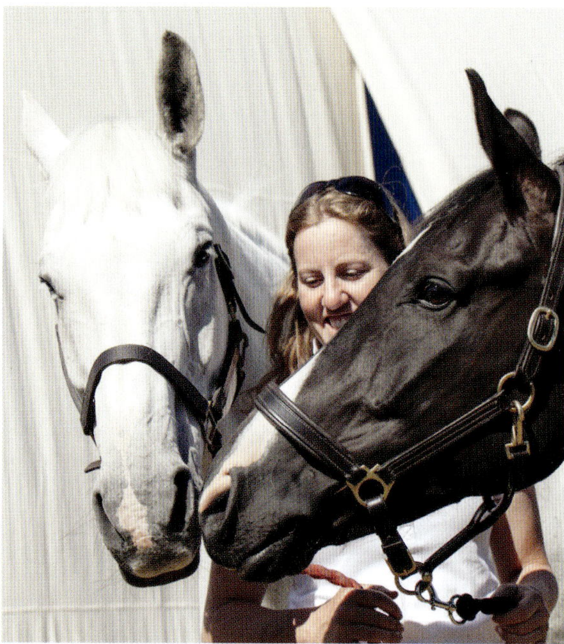

Nosebands were originally cruel pieces of equipment, often barbed and used to control the horse and prevent dislocation of the jaw! Today they are an integral or aesthetic part of a bridle. There are many different types. The simplest is the cavesson.

A noseband that is too tight can cause pain and may push the cheek against the teeth, which can cause abrasions. It can also restrict tongue and jaw movement which can lead to muscle tension throughout the flexor and extensor muscle chains.

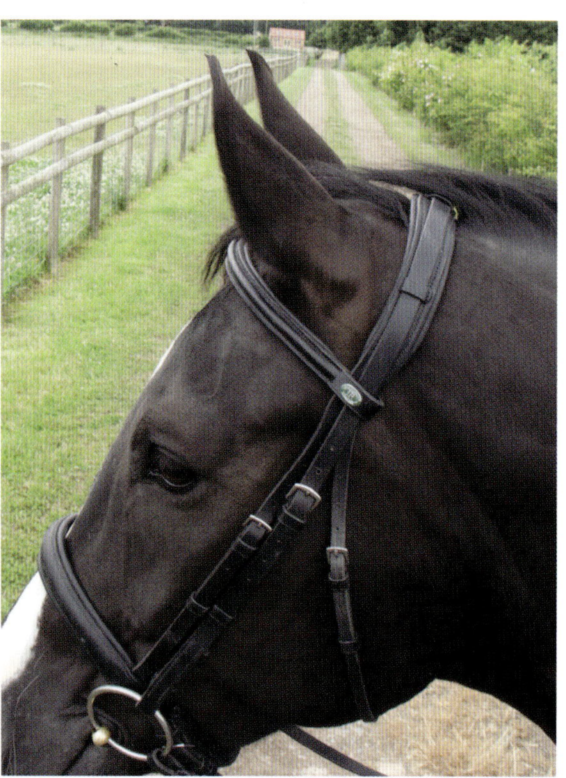

*LEFT Some bridles, either with bits or bitless, work by varying degrees of pressure on the poll. It is important that the headpiece fits comfortably and does not press on the back of the ear or on the bony prominences around the TMJ which may lead to discomfort, headaches, headshaking and the inability to work correctly. A major goal for trainers and riders is compliance and athletic flexion at the poll. This indicates acceptance of the bit.*

*A correctly fitting noseband should be fitted below the rostral end of the facial crest, the infraorbital foramen, which is the exit point for the facial nerves, and the vasular notch where the major facial nerves and blood vessels cross over the rim of the body of the mandible. As the horse can only breathe through his nose, in order to avoid restricting the airflow, nosebands should always be fitted above the nasoincisive notch.*

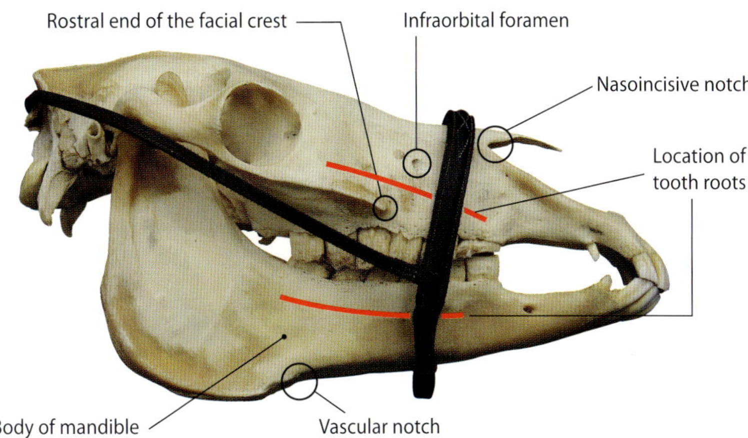


If the horse is trained anatomically and correctly a restrictive noseband shouldnot be necessary.

Unlike a poorly fitting saddle, damage from badly fitting bridles often goes unnoticed. Cheekpieces lie on either side of the face and should be above the superficial facial nerves which cross the masseter muscle and well behind the facial crest, zygomatic arch and temporal bones. The masseter muscle, which attaches to the full length of the facial crest, may be irritated by an inappropriately placed or tight cheekpiece.

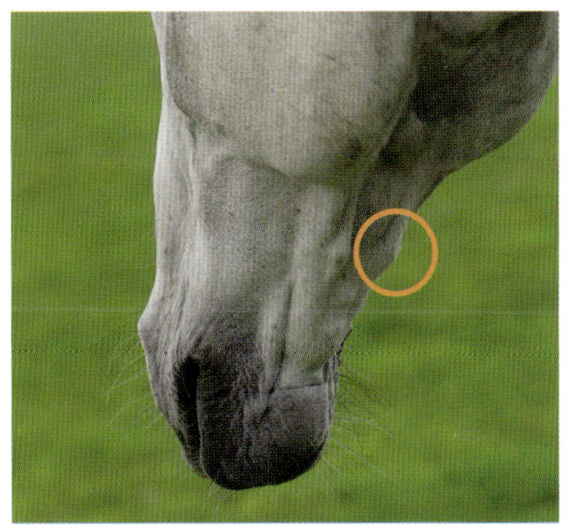

**RIGHT** *Damage to the bone on the body of the mandible or nasal bone, often as a result of too tight a noseband, can be felt as extra bony lumps.*

## BITLESS BRIDLES

**B**itless bridles are chosen for a variety of reasons. Some riders consider them kinder, some horses go better in them and they are a good alternative option for horses who have suffered mouth or tongue injuries. Some bitless bridles spread the pressure over the entire head; others work by putting pressure on the nose or poll. As with traditional bits, bitless bridles can be mild (for example the Doctor Cook) whereas the mechanical hackamore with long shanks is harsh.

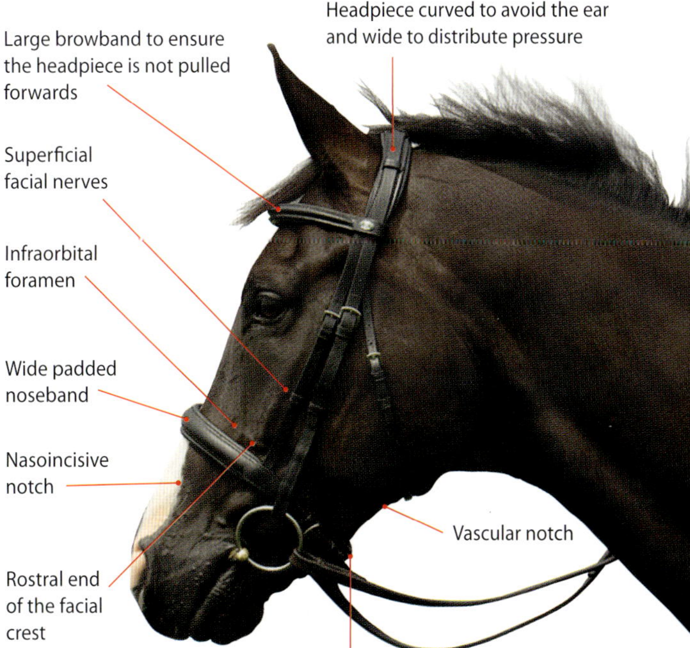


**RIGHT** *It is important to consider the fit, shape and design of the bridle with comfort and anatomy in mind. A poorly fitting bridle can have far-reaching negative effects on movement, balance, general comfort and behaviour.*

## Inner head structures

The horse's mouth is a very sensitive. It consists of the lips, between 36 and 44 continuously erupting teeth, the hard and soft palates, tongue, salivary glands and related muscles.

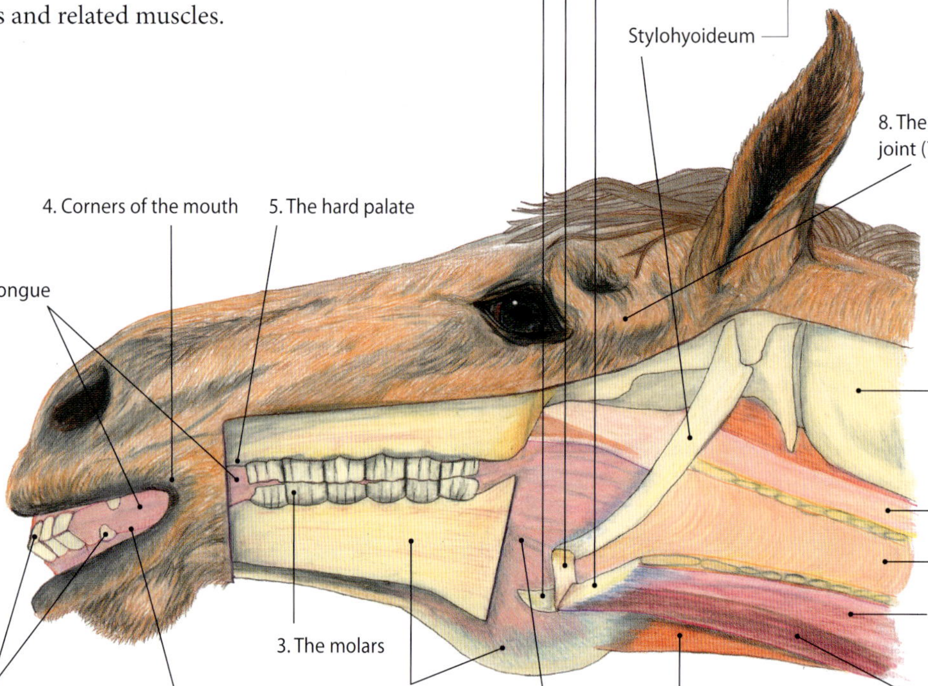

The anatomy of each horse's mouth is unique. Bit comfort is of paramount importance. Simply put, straight bits put more pressure on the tongue; shaped or jointed bits put more pressure on the bars. If a bit causes pain or discomfort, communication breaks down and both performance and the mouth suffer. Problems with a bit do not generally come from the bit itself but more from the rider's hands and how it is used. The bit must be neither too high nor too low, and because mouth conformation varies so enormously between breeds and individual horses, in order to find the correct bit it is advisable to engage the services of a professional fitter.

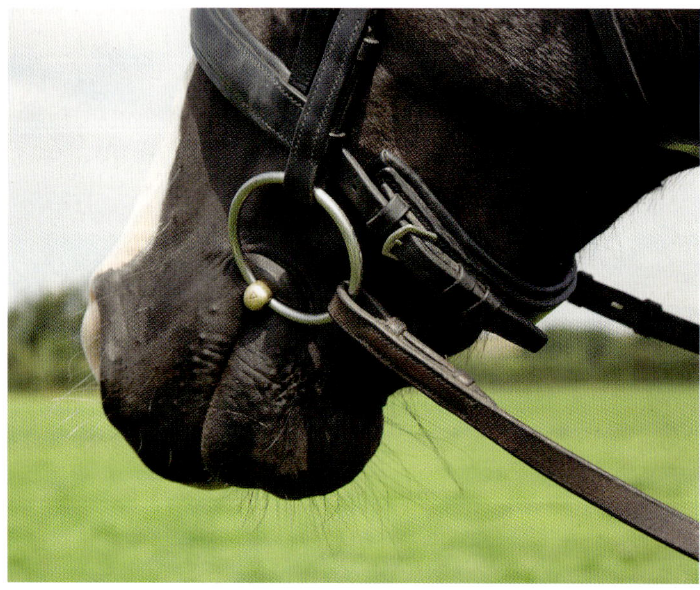

## 1. The incisors and tushes

These teeth should not be affected by the bit unless it is too low.

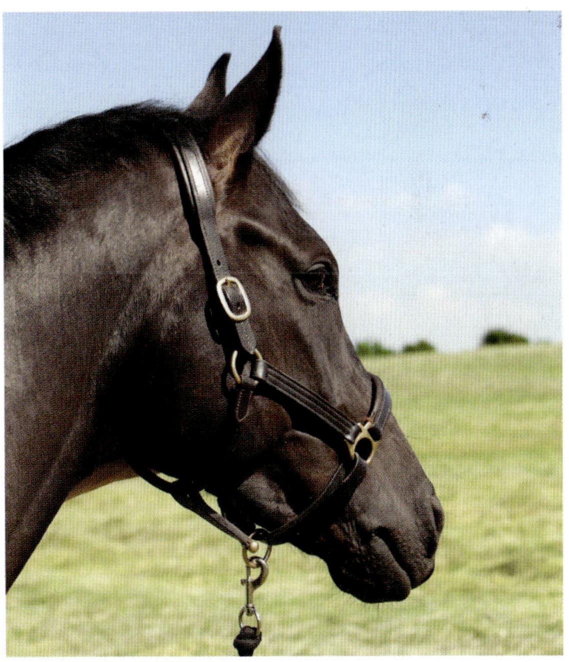

Tongue

Incisors

Tushes

Bars

## 2. The bars

Between the incisors and the molars lie the bars, the interdental, toothless area of gum-lined bone, on which the bit sits. This is a sensitive area susceptible to bruising. Some horses develop thickening of the bone and very occasionally bony spurs as a result of bit pressure.

## 3. The molars

The upper jaw, the maxilla, is wider than the lower jaw, the mandible. The different widths and elliptical chewing motion leads to the formation of sharp edges on the outside of the upper molars along the cheek which, in order to keep the horse comfortable in his mouth and able to perform at his best, require regular six-monthly visits from the dentist. Maintaining correct alignment of the jaw is essential.

Sometimes a wolf tooth, a small extra pre-molar, erupts. This can lie in the way of the bit and be uncomfortable for the horse. In these cases bitting options need to be studied and in some cases the tooth may need to be removed.

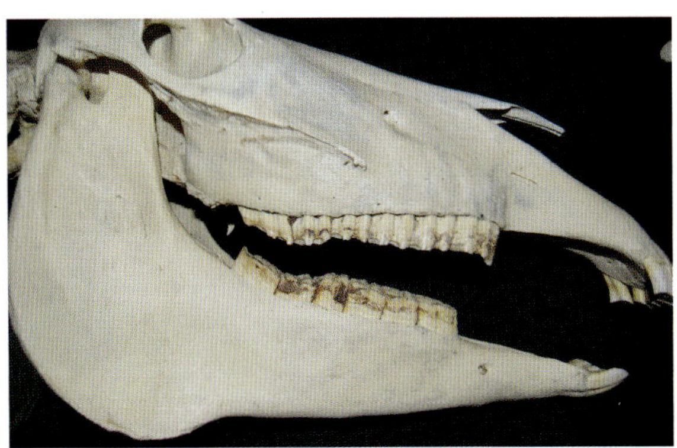

*The corners of the mouth should be checked regularly.*

## 4. Corners of the mouth

The corners of the mouth should be checked regularly. If the bit is too high, poorly fitting, sharp, or the rider's hands are too harsh this can cause splitting, which is very uncomfortable for the horse.

## 5. The hard palate

This is the thin plate that forms the roof of the mouth. The height of the arch varies from horse to horse. Ported bits, although they afford relief for the tongue, put pressure on the hard palate leading to discomfort.

## 6. The tongue

The tongue, a very large muscle, more sensitive at the edges than the centre, is the most sensitive part of the mouth and the most prone to injury. The size varies between breeds, but as a rule of thumb, a large tongue will be seen bulging through the teeth at the bars. (See page 75) Like any other muscle, restriction or tension within it can induce a muscular chain reaction.

## 7. Hyoid apparatus

The hyoid apparatus, sometimes referred to as the tongue bone, is made up of five bones which are located at the base of the skull between the mandible and the larynx. It provides attachments for the tongue and some muscles, tendons and ligaments of the pharynx, neck, sternum and even the forelimb. Although not something we touch directly with the bit, because the tongue attaches directly into it, tongue restriction can affect breathing, neck position, posture, mobility and protraction of the forelimb.

### The hyoid apparatus

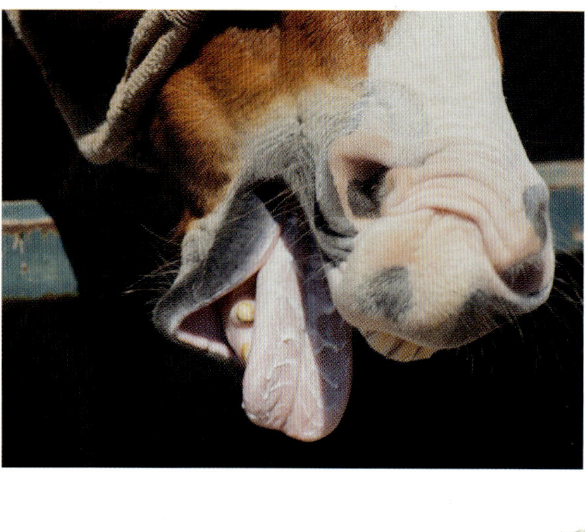

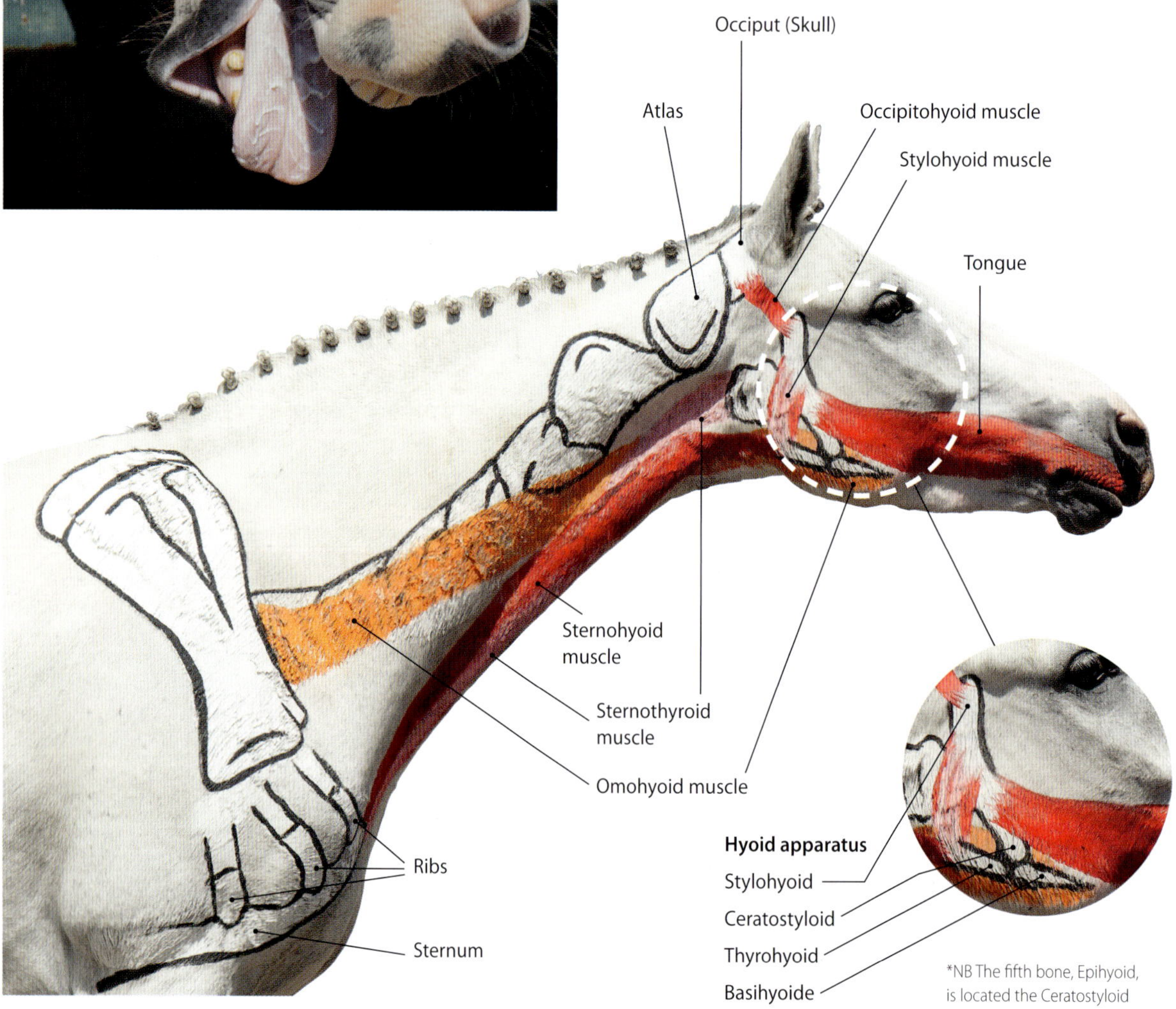

## 8. The temporomandibular joint (TMJ)

The TMJ (see right) connects the lower and upper jaw through the articulation of the temporal bones, the mandible and surrounding tendons, ligaments and muscles. Primary functions include mastication, movement of the jaw and alignment of the teeth. Through the temporal bone, there is a close relationship between the TMJ and the ear which, as with ourselves, is the centre of balance. This affects equilibrium, proprioception and posture. All locomotion is dependent on the relationship between the axial and appendicular skeletons of which, through the muscle chains, the TMJ is key.

Many horses suffer from TMJ pain, often referred to as temporomandibular dysfunction. This involves painful or inflammatory myofascial and/or ligamentous pain, often originating in the misalignment of the teeth or jaw and having a detrimental effect on balance, well-being, attitude, every aspect of performance and overall health. As well as other causes TMJ problems can stem from:

- An ill-fitting bit or overtight noseband
- Pressure and tension applied on the lower jaw through the bit on the bars of the mouth
- Poor equitation skills and over-reliance on the reins for balance.

The masseter, the largest muscle in the face, is the main muscle involved in supporting the TMJ, and closing the jaw. When the horse opens his mouth and 'fixes' his jaw to resist the hand and bit, he tightens not only the TMJ but also all the muscles of the head and neck. This affects the entire flexor and extensor muscle chains and results in a tense and unhappy horse.

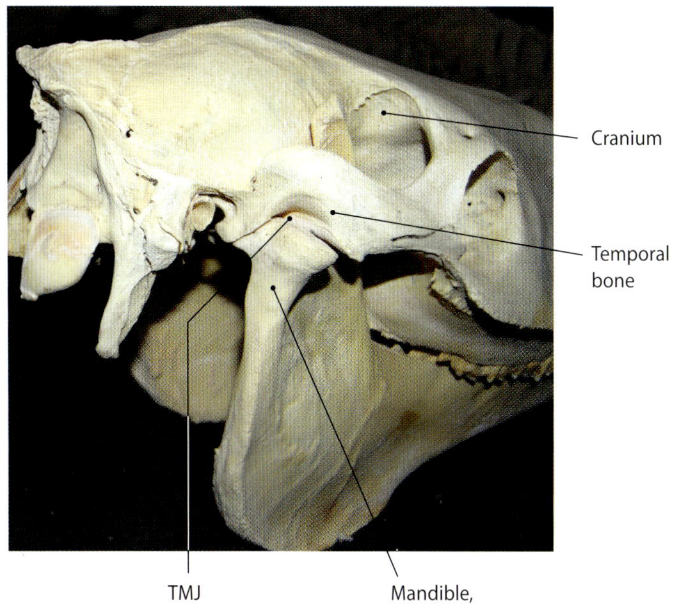


**Rectus capitis muscle group**

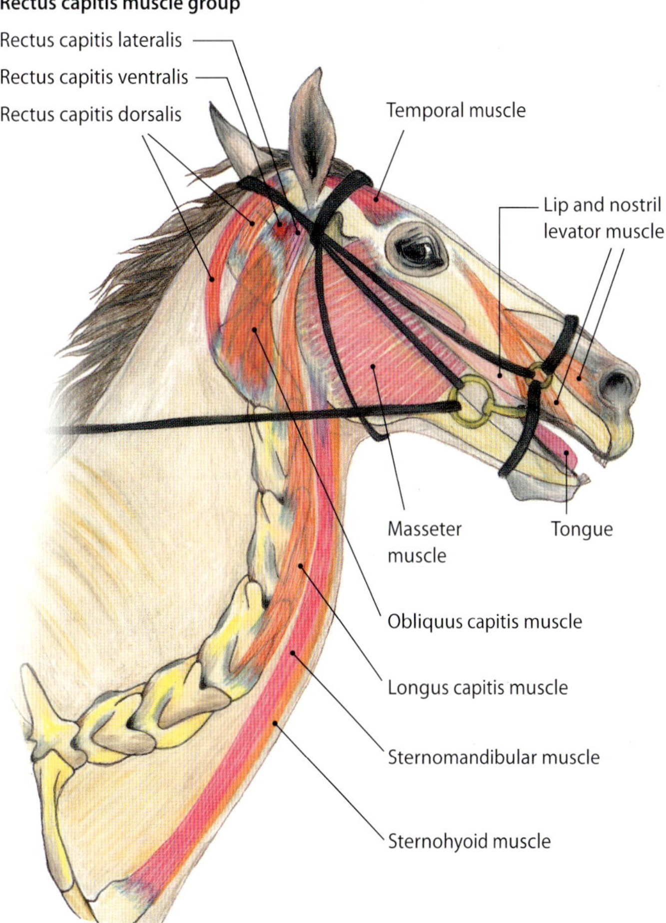

# The Contact

Contact or 'feel' is the connection between the rider's hand and the horse's mouth. It is the means of communication for directional guidance and for the regulation of pace, straightness and collection. It should be neither too light, which means the horse lacks cues, or too heavy, which can potentially damage the delicate structures of the mouth, cause him to fight or lean on the bit. To maintain a steady contact both horse and rider must have the core stability and the muscular strength to maintain balance and a consistent outline.

Any action on the part of the rider that causes discomfort, lack of balance or focus is counterproductive. This can include:

- Variations in pressure from a loose to a suddenly taut rein
- Continuously 'fiddling' with the rein
- Sudden backward pressure
- A locked elbow
- A collapsed chest and inwardly rotated shoulder
- A fixed, unyielding hand.

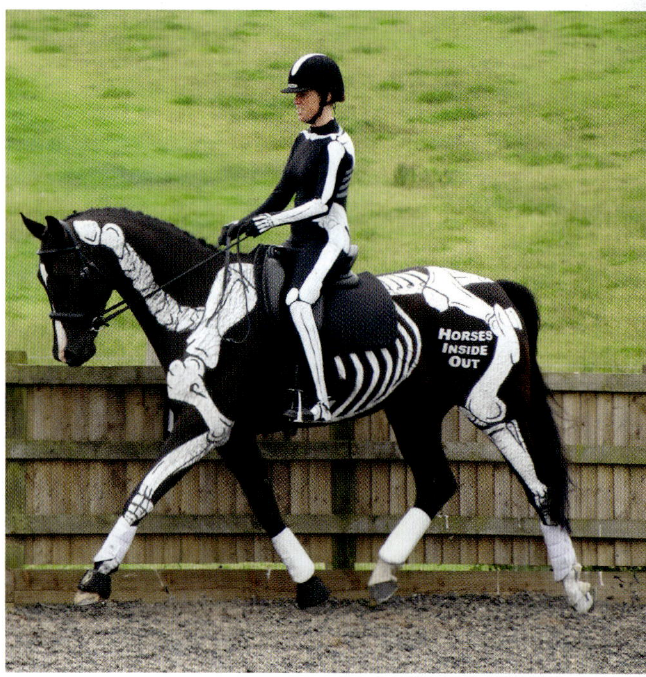


*This horse is demonstrating a soft, consistent, forward contact with the rider sensitively allowing the hands and forearms to follow the movement.*

## SUMMARY

- To reduce the burden on the horse, the rider must maintain a quiet, balanced position whilst applying precise, sensitive, independent aids.
- It is important to understand the anatomy and physiology of the structures on which we sit.
- Attending to posture, looking after our own bodies and keeping fit makes it easier for the horse to carry our weight.
- We use the head more than any other structure to influence and control thehorse.
- It is important to ensure that the saddle, bridle and bit fit correctly and comfortably.
- Contact, the connection between the riders' hands and the horse's mouth must be light, balanced and consistent.

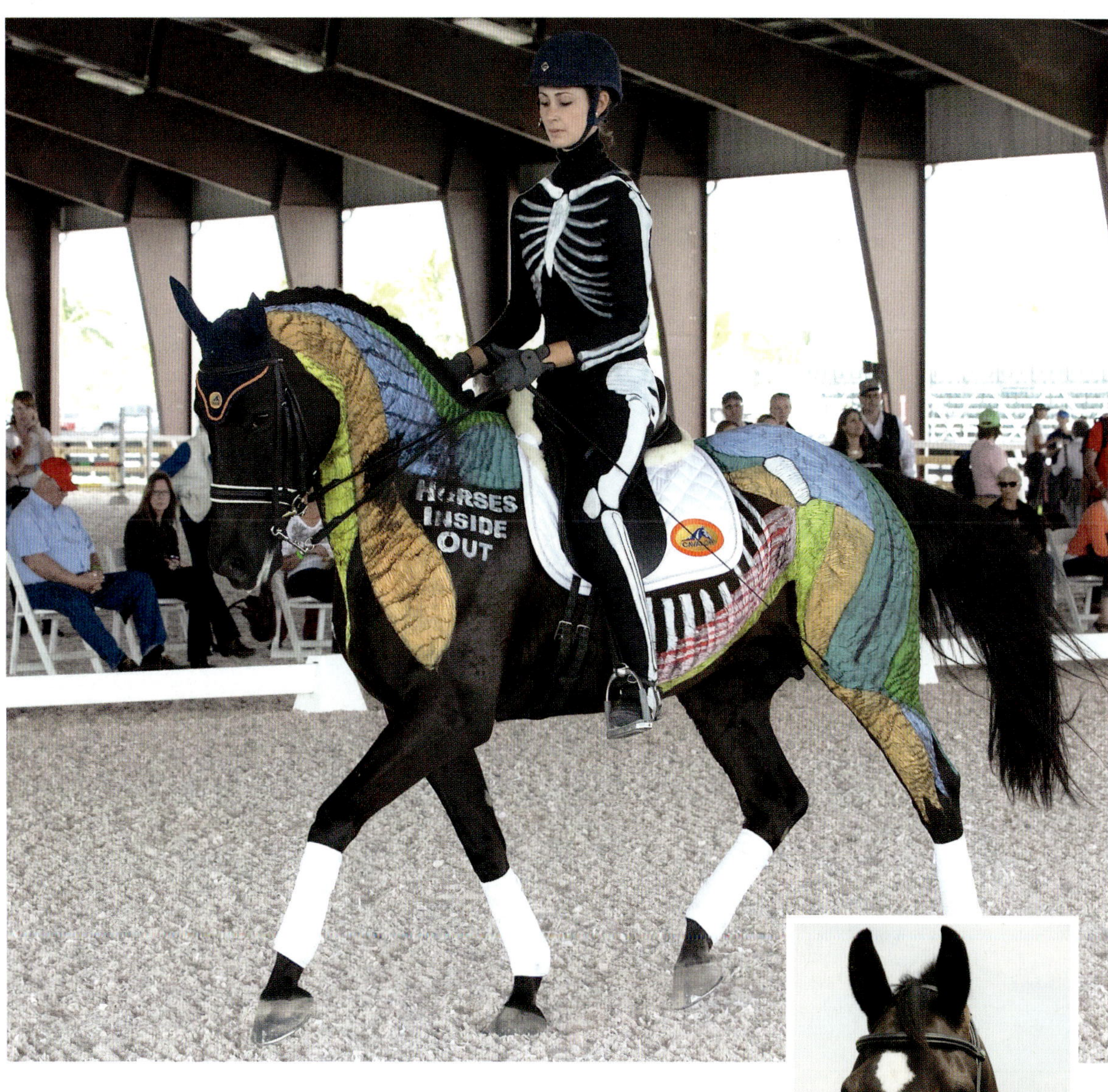

## Symmetry

When considering symmetry in horses we are looking at bilateral musculoskeletal symmetry where the two sides are the same or very close in size, shape and position. Symmetry of movement is where stride length or performance is the same on both reins. This is the ideal.

*No skeleton, frame or muscular system in either horse or human is completely symmetrical.*

## Laterality

This refers to left- or right-brain dominance. In humans this presents as left- or right-handedness. Horses too have dominant brain hemispheres. This laterality, of little consequence until the horse is ridden, can be seen as a preference for working on the left or right rein. Translated into practical application, some horses are more successful or safer when competing or performing on a right-hand track, some on a left.

## Rider Asymmetry

Approximately 80 per cent of people are right-handed and left-brain dominant. This means the left side of the body specialises in balance and support whilst the right side is responsible for motor function. This pattern is continually reinforced by the cellular memory of the muscles and fascia involved in repeated actions, for example always writing with the right or left hand.

All physical activities, whether gymnastics, running, dancing or riding, require specific neuro-motor training in order to minimise the inherent asymmetry. In the case of equestrian sport, asymmetry is further complicated as it involves interaction between horse and rider. By visiting a physiotherapist it is possible to identify and assess myofascial imbalances, recognise asymmetries and, with repeated exercises, improve posture and redress faulty movement patterns. Horses do not have this ability, so it is up to us, as their personal trainers, to devise a programme to minimise both our own and our horses' asymmetries.

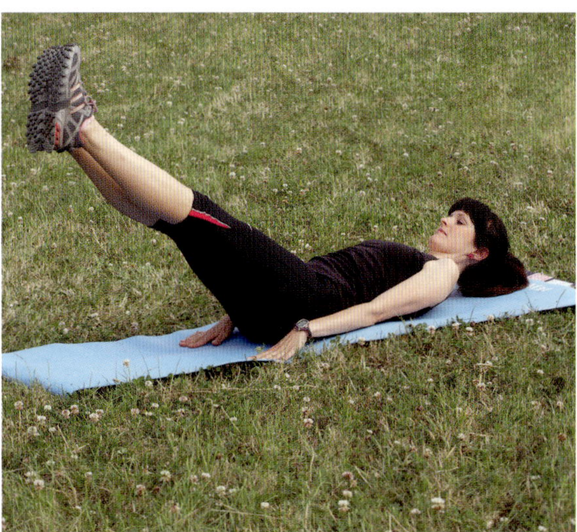

**BELOW**
*Here the strong side is being continually strengthened whilst the weak side is continually weakened.*

**RIGHT AND BELOW RIGHT**
*Stretching and strengthening exercises for horses and Pilates, yoga or the Alexander Technique for ourselves are a good starting point for correcting asymmetry.*

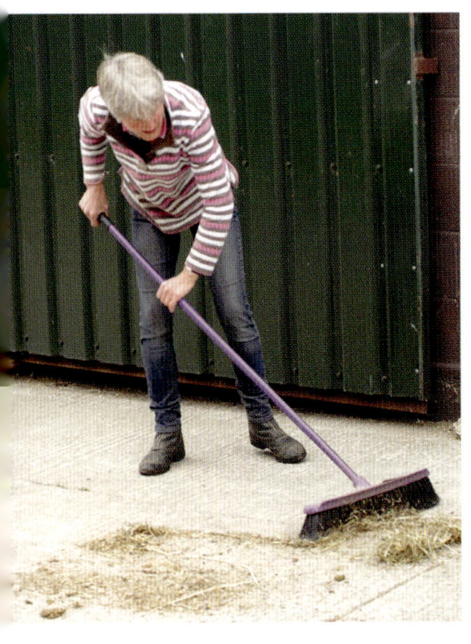

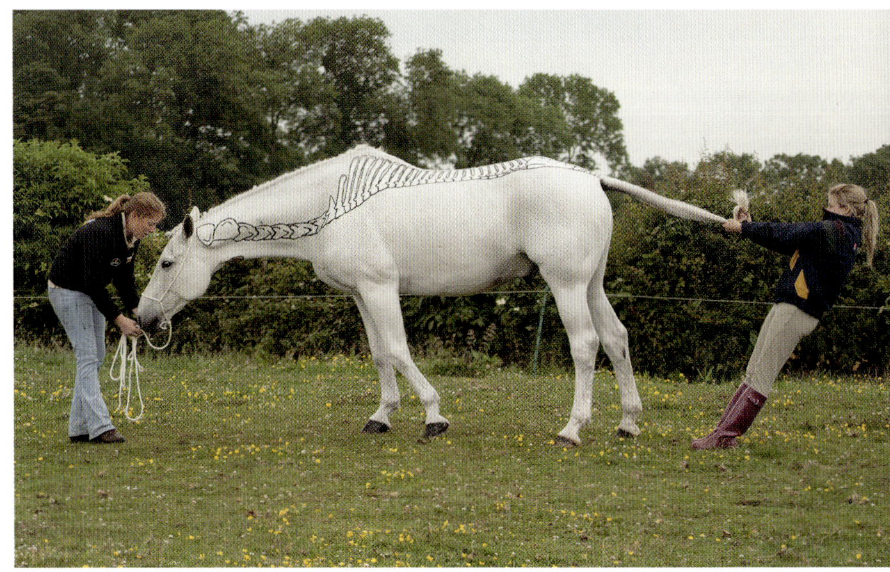

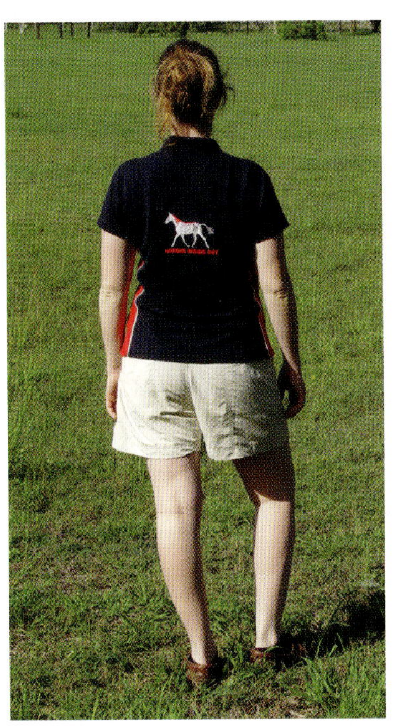

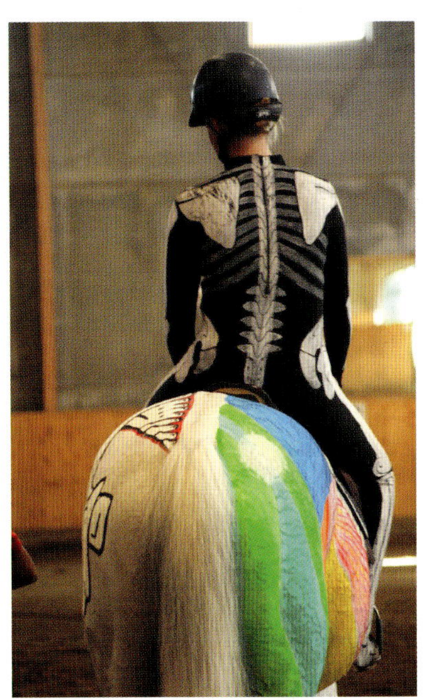

*Good postural symmetry is a desirable quality which should fulfill several criteria. It should allow efficient movement, with minimum energy expenditure to ensure a smooth transition from one movement to the next and not inhibit any ongoing activities. Although this is ideal it is not always the case as many riders do tend to be asymmetrical. Maintaining an asymmetrical stance will, over time alter the musculoskeletal and nervous systems so the adopted position becomes the norm. This will then affect energy expenditure making activity more labored and tiring and may even inhibit movement. If the muscles that attach to the pelvic girdle, mainly the psoas, adductors, piriformis, hamstrings and pelvic floor muscles are uneven in their development, this will affect the rider's seat, aids and balance.*

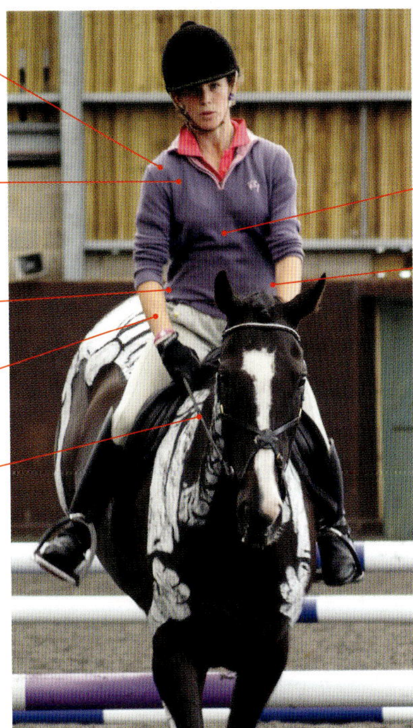


*If the rider is exceptionally left or right dominant or has a particularly one-sided occupation leading to a 'stronger' and 'weaker' side, this will affect their riding. This rider will have stronger hand and leg aids on one side than the other and sit with uneven weight distribution. In response, the horse may lean on one side of the bit, jump crookedly, be 'unwilling' to flex to the opposite side, fall out through the shoulder and bend and work differently on each rein.*

## SEAT AIDS

Effective use of the seat is one of the more difficult aids to achieve. The rider must first learn to relax, align his centre of gravity with that of the horse, recruit the core muscles and sit perfectly still without 'bouncing' or interfering with the movement. When the rider is asymmetrical he may use the weight of his head, arms or legs inappropriately to stabilise his position. This will in turn affect the horse's balance, posture and performance. Achieving a balanced seat allows riders to develop independent hands, good riding posture and supple legs. As the horse learns to respond to the subtle changes of the seat, communication becomes invisible.

# Horse Asymmetry

As with a near symmetrical rider, a near symmetrical horse is more likely to be straight, move efficiently and correctly, expend a minimum amount of energy and distribute his weight evenly. Conversely, an asymmetrical horse will exhibit uneven wear and tear through the limbs and body, uneven gaits and eventually varying degrees of lameness. Asymmetry can be congenital or as a result of trauma, conditioning, uneven muscle development, conformational discrepancies or lameness. It can be exacerbated by always pulling hay from a haynet in the same direction, being led, saddled or mounted from the same side or by working more on one rein than the other when schooling. Horses will always move in the way that is most comfortable and easiest for them. Asymmetry is often exacerbated by repeatedly, generally unintentionally, strengthening the already strong muscles and weakening the weak. This results, often from an early age in:

- Uneven conditioning of muscle tone and body mass
- Uneven development of the musculoskeletal system and
- Asymmetrical movement patterns.

Asymmetry manifests itself in:

- Imbalanced musculature
- Unequal pushing from behind
- Uneven hindlimb protraction
- Reduced range of movement and difficulty bending in one direction
- Consistently falling out through one shoulder
- A preference for working on one rein
- A preferred canter lead or favoured landing limb from a jump
- Working on three tracks as opposed to two.

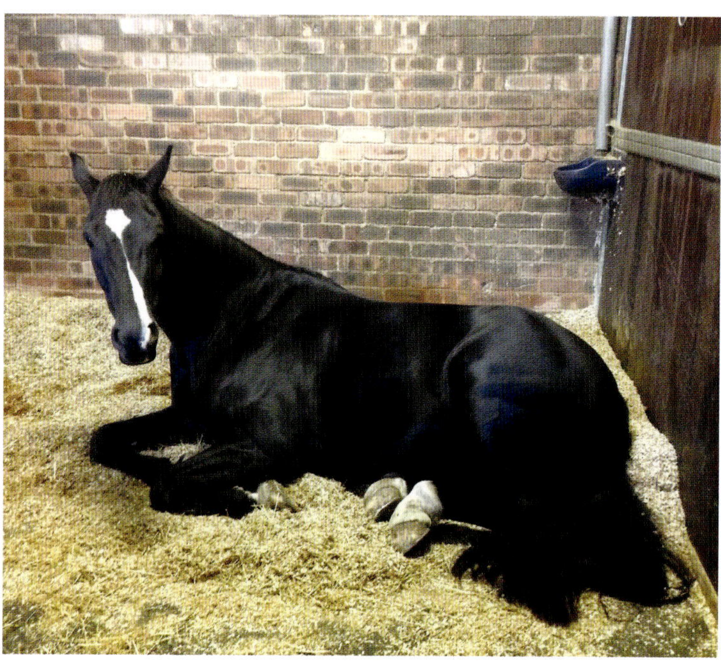

**ABOVE** *Horses generally lie on the same side and most are more adept at rolling from one side to the other. This horse who prefers lying in the right side with his legs tucked to the left, works better on the left rein.*

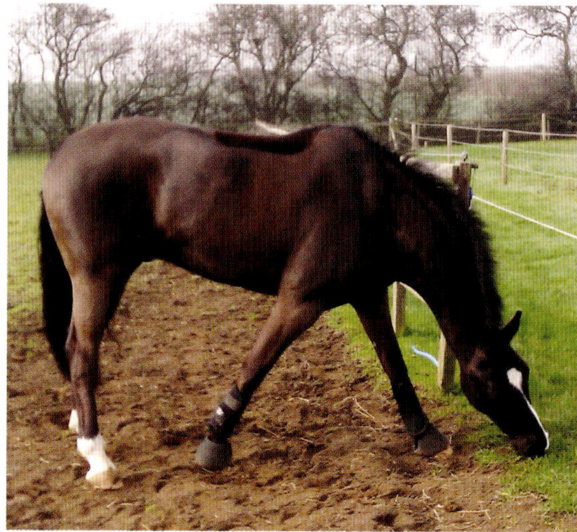

**ABOVE** *Horses that constantly adopt an asymmetrical grazing stance will be prone to uneven muscle development which may ultimately affect movement and stride length. It may also affect the bones of the forelimb, hoof capsule and hoof/ pastern axis as the horse grows.*

The reasons for asymmetry are not always readily obvious. The pony spine seen in the photo below had an extra vertebra between the 18th thoracic vertebra and the 1st lumbar vertebra. This vertebra sported a thoracic rib on the right and a lumbar transverse process on the left. This asymmetrical anatomical anomaly would almost certainly have had an effect on the ability to bend and move symmetrically.

Assessing straightness and symmetry during movement is as important as the static assessment. A qualified practitioner can identify the movement patterns that we would like to change and the factors that are interfering with the movement we would like to achieve. We can then learn new movement patterns that are more productive for both horse and rider.

**RIGHT** *If a well-fitting saddle constantly slips to one side, this could be as a result of hindlimb lameness transferring unequal forces from the hind legs to the back. Other causes of saddle slippage include asymmetrical muscle development of the back, uneven flocking of the saddle, unlevel stirrups and/or an asymmetrical rider.*

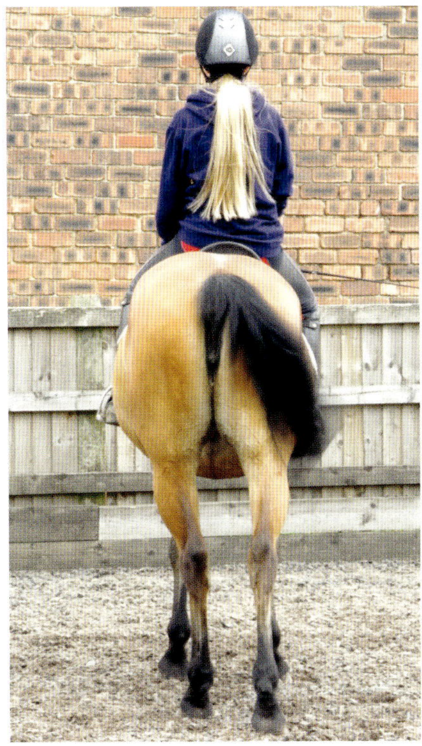

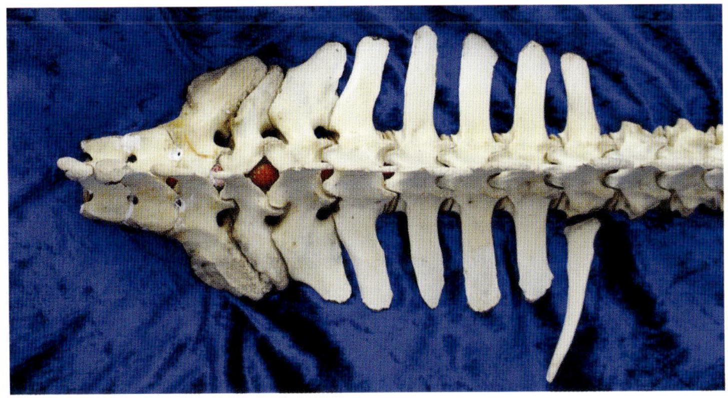

**LEFT** *This pony had an extra vertebra between the 18th thoracic vertebra and the 1st lumbar vertebra.*

**BELOW** *Assessing straightness and symmetry during movement is as important as the static assessment.*

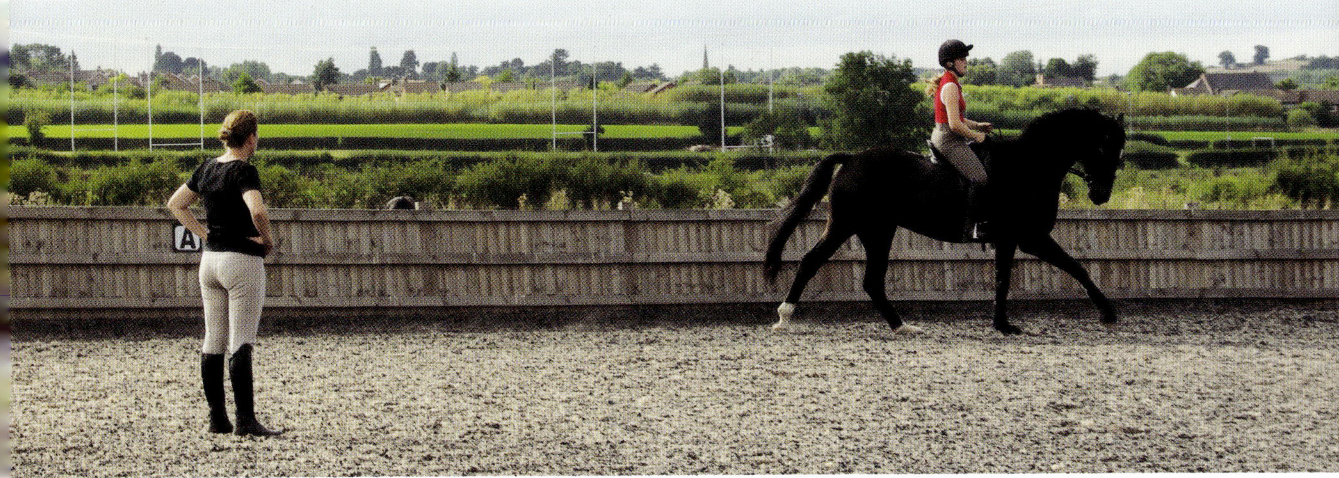

## Compensating for Asymmetry

When compensating for asymmetries in any part of the body, the effects may present as altered movement patterns in sites far removed from the original problem. For example, if the horse experiences pain in the jaw, this can have a causal effect on the poll, neck, forelimbs, back and associated movement patterns. This complex scenario varies from horse to horse.

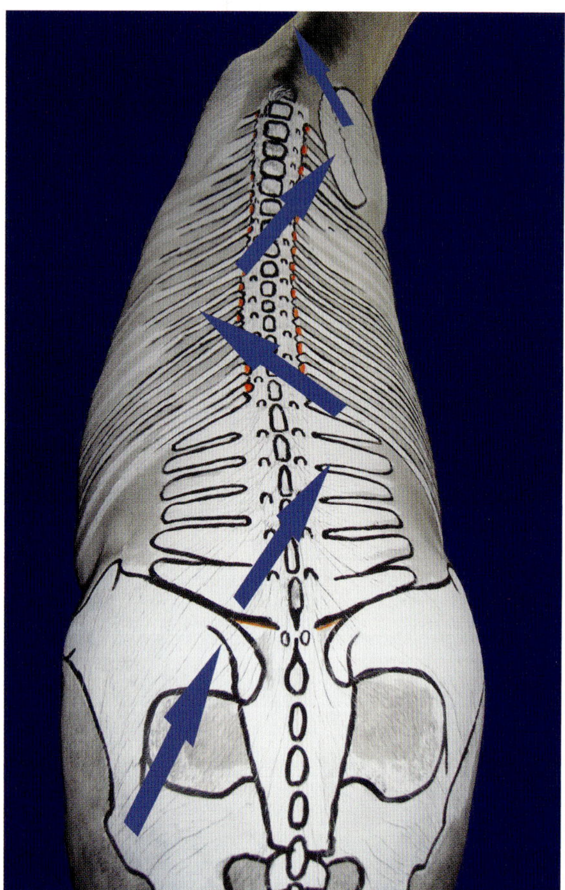

**ABOVE** *Where the horse pushes unequally from behind, the forces being transferred forward will also be unequal. The arrows on the photograph indicate the possible flow of compensatory forces and this explains why horses can develop back pain as a secondary symptom of hindlimb lameness.*

**RIGHT** *Advanced level dressage requires the horse and rider combination to be straight. Exercises to enhance straightness and balance, minimise asymmetry and encourage the horse to push equally from behind can be found in Part 2.*

## Straightness

Once we recognise and accept a degree of asymmetry and imbalance present in our horse we can take action to counter its effects. By training the muscles and straightening him it is possible to achieve optimum movement, posture and performance. A straightened horse will be physically and mentally in balance, muscularly and symmetrically fit, supple, strong, able to round the back and carry the rider with ease.

Straightness refers to the muscular symmetry and even development of the horse from side to side. When the horse is straight, that is when his longitudinal axis is aligned with and can follow a straight or curved track and when he can bend or flex equally on either rein, performance will be maximised. Regardless of activity, stage of training and head position, whether we are asking for a free or collected walk, leg-yield or advanced dressage movements, weight will be transferred equally, the hind legs will push in the direction of the centre of mass and wear and tear on the joints will be minimised.

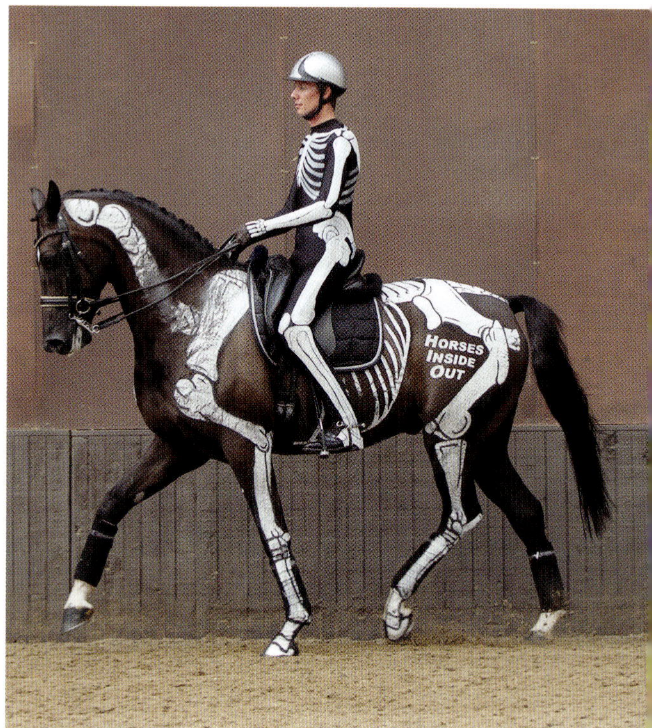

## HOW TO ASSESS ASYMMETRY

This simple twenty-point checklist of physical indicators can be used to assess symmetry. When standing square on a flat firm surface:

1. Are the false hips (tuber coxae) level?
2. Is the jumper's bump (tuber sacrale) horizontal?
3. Are the hindquarters equally muscled?
4. Are the point of buttocks (tuber ischia) the same height?
5. Is the tail centred or is it carried to one side?
6. Is the spine straight from tail to ears?
7. Are the ears level?
8. Are the withers and tops of scapulae equal on both sides?
9. Is the back musculature the same on the left and right sides?
10. Are the thighs equally muscled?
11. Are the hocks level?
12. Are the chest (pectoral) muscles equal?
13. Are the muscles at the base of the neck and shoulder the same left to right?
14. Are the points of shoulder level?
15. Are the forelegs equally muscled?
16. Are the hooves the same shape and the hoof/pastern axis the same angle left to right?
17. Are the hooves worn evenly?
18. Are the fetlocks symmetrical?
19. Is the barrel of the ribs equal on both sides?
20. Is the head and neck the same shape on both sides?

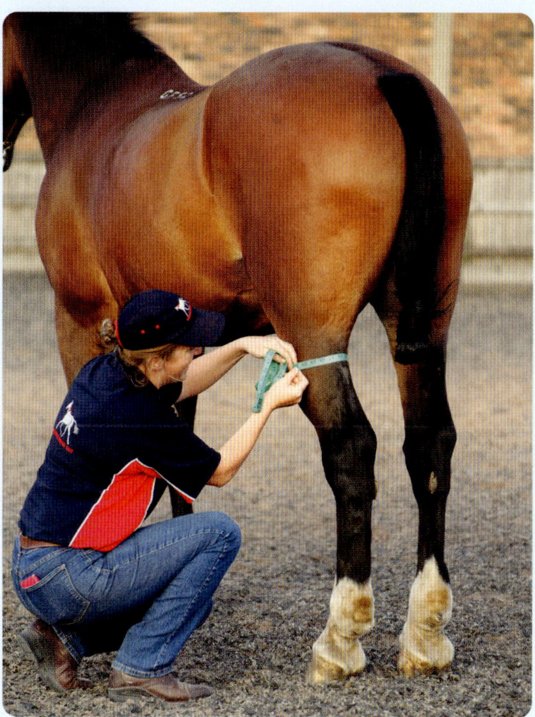

*The development of this horse's hindquarter and thigh muscles is asymmetrical. This could be as a result of uneven movement, discomfort, conformation, training or management.*

## SUMMARY

- Neither horse nor human is completely symmetrical.
- A nearly symmetrical horse is more likely to be straight and move correctly with even weight distribution.
- Asymmetrical forces from the hindlimbs may result in saddle slippage.
- Horses have a preferred rein influenced by their right- or left-handedness.
- Compensating for asymmetry can be seen as altered movement patterns.

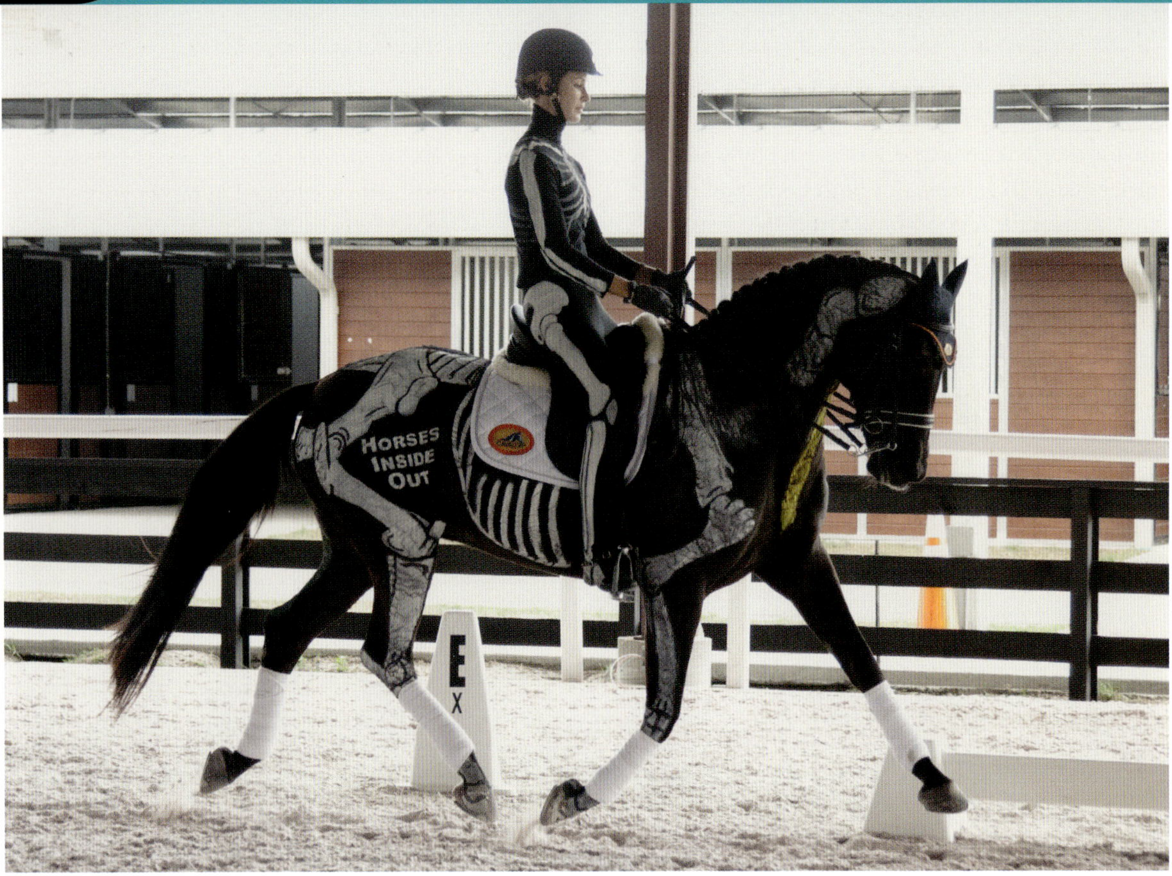

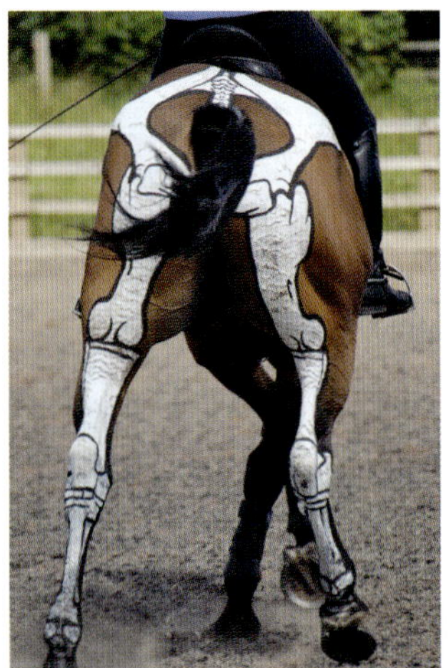


This section will consider the basic natural gaits of walk, trot, canter and gallop, compare their biomechanical properties and look at the benefits of fast work. The gaits can be subdivided into working, medium, extended and collected trot and canter, with free, medium, extended and collected being applied to walk. There are further 'artificial' gaits such as pace, running walk, tølt and many others. Some horses, for example the Tennessee Walking Horse, are bred to perform specialised gaits. Perfecting the correct execution of walk, trot and canter enables the rider to use them as an exercise in their own right and forms a sound basis for future training.

**Half-pass right in trot**   **Half-pass right in canter**

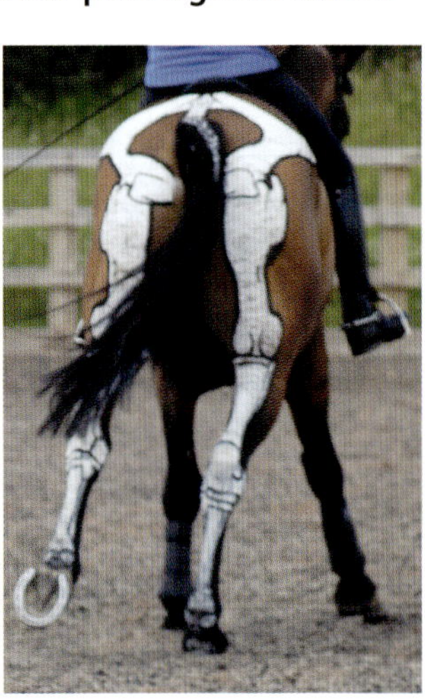

*Performing the same exercise in different gaits will have a different influence on the horse's musculoskeletal system.*

# 1. Walk

Walk is a regular four-beat gait. Generally, the advancing rear hoof overtracks the spot where the previously placed front hoof made ground contact. Walk steps must be regular and rhythmical and the gait must be ridden with impulsion and engagement. To achieve this both horse and rider must be relaxed. A good walk forms the basis of all training. Young horses begin their training with free walk on a long rein. With a light contact this allows them to mentally relax, look around, work through the back, stretch the topline, strengthen the muscles and skeleton and develop a long even stride. Once achieved, the rider can then generate more power from behind, pick up a light contact and introduce and progress through the different types of walk. Whenever the horse is engaged in muscularly hard work or introduced to a new movement, it is important to return to free walk on a long rein.

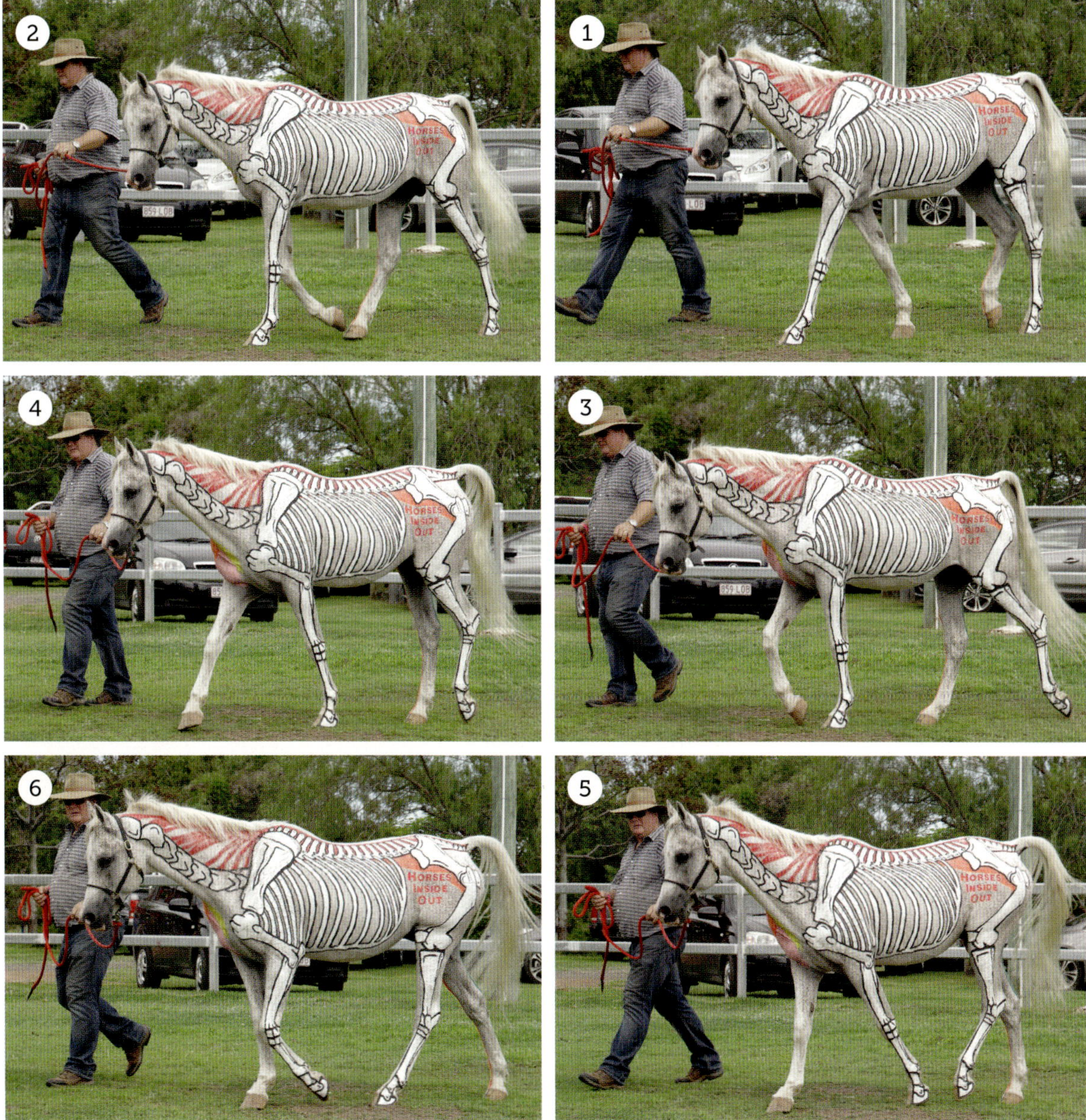

## Back movement in walk

There are many different types of walk which vary in stride length, speed, impulsion and tempo. With no moment of suspension these factors are influenced by flexibility and range of movement in the hip joint, pelvis and back rather than by momentum. Of all the gaits, walk uses the greatest range of rib movement and rotation through the thoracolumbar spine. As the left fore and left hind come together (Picture 5) the ribs swing to the right. As the left fore and left hind move away from each other (Picture 1) the ribs swing to the left. As the pelvis is fixed onto the sacrum at the sacroiliac joint, movement of the pelvis causes spinal rotation and lateral flexion. Contributing to athleticism and flexibility, walk is a superb gait to help release tension in the back and mobilise the thoracolumbar vertebrae.

## Benefits of walk

As a low-impact gait with a relatively low risk of repetitive strain injury the benefits of walk are often underestimated. It is particularly good for:

- Warming up
- Suppling and mobilising spinal joints
- Improving spinal rotation and lateral flexion
- Improving stride length and joint range of movement
- Encouraging relaxation
- Improving muscular control and strength
- Introducing new exercises.

## Irregularities in walk

An even, rhythmical, relaxed walk is difficult to achieve. Tension, either physical or psychological, anticipation, rider influence, lameness, neurological problems or demanding too much collection too soon will result in a loss of regularity and rhythm of the footfalls, jogging or an uneven incorrect walk.

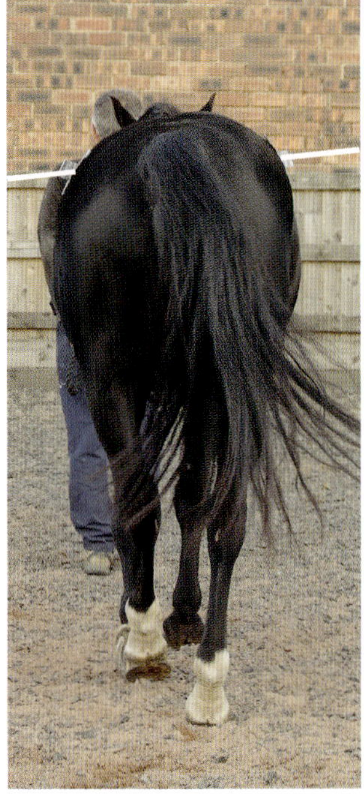
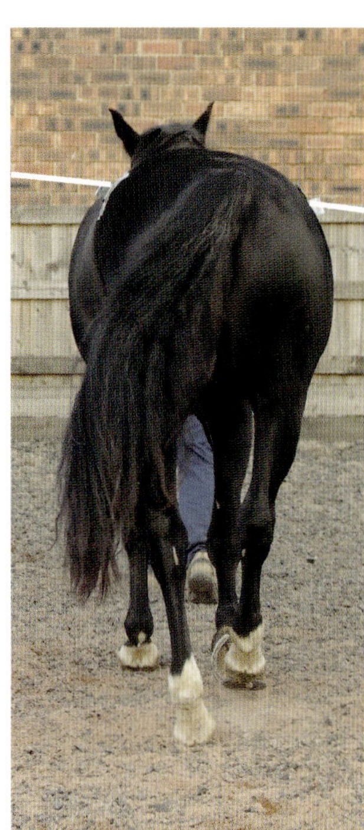

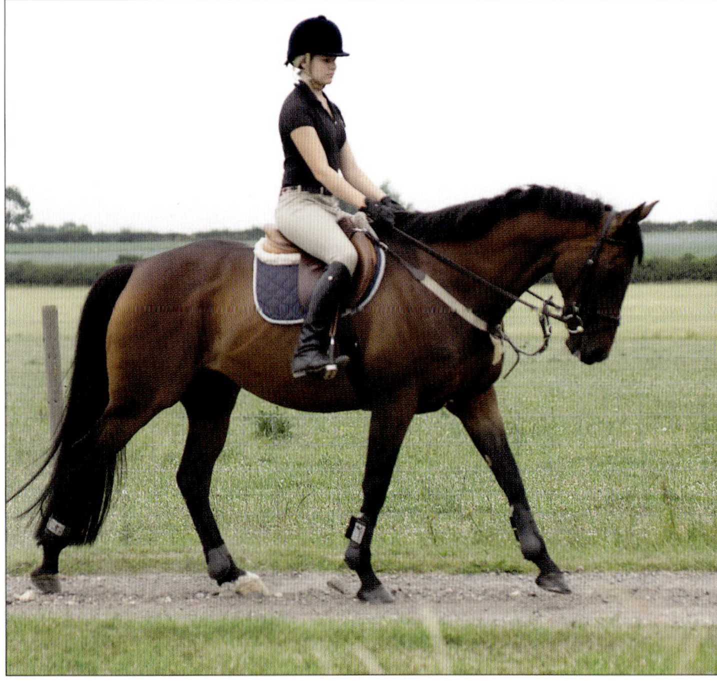

*The term 'lateral walk' describes a gait irregularity whereby the limbs, instead of moving correctly in a four-beat rhythmical sequence (1..2..3..4..), tend towards a two-beat sequence, for example inside hind and inside fore followed by the outside hind and outside fore in the form 12...34.*

## Improving the walk

The quality of the walk can be improved by:

- Encouraging relaxation and confidence with plenty of free and extended walk on a long rein
- Riding regular transitions between medium and free walk on a long rein
- Working on concentration and coordination with lateral exercises such as leg-yield and shoulder-in
- Walking over poles to improve regularity and coordination
- Gradually introducing a few steps of collected walk once an even, consistent medium walk is established.

## Types of walk

### Free walk on a long rein

This horse is demonstrating an elongated frame and good range of movement. The hindlimbs especially indicate an extended gait. He is relaxed and the muscles are sufficiently supple to allow this.

### Collected walk

This horse has well-conditioned gluteals, is engaging the hindquarters and has well-toned neck muscles.

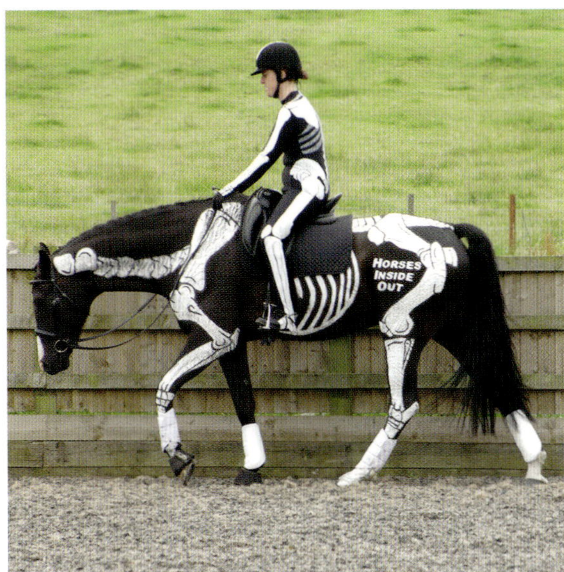


*Free walk on a long rein.*

He is demonstrating good eccentric muscle contraction. The frame is shortened and the neck slightly arched and elevated. This is tiring for the horse so it is important to allow him to regularly stretch down to relax. Note: in collected walk the frame and stride length shorten so the horse does not track up.

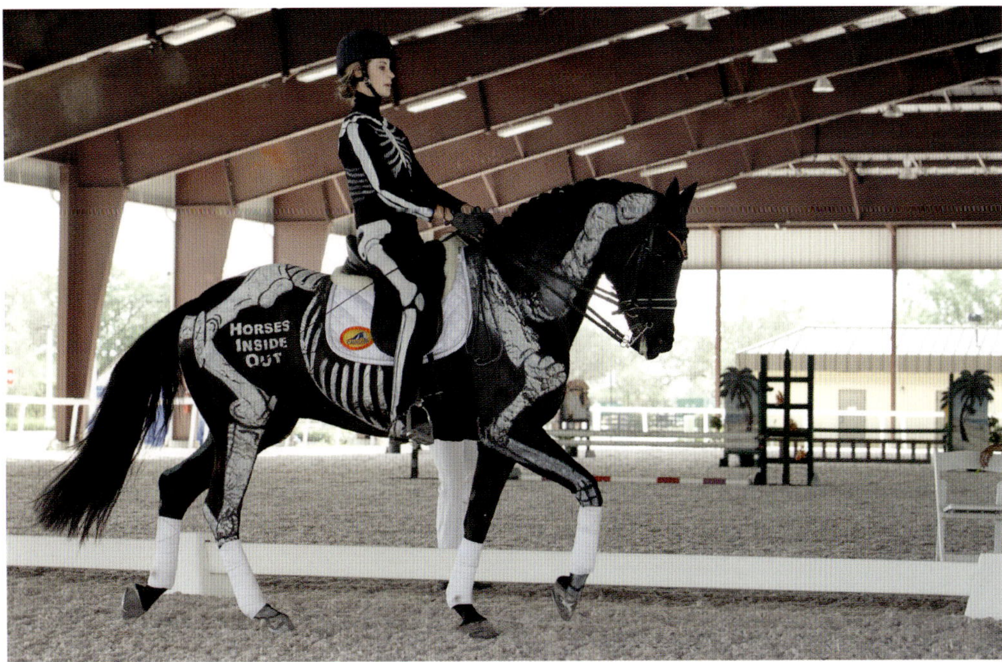


*Collected walk.*

## 2. Trot

Trot is a two-time symmetrical, rhythmical gait whereby the horse springs from one diagonal pair to the other with the hind legs at opposite phases of the stride at any one time. The moment of suspension causes an increase in the stretch of muscles, tendons and ligaments, which have to absorb the extra load as the fetlocks sink following impact. The subsequent recoil plays an important role in contributing to momentum. The qualities of a good trot are rhythm, regularity, cadence, mental and physical relaxation, harmony and impulsion. This is achieved through:

- Correct posture
- Balance
- Straightness
- A symmetrical, regular push from behind
- Equal range and elevation of the legs between each stride.

### Back movement in trot

As the horse trots there is a small amount of passive flexion and extension through the thoracolumbar and lumbosacral regions. As he pushes up into the moment of suspension (Pictures 1 and 4) the abdominal contents, approximately 150kg in a 500kg horse, push up against the underside of the back causing it to flex. As this happens the longissimus dorsi muscles contract to counteract this upward pressure and limit back flexion. Conversely during stance (Pictures 3 and 6) the weight of the abdomen pulls down on the back causing it to extend. At this point the abdominal muscles, particularly the rectus abdominis, contract eccentrically to counteract the extension. Adding the weight of the rider will reduce passive flexion and increase extension.

*The sequence of the footfalls in trot, and contraction of the spinal flexor and extensor chains of muscles working alternately on the left and right sides, cause a small amount of spinal lateral flexion and rotation. This is reflected in pelvic movement.*

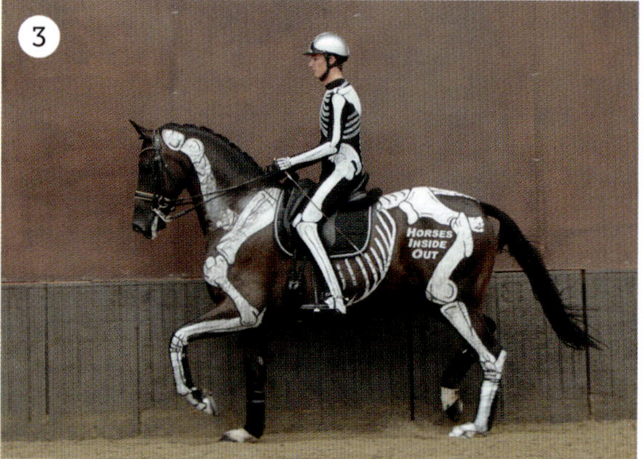


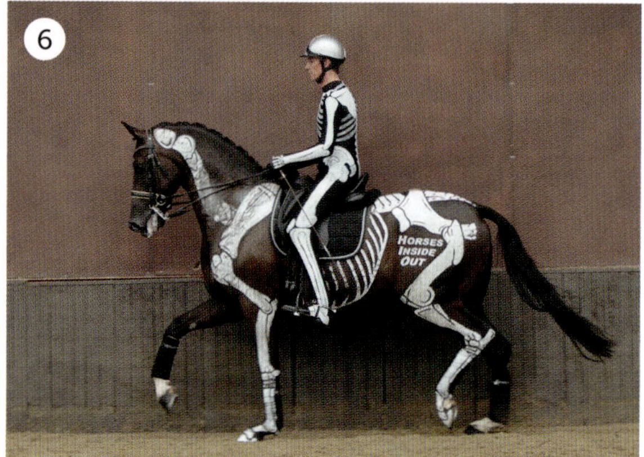


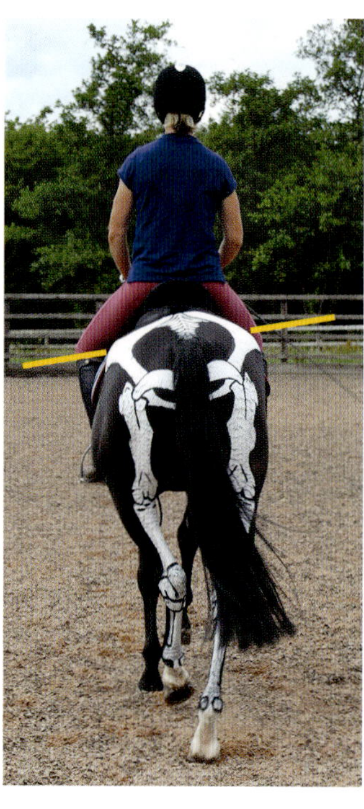

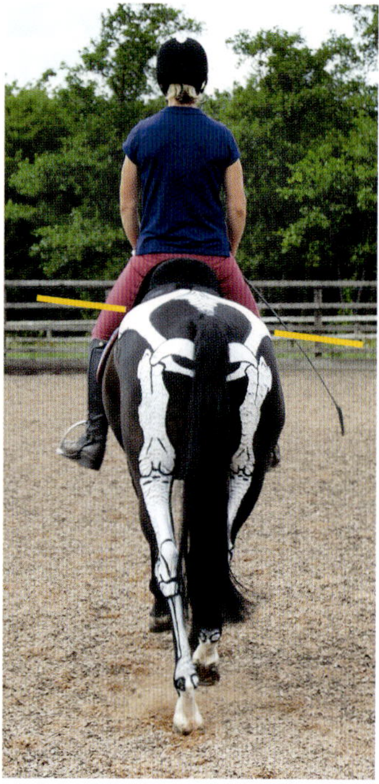

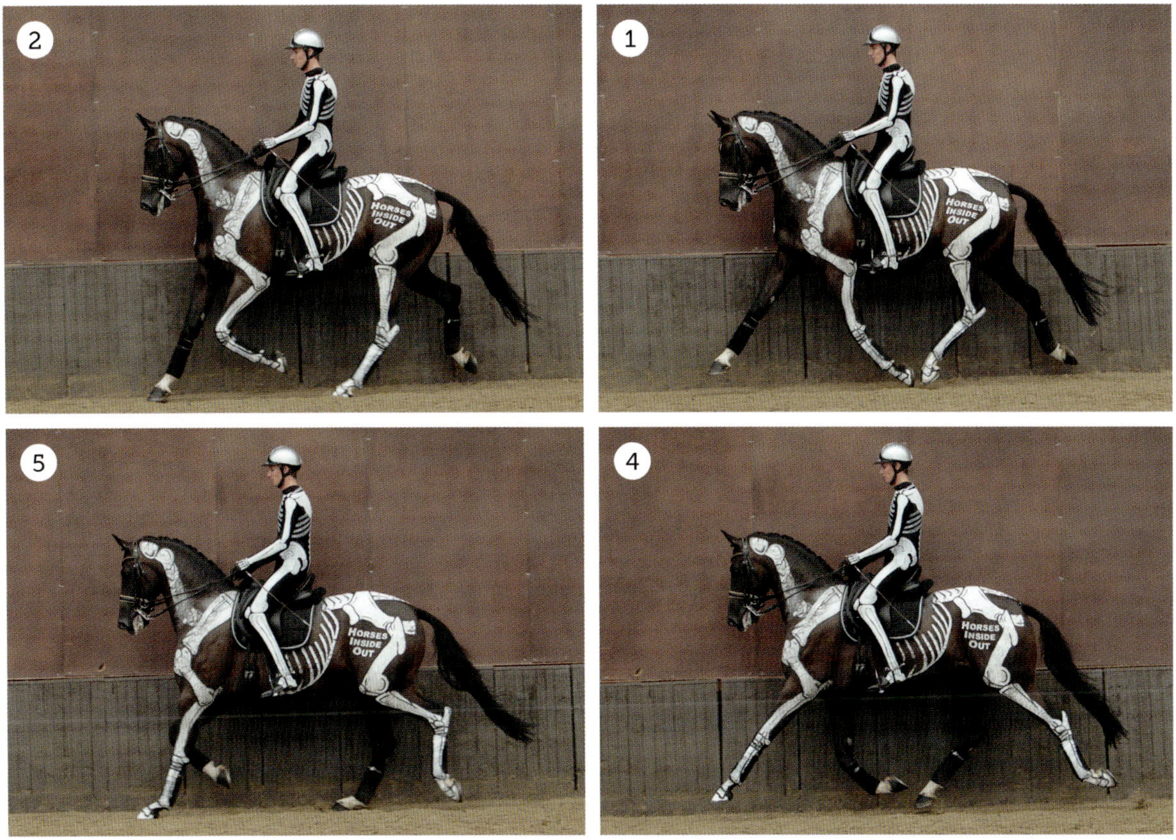

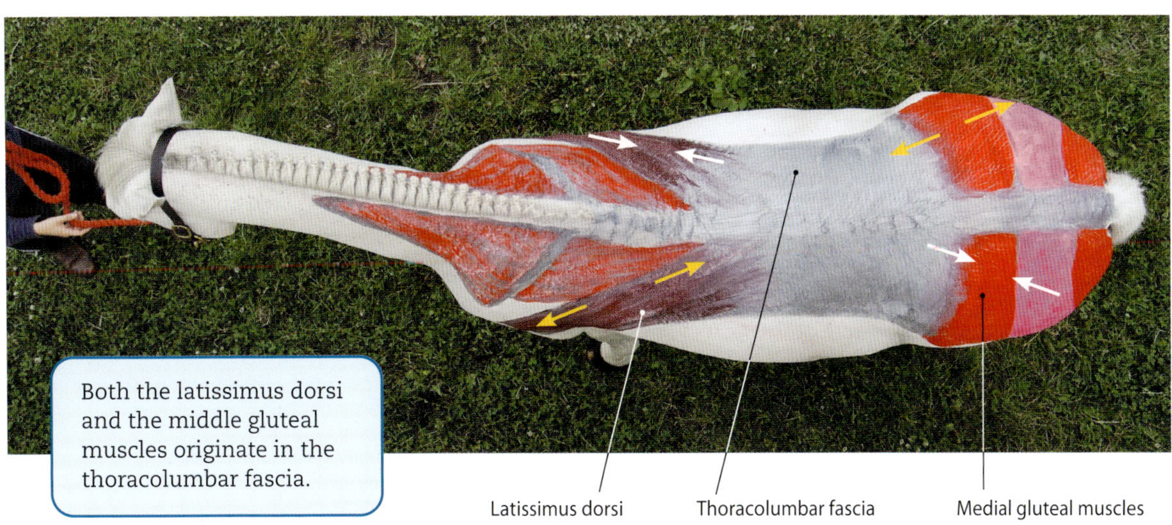



*During the stance phase, as the left hind hoof is on the ground and the left gluteal and right latissimus dorsi muscles contract, the right gluteal and the left latissimus dorsi elongate. This results in diagonal tensioning across the thoracolumbar fascia during the pushing phase of the stride. If the horse pushes asymmetrically from behind this will directly affect the forelimbs, explaining why a problem in the hindlimb can be reflected in the diagonally opposite forelimb.*

## Benefits of trot

Trot is a particularly useful gait for:

- Improving rhythm
- Assessing symmetry
- Identifying lameness
- Improving muscular strength, expression and cadence
- Improving balance and core control.

## Types of trot

There is a range of trots which vary in power, tempo and stride length. These are dependent on the strength of the gluteal and hamstring muscles, which allow optimal engagement of the hindquarters, and the strength of the forelimb protraction muscles responsible for expression in the forelimbs.

Working trot is the most efficient and sustainable gait for the horse. Once the horse is working rhythmically and consistently with good posture, is tracking up, and when his muscles are sufficiently conditioned, work towards medium and collected trot can begin. As the horse moves up through the grades it is important to return to trotting on a loose rein between bouts of hard work to give the muscles time to stretch, relax and recover.

## Collected trot

As with extended trot, collected trot cannot be achieved, and should not be introduced, before the horse is skeletally mature and has sufficient muscular strength to maintain it. It has several unique characteristics:

- Shortened steps, more elevated and more energetic
- Anatomically there is increased flexion of the hip, stifle, hock and fetlock which generates increased power and thrust
- Muscular strength and control is required as the haunches are lowered and the hind end takes more weight
- A strong core and muscular strength is required to maintain the shortened frame and lightened forehand
- An arched and raised neck contributes to lightness and mobility of the shoulders.

Because collected trot, which is a prerequisite for piaffe and passage, is muscularly tiring, it should be interspersed with a few strides of medium or working trot at regular intervals. Periodically introducing a few strides of basic collected trot within the working trot is an effective strengthening exercise for young horses.

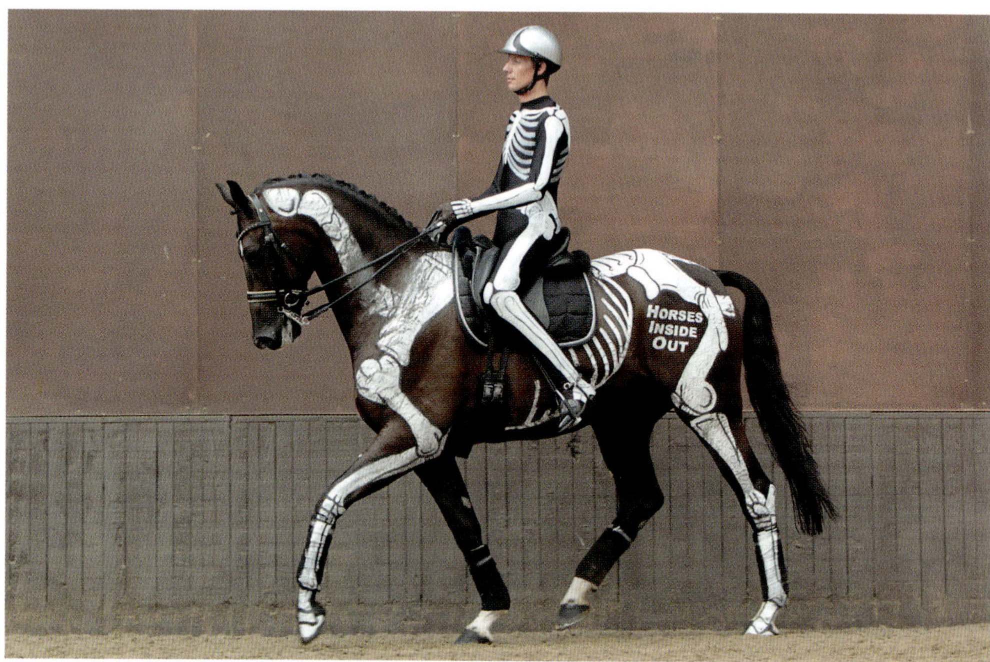


*Collected trot.*

## Extended trot

Extended trot cannot be achieved before the horse is strong and the musculoskeletal system is mature. It requires an elongated frame, a strong core, muscular strength, power and elasticity. With this trot there is more spinal lateral flexion and rotation, a longer stride length, greater overtrack and an increased moment of suspension compared to collected trot.

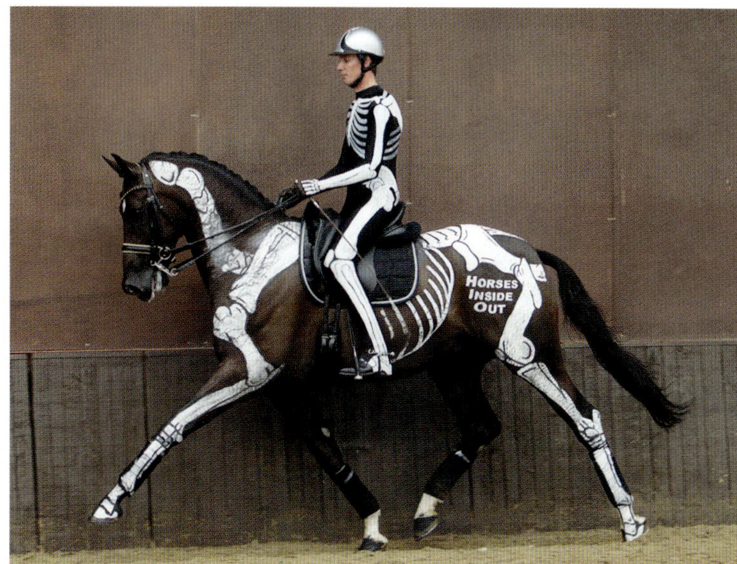


*Extended trot.*

## Diagonal dissociation

This refers to the placing of the diagonal pairs as the horse trots. Ideally the diagonal pairs impact simultaneously. However, this is not always the case. Diagonal dissociation cannot be seen by the naked eye but can be seen in slow-motion video.

**Positive dissociation**, when the hind foot hits the ground slightly before the diagonally opposite forefoot, indicates a good 'uphill balance'. This enables greater forelimb protraction and more weight to be carried on the hindquarters. This is often seen in advanced dressage horses.

**Negative dissociation**, when the forefoot hits the ground before the diagonally opposite hind foot, indicates poor 'downhill' balance. This causes more weight to be carried on the forehand or the horse to pull himself along from the front rather than pushing from behind. Many young horses move with negative diagonal dissociation particularly during downward transitions and when they first start carrying the weight of the rider. Basic strengthening and collection exercises (see Chapter 10) are effective in reversing this trait.

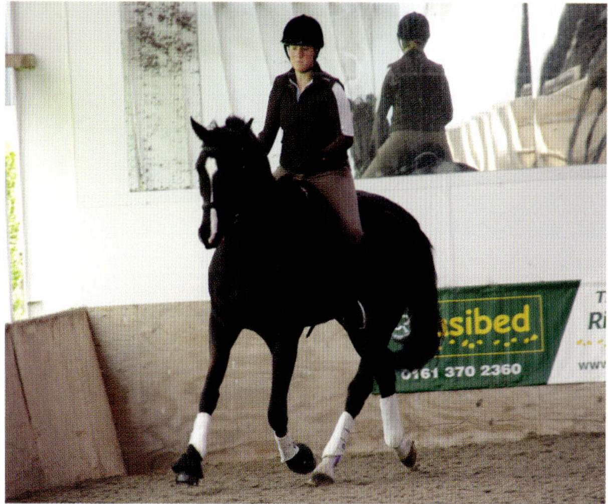


*Positive dissociation.*

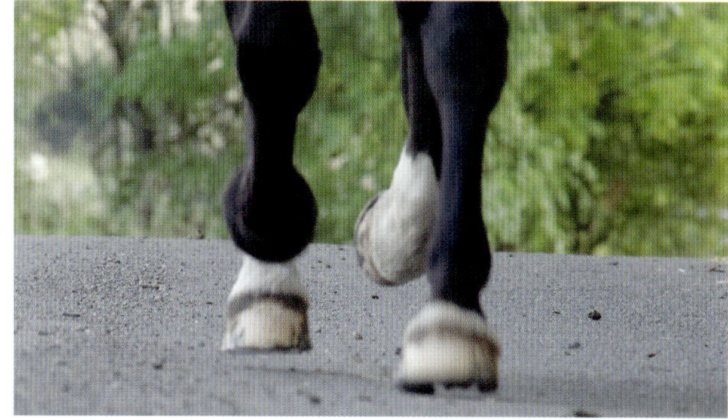

*Negative dissociation.*

# 3. Canter

Canter is an asymmetrical three-beat gait with a moment of suspension. Because the main thrust comes from the outside hind leg it is important that the rider applies the aid to canter when the outside hind is on the ground. A good canter is rhythmical, balanced, powerful and energetic. Practising exercises in canter improves strength, elasticity and mobility of the musculoskeletal system, spring, balance, coordination and expression.

The moment of suspension, speed and the reduced number of hooves on the ground, increases limb loading to more than twice the body weight. This means that the stretch and recoil within the muscles, tendons and ligaments increases, putting them under greater strain.

In canter the body rocks between the hindquarters and the forehand. This makes it the most effective gait for strengthening the thoracic sling muscles. These stretch during the weight-bearing phase (Picture 3) but then rapidly shorten to bring the forehand up (Picture 4). This ultimately creates the moment of suspension. Canter is also the best gait for toning weak abdominal muscles, vital for supporting the back. See sequence opposite.

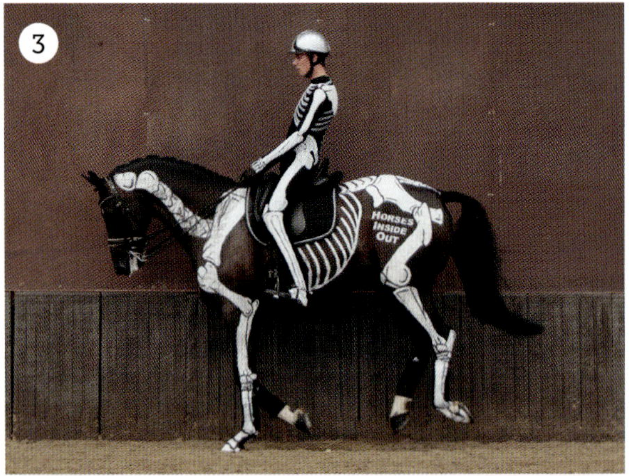


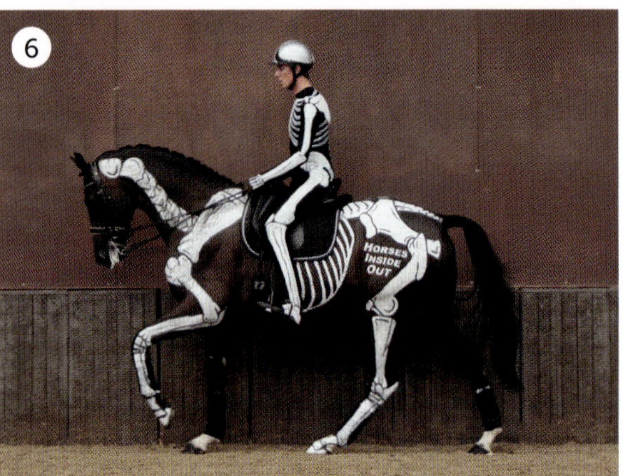


## Back movement in canter

Canter is the gait which creates the most back flexion and extension. As the hind legs come underneath the body nearly together, back and pelvic movement, together with flexion and extension of the lumbosacral junction, results in the tilting of the pelvis and contributes to hindlimb stride length. In canter:

- The back actively flexes and extends with each stride
- Left and right spinal flexor and extensor muscle chains contract almost simultaneously
- The abdominal line shortens with each stride.

### BACK STIFFNESS

Some horses may be stiff or reluctant to canter. This may be as a result of a physical problem such as insufficient muscular strength, back or sacroiliac pain, a behavioural problem, an inexperienced rider or uncomfortable tack. If associated with lameness, bucking, changing behind or an inability to maintain the canter, it is advisable to seek professional advice. Once the cause has been identified and addressed, exercises to reduce stiffness and help supple the back can include:

- Riding variations within the gait – moving between working canter and medium canter
- Backing up
- Forward canter and fast work
- Canter poles
- Counter-canter
- Lateral work.

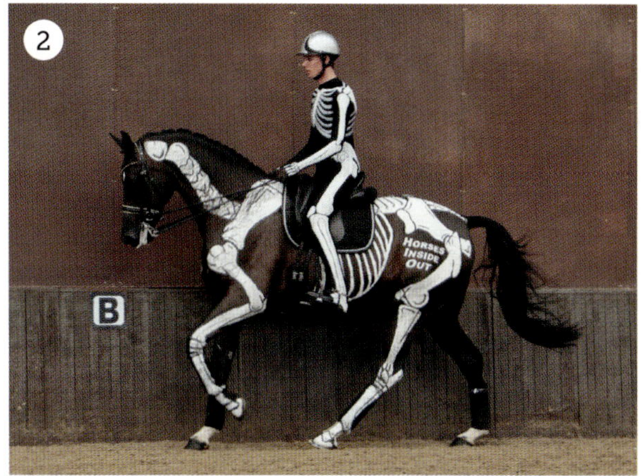

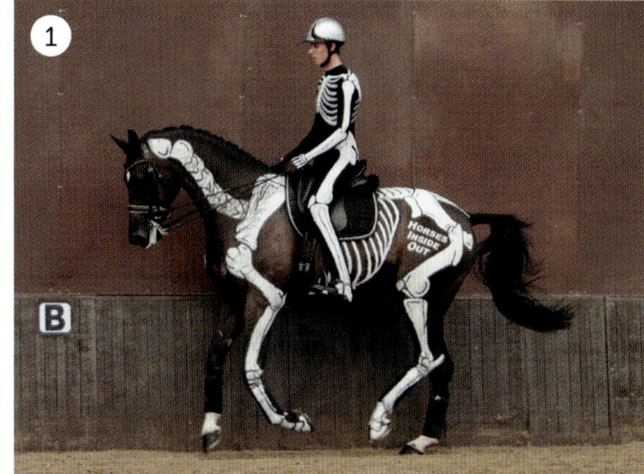

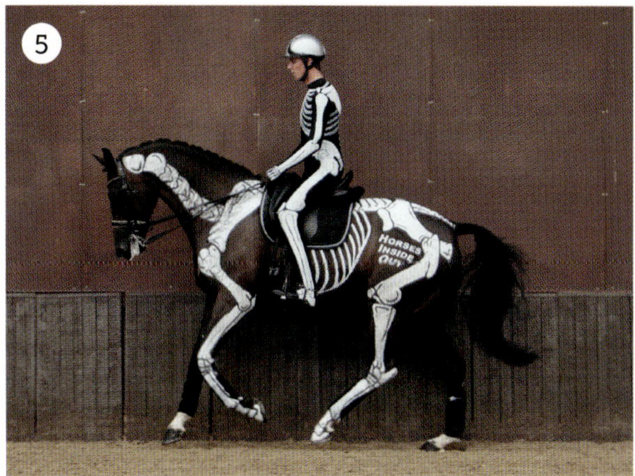

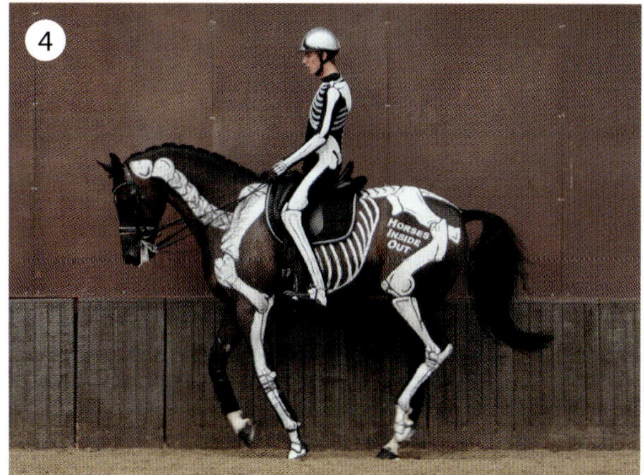

RIGHT *To encourage the abdominal and hindlimb protraction, muscles to contract strongly to provide the engagement required for a good canter, leg aids must be applied during the moment of suspension. As the horse pushes asymmetrically in canter there will be slight rotation and lateral flexion towards the leading leg. It is therefore important to canter equally on both reins.*

## Benefits of canter

Canter is a particularly useful gait for:

- Warming up and suppling the back
- Conditioning the cardiovascular and musculoskeletal systems
- Encouraging positive forward motion
- Strengthening and toning the abdominal muscles
- Improving back suppleness
- Improving muscular strength and power
- Creating enthusiasm and *joie de vivre*.

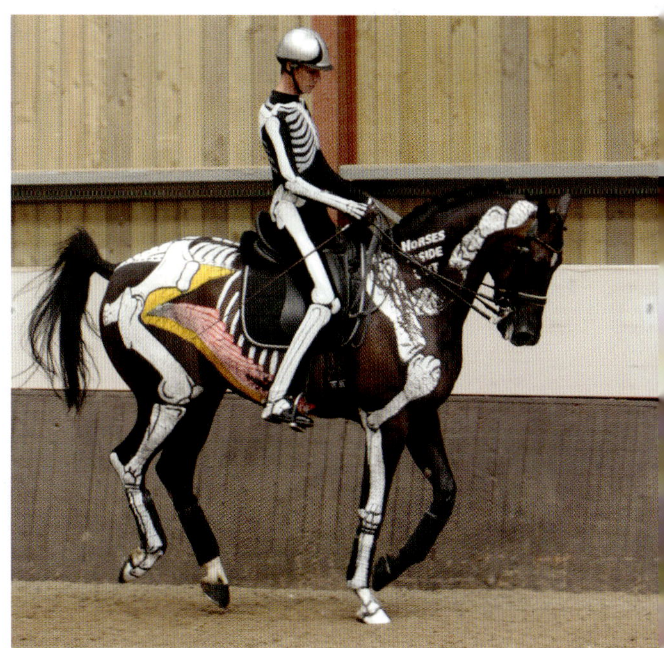

## Types of canter

As with walk and trot, there are many variations of canter. It is important that a rhythmical, balanced working canter is firmly established before progressing to more advanced canters.

## Collected canter

Collected canter is characterised by shorter, springier steps and increased flexion of the hind joints. This requires skeletal maturity and good core strength. The frame should be more compressed with the neck raised and arched. As the hindquarters lower they take more weight. This results in greater engagement, back suppleness, strength and lightness of the forehand. As they carry more weight, the hind legs do not push out as far behind (retract) and the muscles work harder to maintain flexion in the back, lumbosacral and hindlimb joints. Collected canter is muscularly tiring for the horse so should be ridden for short periods only.

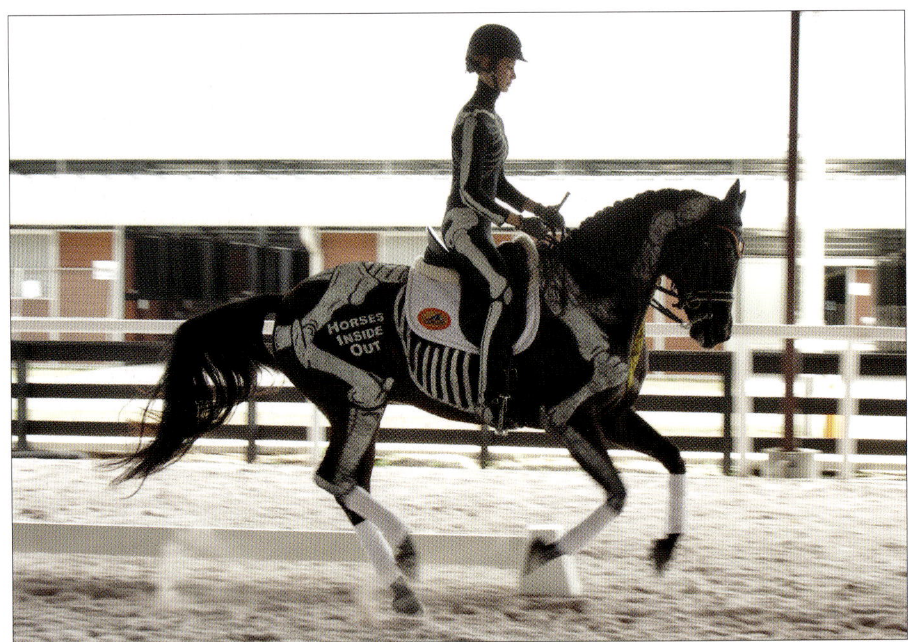


**LEFT** *Collected canter.*

**BELOW** *Extended canter.*

## Extended canter

Extended canter shows the greatest degree of neck extension, stride length and ground coverage. Strides should be long, even and energetic with the hind legs pushing further out behind. This requires greater back and lumbosacral extension, elongation of the iliopsoas muscles and contraction of the longissimus dorsi and gluteal muscle groups. Strengthening these muscles is good for improving power, expression and mobility required for optimum performance in all the gaits.

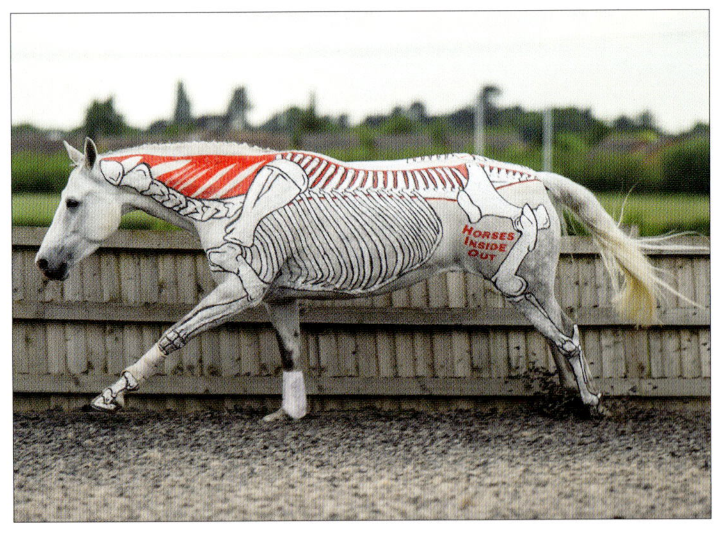

# Fast Work

Covering more ground than canter, the gallop is a naturally extended asymmetrical, four-beat gait followed by a moment of suspension. At full gallop a racehorse can reach speeds of over 30 mph with a stride length of 7–8m and a stride rate of three per second. As breathing is coupled with stride, respiration is governed by the stride rate – up to 180 breaths per minute. At gallop, muscles contract faster than at any other gait; galloping therefore is good for improving muscular and neurological reactions.

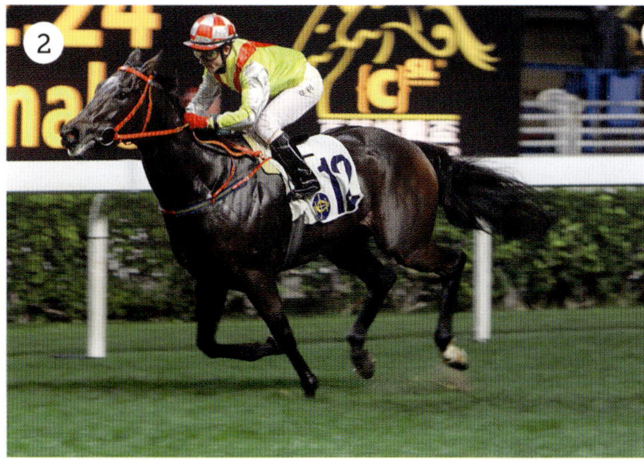
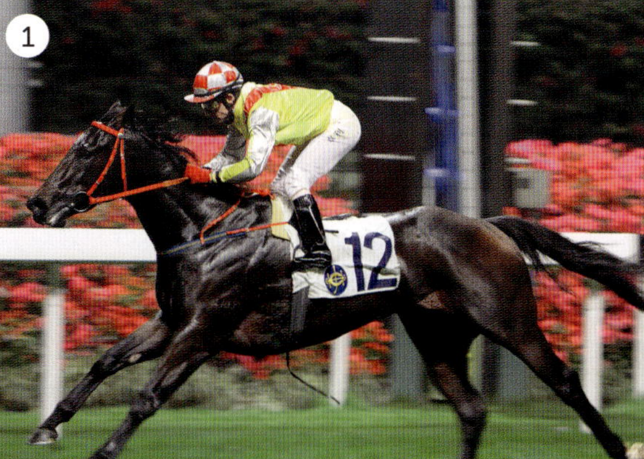
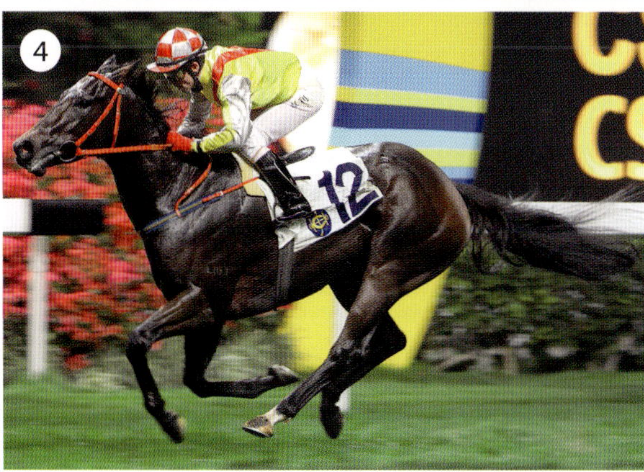
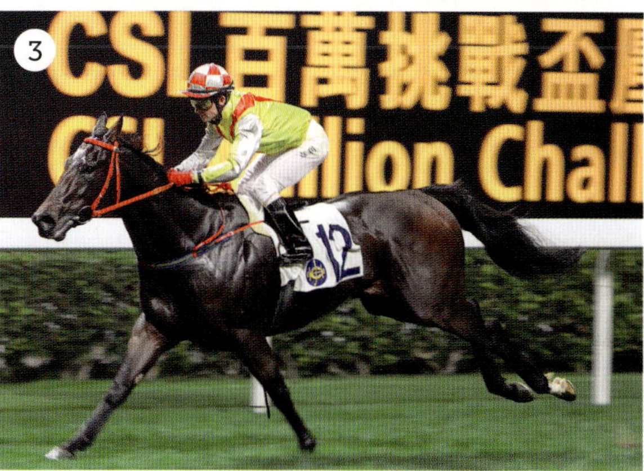

## Biomechanics during gallop

### Head and neck

The head and neck should be stretched out and free to move. This increases momentum, opens the airways for maximum air intake, facilitates dynamic balance and allows for alterations in the centre of mass.

### The back and hindlimbs

Uninhibited hip extension and maximum stride length propel the body forwards. The back flexes and extends more than in canter. This gives some horses an almost 'cheetah-like' action.

## Benefits of fast work

Every horse can benefit from some form of fast work. This is good for:

- Maximising lung capacity and improving cardiovascular fitness
- Improving coordination and speed of muscular reaction and contraction
- Suppling the hip and vertebral joints
- Toning the pelvic, back and abdominal muscles
- Improving muscular strength, power and fitness.

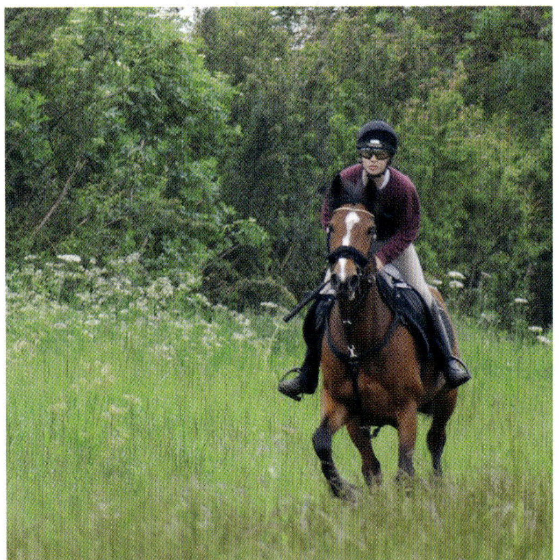

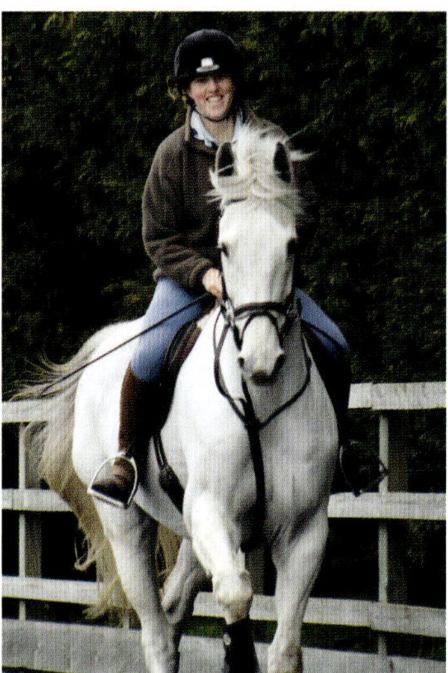

**LEFT** *Fast work can encourage the horse to think and move forwards with enthusiasm. This can prevent him from becoming stale in his work.*

**RIGHT** *If suitable conditions are not available, interval training and fast work in the form of extended canter can be performed in a school. This may also be more appropriate for over-excitable horses or nervous riders.*

## THE RISKS OF FAST WORK

Galloping increases the forces that must be absorbed through each limb to more than three times the body weight. The muscles and soft tissue structures are put under greater strain, stretch and recoil. The greatest risk of injury occurs when the core is weak, the muscles tire and strain is taken up by the connective tissue. To minimise the risk of injury:

- Only gallop if horse and rider are fit, confident and can stay in balance and control
- Warm up thoroughly before galloping
- Ensure that the environment is safe and the surface consistent and appropriate
- Only gallop for short periods of time relative to fitness and condition
- Do not gallop a tired horse
- Pull up slowly in a straight line and decelerate through the gaits to allow the muscles to adjust
- Walk for at least twenty minutes after the heart rate has returned to normal to allow the complete removal of toxins from the blood.
- Leave at least four days between fast work sessions to allow muscles to recover.

## SUMMARY

- A good walk forms the basis of all training.
- Walk is a low-impact gait with no moment of suspension.
- Walk is the gait with most rotation in the thoracolumbar spine.
- The moment of suspension in trot increases stretch and recoil in muscles and in the tendons and ligaments of the lower limb.
- There is passive flexion and extension of the back in trot.
- Canter is an asymmetrical gait with a moment of suspension.
- Canter is good for strengthening the thoracic sling and toning long, weak abdominal muscles vital for supporting the back.
- In canter and gallop there is active back flexion and extension with each stride, which is good for keeping the back supple.
- Fast work is good for respiratory and cardiovascular fitness.

# Exercises for Performance

Some suggestions for improving outline, gait, posture, flexibility, core stability and musculoskeletal health.

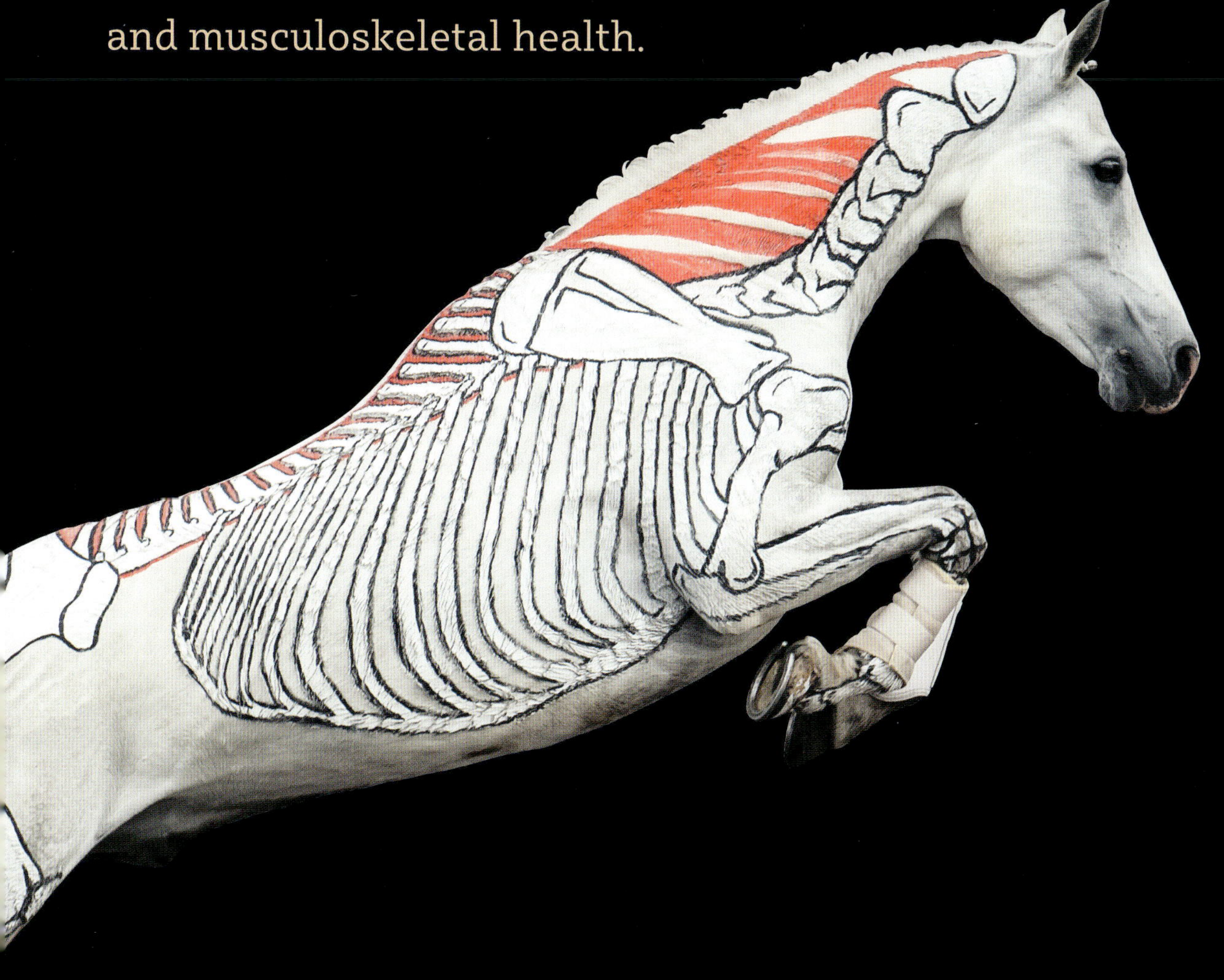

# Positioning of the Head and Neck

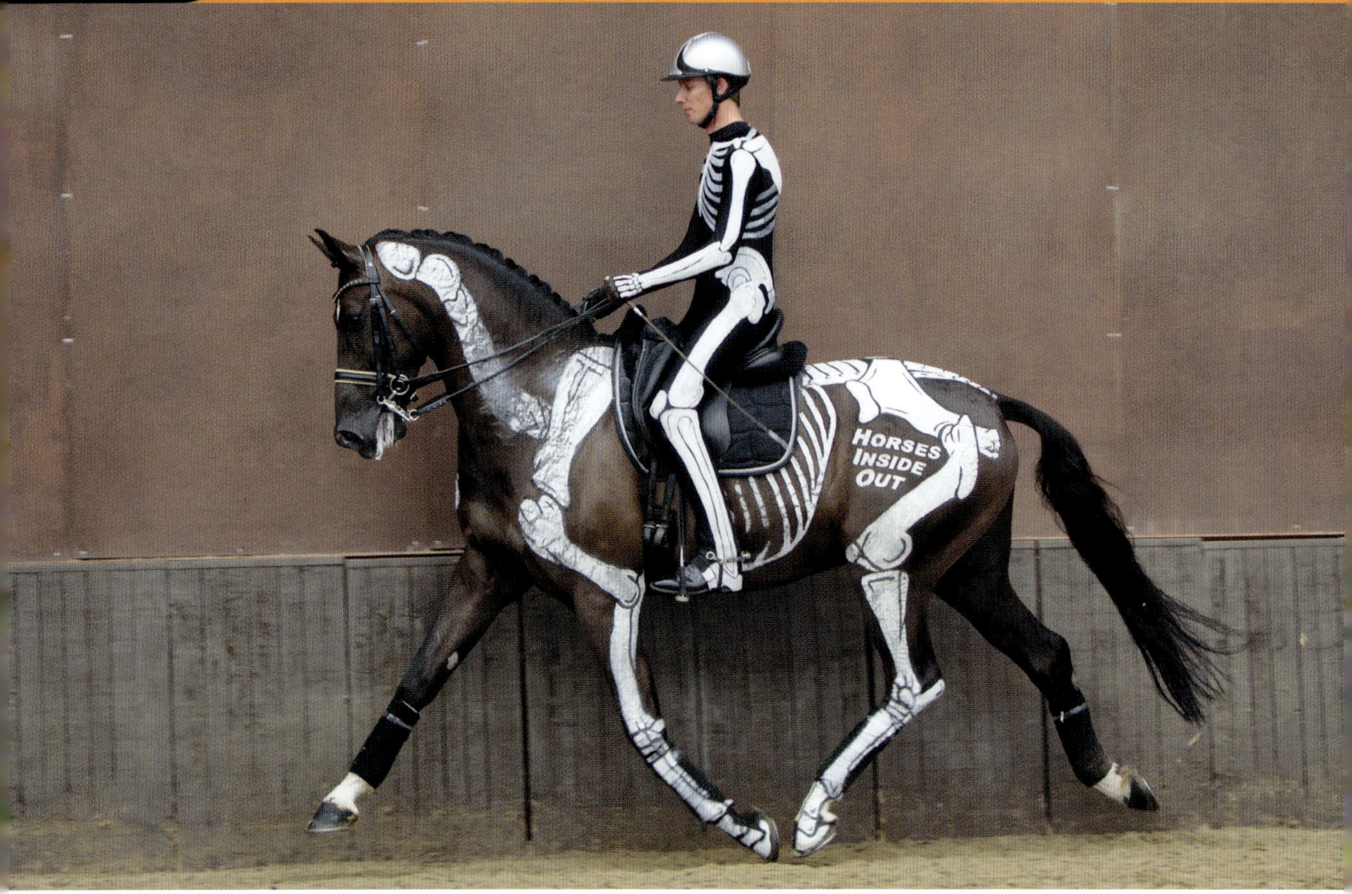

To ensure efficient movement with free, regular gaits, the horse must be permitted to carry his head in a relaxed, comfortable manner without restriction. Understanding how the horse uses positioning of the head and neck to affect the back via the spinal ligament system (see page 36) is probably the most important factor in achieving a balanced, well-adjusted horse. It also influences all other aspects of movement and performance both physically and psychologically.

Understanding the structure and function of the neck helps us to train with empathy and select suitable exercises and an appropriate neck outline for age, muscle condition and stage of training.

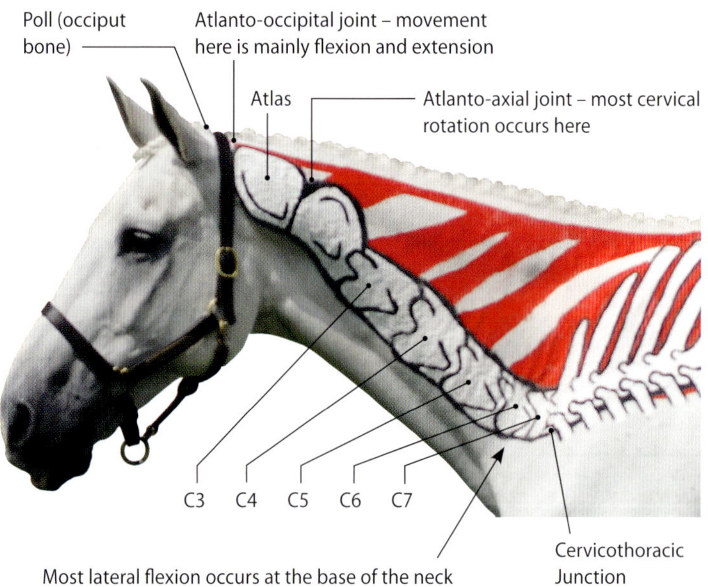

# How Positioning of the Head and Neck Affects Balance

As the head is a weight on the end of a long lever, neck position will affect the centre of balance. This point is dynamic. In trot, canter or gallop, when accelerating or jumping, it shifts forward. In collection it moves back. For the best performance horse and rider should be in perfect equilibrium with the rider's weight positioned above the centre of balance of the horse.

*1. As the horse reaches forward the centre of mass moves forwards. 2. As the horse lifts his neck the centre of mass moves backwards. 3. As the head is lowered and more weight is carried on the forehand the centre of mass moves forward. 4. Lowering of the head as the horse is in flight contributes to raising the centre of mass, which enables the horse to clear the obstacle. 5. When the head, neck, shoulders or quarters move to the side, the centre of mass will also move sideways. 6. This horse is using his head and neck to regain balance. In this situation the head and neck are sometimes referred to as the 'fifth leg'.*

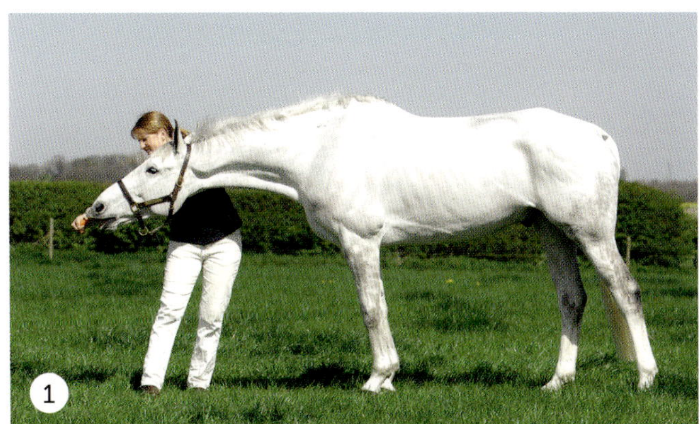

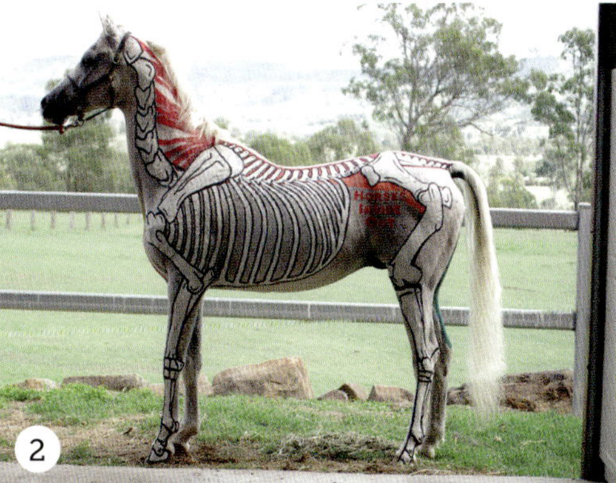

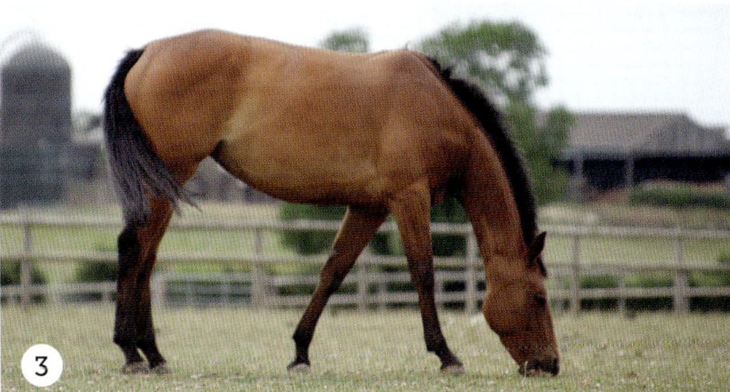

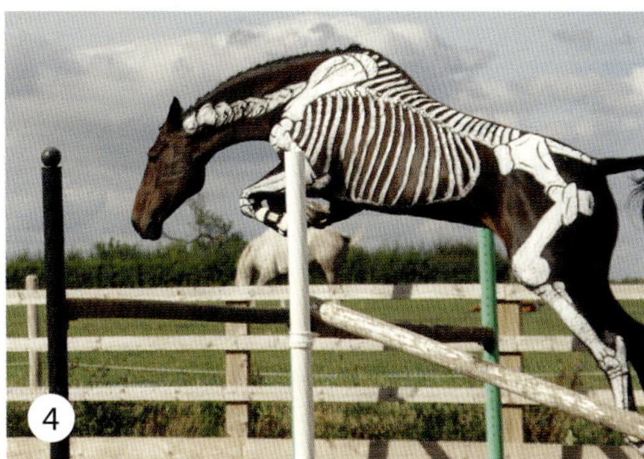

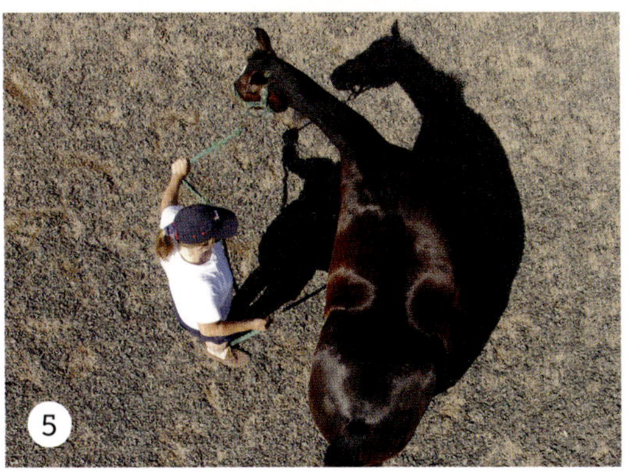

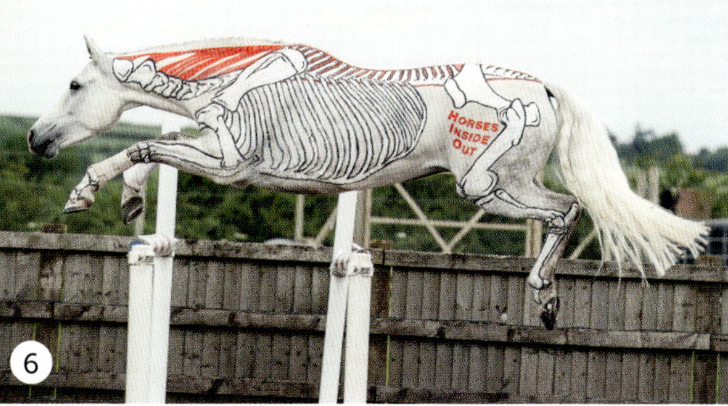

# How Positioning of the Head and Neck Affects Hindlimb Movement

Unrestricted hip extension when galloping or taking off for a wide fence can only be achieved if the rider's hands are pushed forwards, allowing the head and neck to be telescoped outwards. Hip extension is also an important requirement for good expression, power and stride length during extension in a dressage test.

A shortened neck position will restrict hip extension. This will result in loss of performance in the extended movements in dressage, a reduction of speed when galloping, and will limit restriction of the frame when taking off for a jump.

When the head is raised, this causes the hindlimbs to 'trail'.

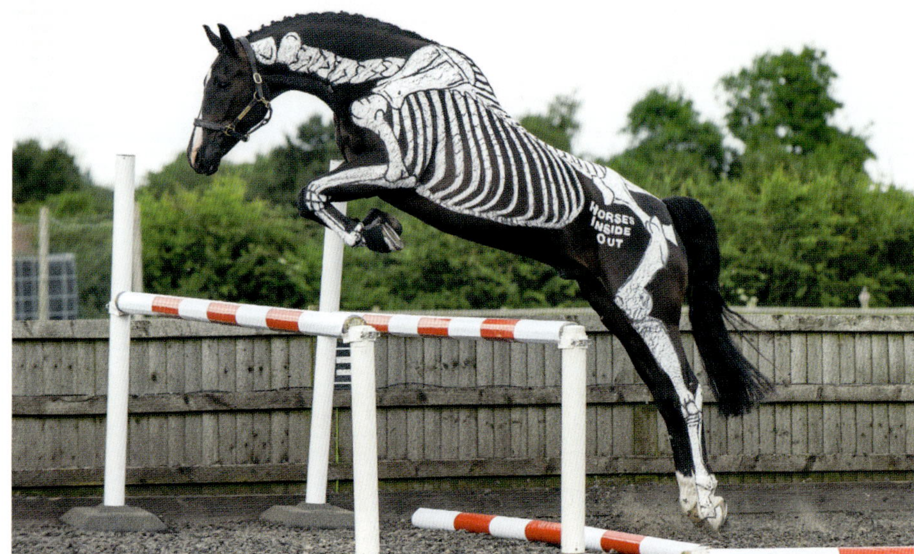


RIGHT *Head and neck telescoped outwards.*

BELOW LEFT *A shortened neck position.*

BELOW RIGHT *The head raised.*

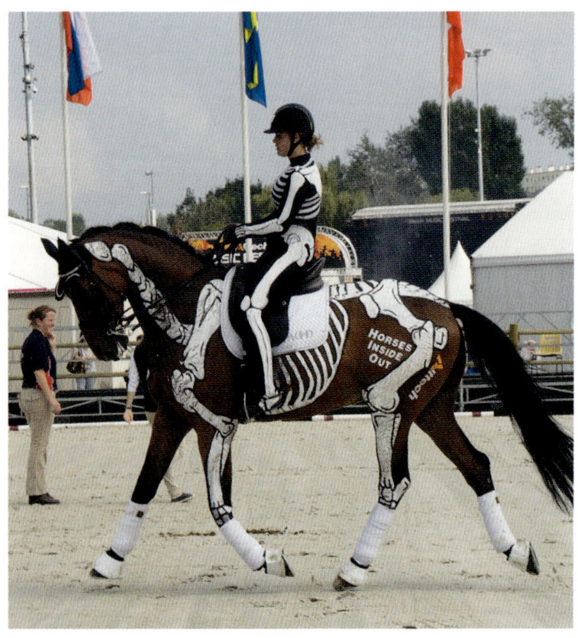


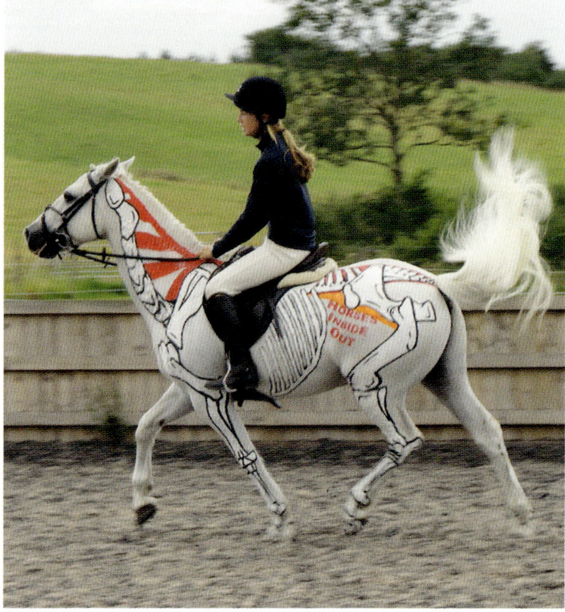

# How Positioning of the Head and Neck Affects Forelimb Movement

When the head is up the forelimbs extend. Although this is useful in some circumstances it is detrimental in others. For example if the head is up in dressage this will inhibit forelimb elevation and expression.

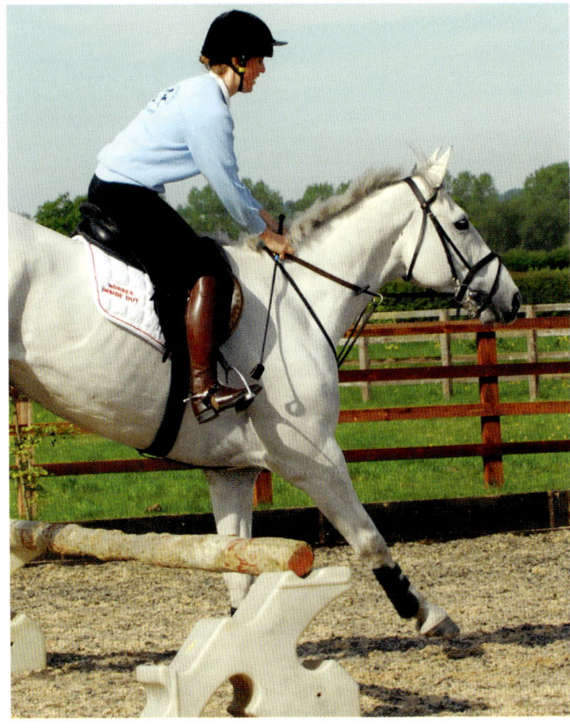

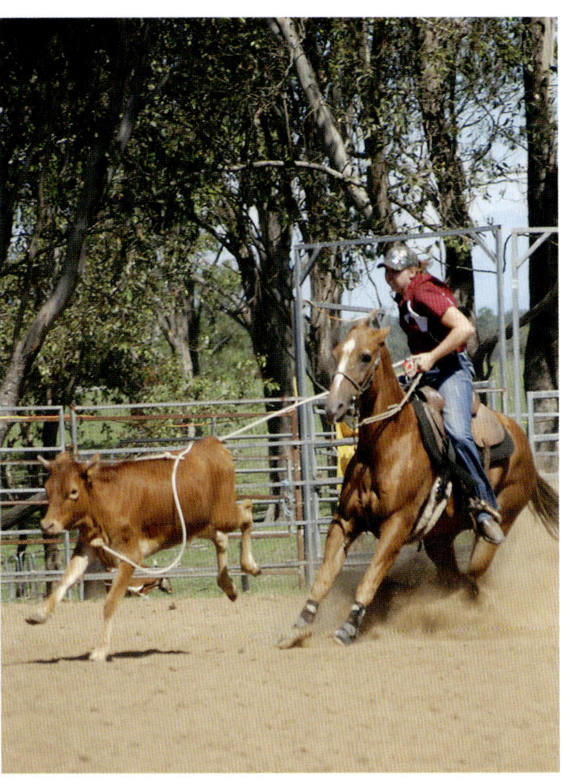

**LEFT AND ABOVE** *When the head is up the forelimbs extend.*

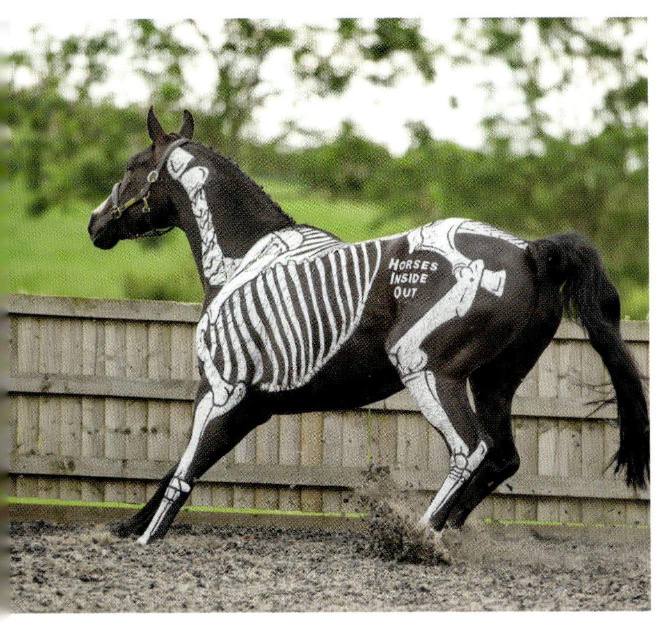


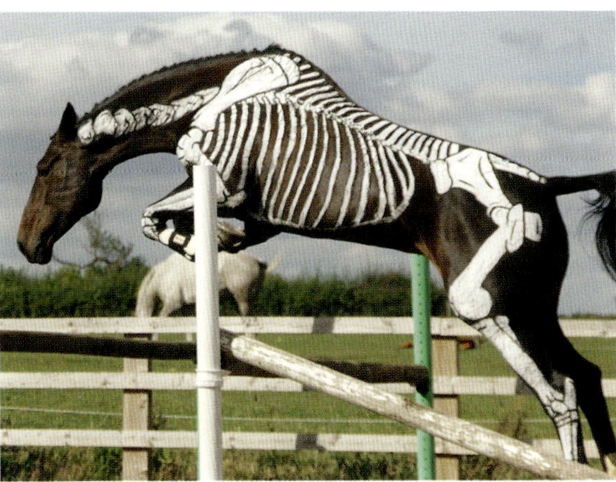

**ABOVE** *Flexion of the head and neck is related to flexion of the forelimbs. This can be seen in the photo – a bascule over a jump. This head and neck position allows the horse to lift the base of the neck and withers and contributes to freer shoulder movement.*

# How Positioning of the Head and Neck Affects Breathing

For maximum efficiency, the airways need to be unrestricted and open. Any artificial head positions, whether created by restraining tack or the rider's hands, will cause some restriction, making it difficult for the horse to breathe. This is a particularly important consideration when training horses with upper respiratory tract dysfunction.

A forced bend at the throat always causes some resistance as the pharynx is compressed and the trachea flexes and shortens. When extremely overbent, the horse may struggle to breathe, 'make a noise' as the vocal cords vibrate, or resist the rider's demands by dropping the head or coming behind the bit. In this case performance and comfort may well suffer. We could not run a marathon with our chin on our chest!

*For maximum airflow the pharyngeal diameter is at its greatest when the neck is extended.*

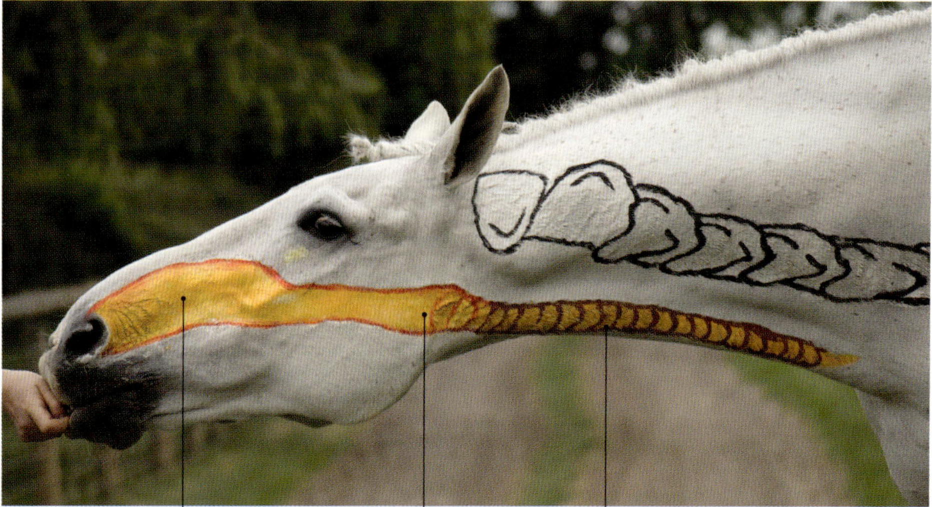


*The diameter of the pharynx is reduced when the head and neck are flexed. The varying degrees of flexion deemed necessary by some showjumpers or dressage riders reduces the airflow.*

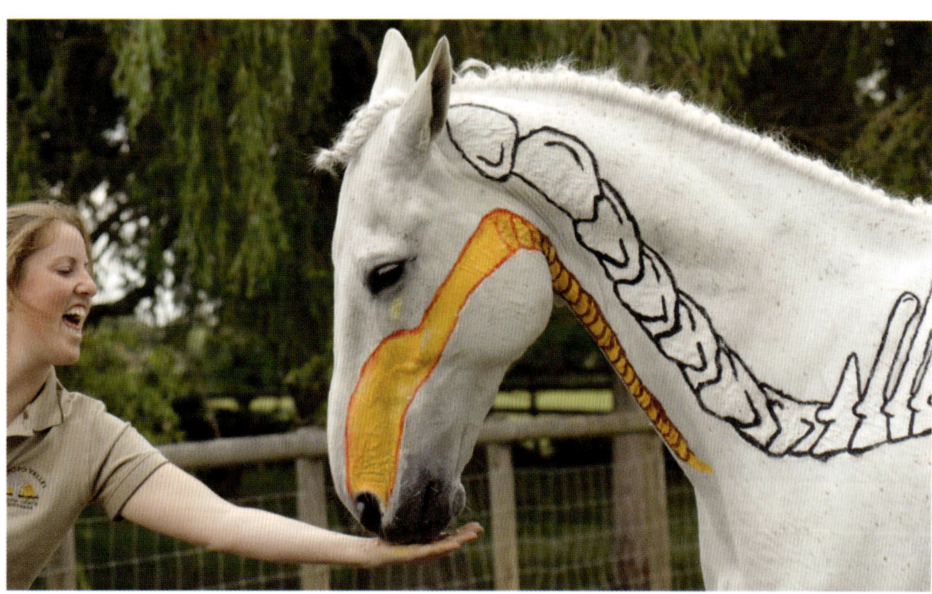

## How Positioning of the Head and Neck Affects Vision

The horse needs to position his head in order to focus. Monocular vision allows him to see different things from each eye whilst binocular vision allows him to judge distance.

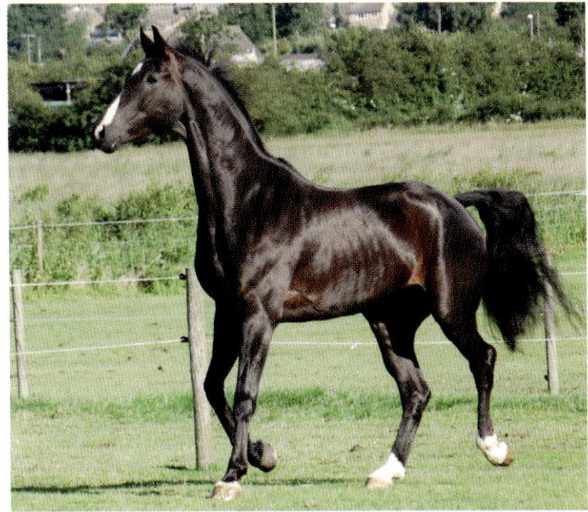

**ABOVE** *In order to focus on something in the distance the horse will raise his head. A horse approaching a jump needs to lift his head in order to assess the height and depth of the obstacle.*

**BELOW** *When a horse is over-flexed, his field of vision, which is then directed towards the ground (or in some cases back towards his feet) is considerably curtailed. With no forward view, and a blind spot in front of him, the horse is forced to put all his trust in the rider. This horse will also find breathing difficult as the trachea is severely restricted, thereby increasing pressure and reducing air flow.*

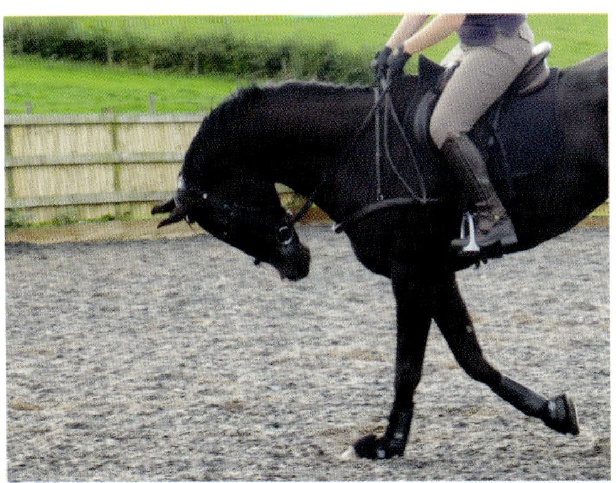

## How Positioning of the Head and Neck Affects Behaviour

With both humans and horses, physiology can influence psychology, with mood and performance being influenced by physical condition. Overall body language and the position of the head and neck are good behavioural indicators. An excited, tense or nervous horse, in the fright/flight pose, will have a high head-carriage whereas a relaxed horse, comfortable in mind and body, will hold his head lower, move in a relaxed 'easy' manner and be much easier to handle and train.

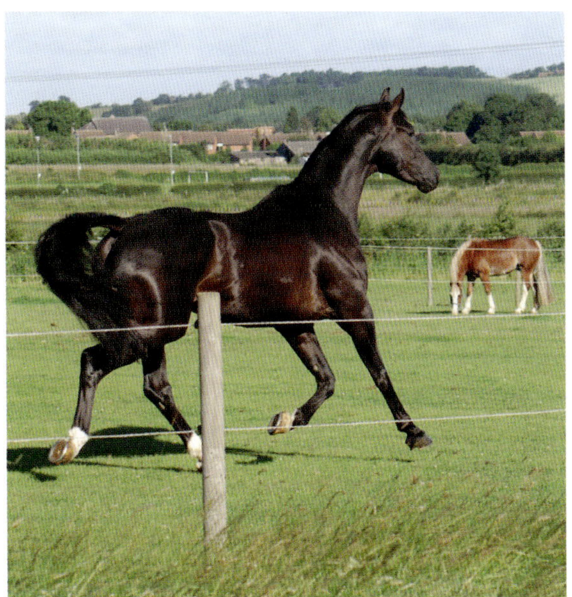

**ABOVE** *Tense/excited posture.* **BELOW** *Relaxed Posture.*

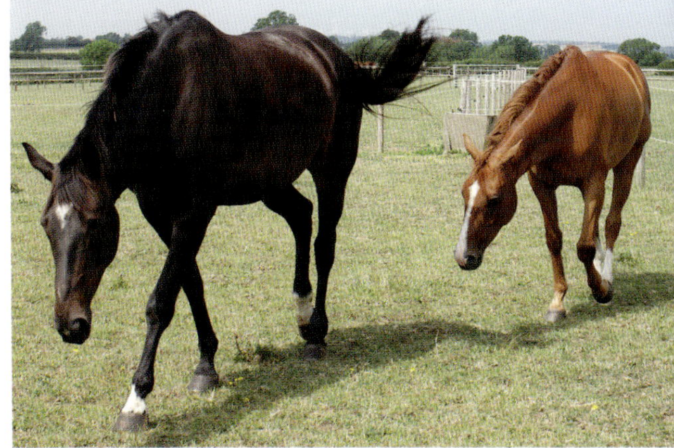

# Forwards and Down Neck Position

With the lowered head position:

- Traction within the nuchal ligament supports the back via the supraspinous ligament
- There are larger spaces between the thoracic spinous processes and greater flexion through the thoracolumbar region. This makes it easier to support the weight of the rider
- There is increased rotation and lateral flexion within the caudal thoracic and lumbar region
- Correct alignment of the vertebrae allows unrestricted passage of spinal nerves through the vertebral canal
- Thoracic sling muscle recruitment is increased and the muscles at the cervicothoracic junction involved in raising the base of the neck and supporting the forehand are strengthened
- Back problems can be alleviated or in some cases avoided. This is as an effective analgesic position particularly useful for older horses and those with kissing spines or other back problems
- There is increased abdominal muscle recruitment
- This way of going encourages mental relaxation.

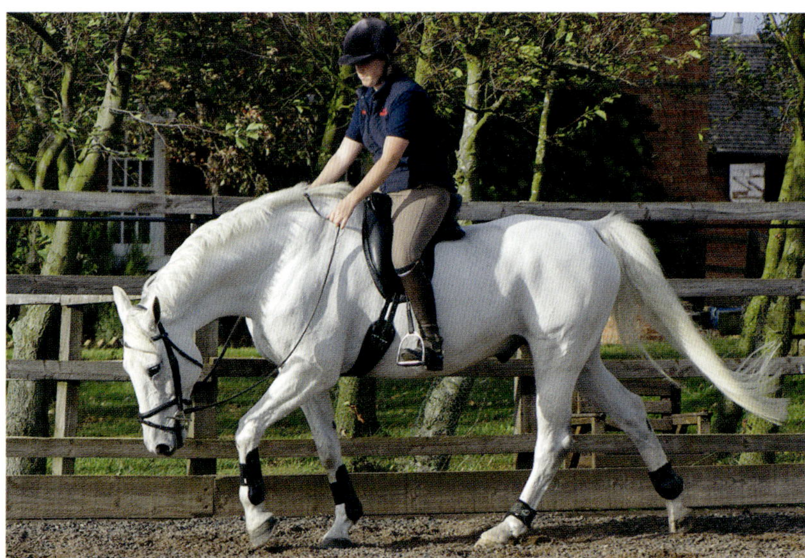

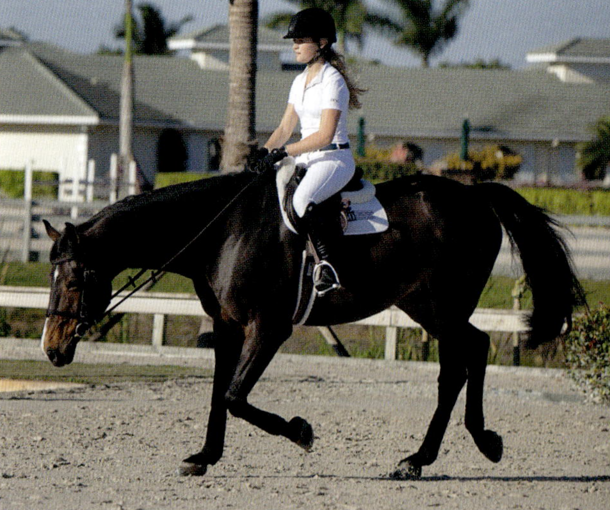

*BELOW, RIGHT Working a horse in a forward and down neck outline increases the weight and forces through the forelimb joints, tendons and ligaments. To counteract this, especially if he is already heavy on the forehand, tends to lean on the bit, has structural weaknesses or an old injury, it is important to encourage him to carry more weight behind and to limit the length of time he is required to work in this position, reduce the pressure and lighten the forehand by encouraging him to push from behind.*

*ABOVE AND BELOW As positioning the head and neck affects the back, which in turn affects posture, all training sessions, whether ridden or on the lunge, should begin with working in a forward and down outline. This has many benefits for all horses and is essential for young or weak horses.*

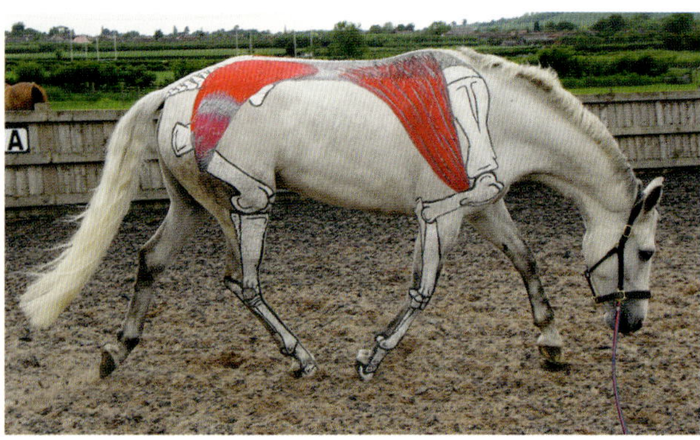

# Raised and Round Neck Outline

Once the horse is relaxed and working over the back it is time to work with more energy, pick up the contact, engage the hindquarters and raise the base of the neck. The resultant higher neck position is sometimes described as raised and round. This outline, appropriate to age, stage, (the horse in the photo below is a 7-year-old novice dressage horse) conditioning and level of training, should be maintained with suppleness and relaxation.

As the head and neck is raised:

- The nose should be either on or slightly in front of the vertical
- A greater proportion of isometric and eccentric muscular contraction is required to support the neck and back

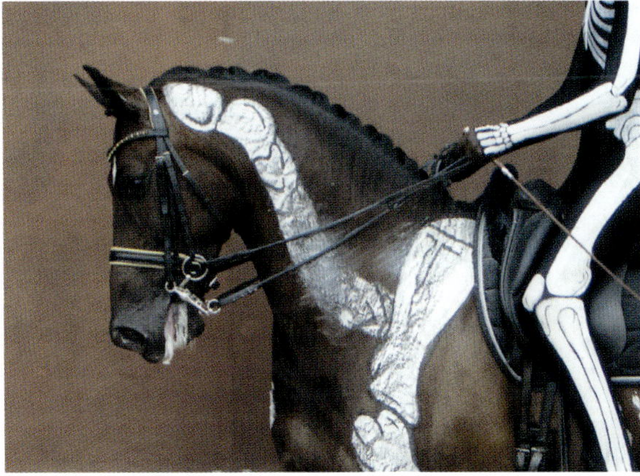

- The splenius and topline muscles use isometric muscular contraction to maintain flexion in the neck
- The base of the neck is retracted (raised) and the thoracic sling muscles work in a shortened position to provide a stable base for expressive forelimb movement
- There is increased flexion at the lumbosacral junction, greater engagement and more weight carried by the hindlimbs.

Progression to, or maintaining a raised and round neck position requires:

- Patience, as this outline can only be achieved gradually
- Preparing the muscles for each training session by working long and low
- Working with impulsion, engagement and straightness
- Sitting up to reduce strain on and lighten the forehand
- Shifting the centre of mass backwards by strengthening the hindquarter, back and neck muscles
- Working from behind using collection exercises such as transitions and backing up
- Incorporating periods of stretching to relieve tension in muscles.

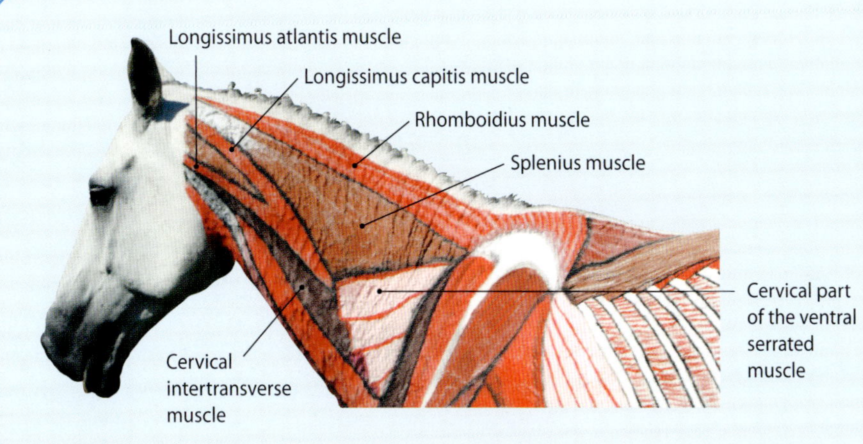


When the horse is worked in a raised and round neck outline the neck extensor muscles (left) work isometrically and eccentrically to maintain flexion.

## On the bit

If the horse is working in self-carriage without leaning on the rider's hands and is holding his head slightly in front of the vertical he is said to be working correctly 'on the bit'. To accomplish this it is essential that his muscles are strong enough to support his head and he is pushing evenly from behind. Achieving a beautiful, correctly muscled arched neck outline is an ultimate training goal. In practice however, there are many undesirable outlines.

## Above the bit

If the horse is 'above the bit' with the head in a high extended outline and the back hollow, the muscles and ligaments will be put under strain and the spinous processes may begin to impinge. This can be caused either by incorrect training or poor conformation, with the neck being set low. In this case the horse will be unable to raise his shoulder, and will find it difficult to maintain a positive connection from the hind leg through to the hand. Not every horse has ideal conformation and working consistently through from behind will help gain muscle strength and allow him to perform to the best of his ability.

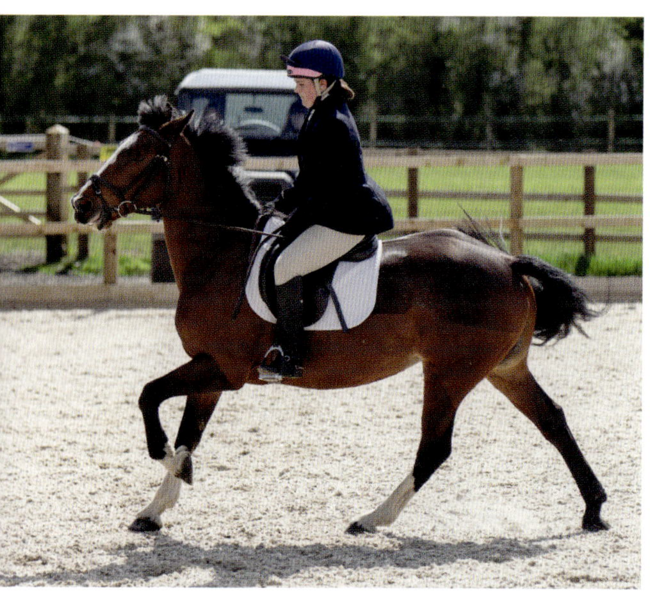

*'Above the bit' with the head in a high extended outline and the back hollow.*

## Overdeveloped flexor chain neck musculature

Overdeveloped muscles on the underside of the neck are indicative of incorrect riding, training, tension and resistance. They are often seen in horses that pull heavy loads or pull themselves along from the front rather than pushing from behind. A concave curve locks the neck, prevents lateral flexion and leads to a downward spiral of poor movement, resistance, lack of concentration, further incorrect muscle development and tension.

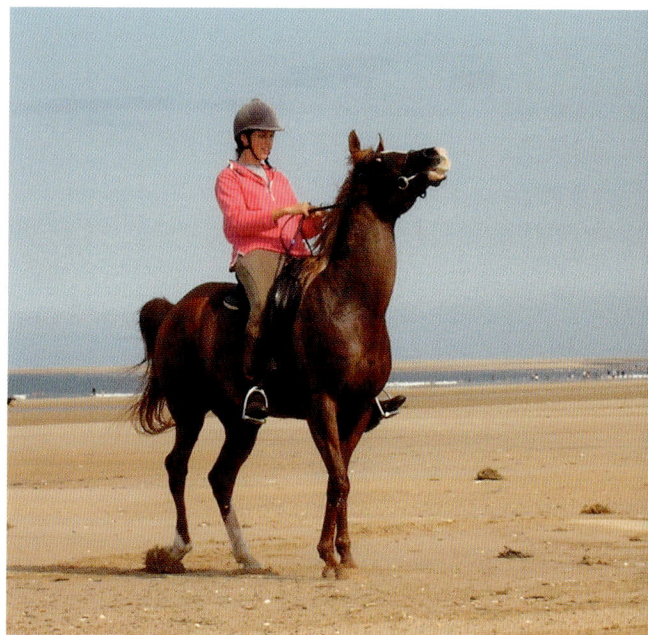

**ABOVE** *Overdeveloped muscles on the underside of the neck.*

## High and protracted

Although the horse at the top of page 109 is working with the poll at the highest point and his nose on the vertical, he has dropped through the base of the neck and is displaying an exaggerated 'S' bend within the vertebrae. Shortening in this way causes the upper cervical vertebrae to flex whilst the lower vertebrae hollow This can lead to upper respiratory constriction, strain and stiffness through the thoracic region and extra tension through the topline. This makes working correctly over the back impossible.

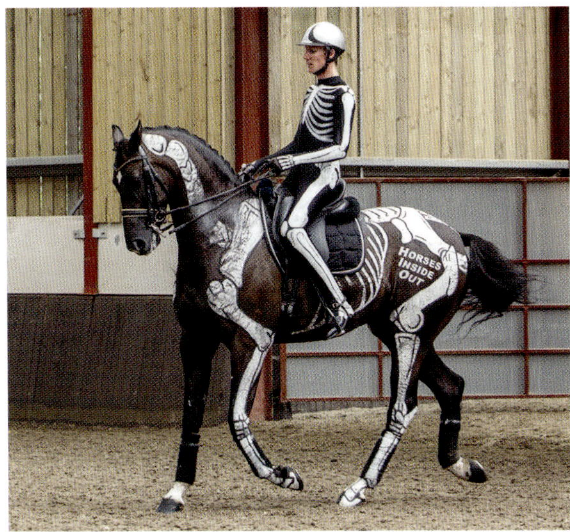

*High, protracted neck outline.*

## Behind the bit

The horse pictured below is being ridden incorrectly. The rider is pulling the head in rather than focusing on impulsion, engagement and working from behind. A horse that is permanently worked in an overbent outline will struggle to raise the forehand. This is a difficult problem to overcome.

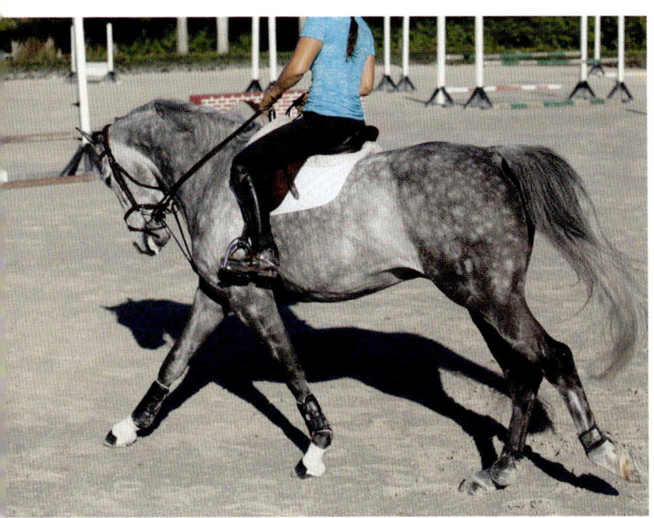

**RIGHT** *A Western horse in hyperflexed neck position. The leverage created in this position is often painful for the horse and puts an unacceptable amount of pressure on the small atlanto-occipital joint.*

## Hyperflexed neck position

The leverage created in this position is often painful for the horse and puts an unacceptable amount of pressure on the small atlanto-occipital joint. Any disruption to the mechanics of this joint can affect the posture of the entire spine. It is used by insensitive riders wanting complete submission from their horse. Disadvantages include:

- Tension, strain and potential damage to the nuchal ligament particularly in the upper cervical region
- A severely restricted windpipe
- Crushing of the soft tissue structures on the underside of the neck
- Pressure on the bars of the mouth
- Restriction in circulation to the tongue
- Excessive recruitment and shortening of the scalene, longus colli, brachiocephalic, sternomandibular and some of the thoracic sling muscles
- Constricted intervertebral foramina (spaces through which the spinal nerves exit from the spinal cord) potentially affecting neuromuscular control
- Reduction of weight carried on the hindquarters, making the horse heavy on the forehand
- Prevention of true collection by restricting the ability to step under, causing the hocks to trail
- Reduced hindlimb protraction
- Restricted vision.

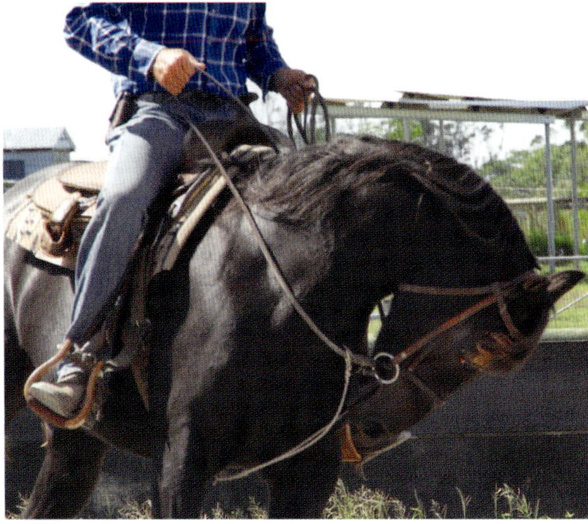

## AN ANATOMICAL REACTION TO OVER-FLEXION

The nuchal ligament has its strongest attachment into the second cervical vertebra and the poll. Riding a horse in an extremely overbent position increases the strain on the axis, atlas and occiput. This increases the risk of injury to the nuchal ligament in this area. Ridden in an overbent position, the jaw, TMJ, atlanto-occipital joint and atlanto-axial joint often become fixed, acting as one unit. Lateral flexion at the poll becomes difficult and the horse will try to compensate by using the less flexible mid-section of his neck to create bend. As the nuchal, supraspinous and dorsal sacroiliac ligaments are all connected, the entire dorsal chain will be adversely affected thus creating an imbalance that inhibits engagement, posture and performance.

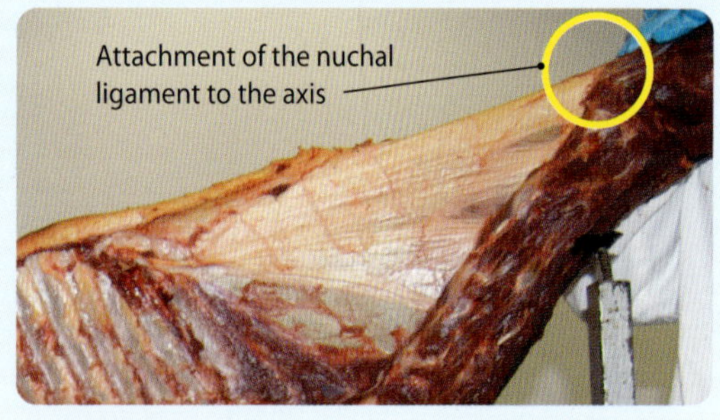


## Avoiding or correcting undesirable head and neck outlines

To reduce resistance and tension in the neck and correct the various undesirable neck outlines it is necessary to:

- Ride quietly with still handS and gentle, steady contact
- Work regularly in a stretching forwards and down neck position
- Encourage the horse to support the forehand by working from behind, stepping 'well under'
- Ride forward with purpose (even when on a long rein) ensuring the the horse is 'in front of the leg'

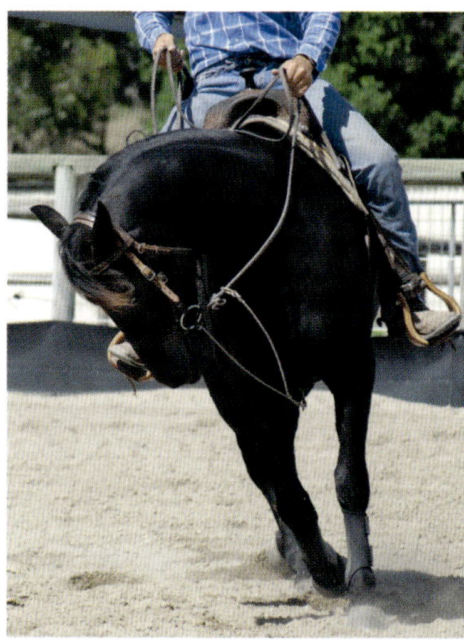

*Gadgets or 'schooling aids' are no substitute for slow, sensitive and correct training.*

- Use lateral neck flexion and bending exercises to promote longitudinal suppleness and submission
- Follow the steps for maintaining a raised and round neck position as explained earlier
- Use exercises such as backing up and lateral work to stimulate the thoracic sling muscles
- Use canter and fast work as tools to encourage the horse to extend the neck.

## SUMMARY

- Understanding the structure and function of the neck helps us to train with empathy and select suitable exercises and an appropriate neck outline for age, muscle condition and stage of training.
- For the best performance horse and rider should be in perfect balance.
- All training sessions should begin with, end with and include some work in a forward and down outline.
- To achieve an outline commensurate with age and stage, it is essential that the muscles are conditioned to maintain that position, strong enough to support the head, neck and weight of the rider, and the horse is pushing evenly from behind.

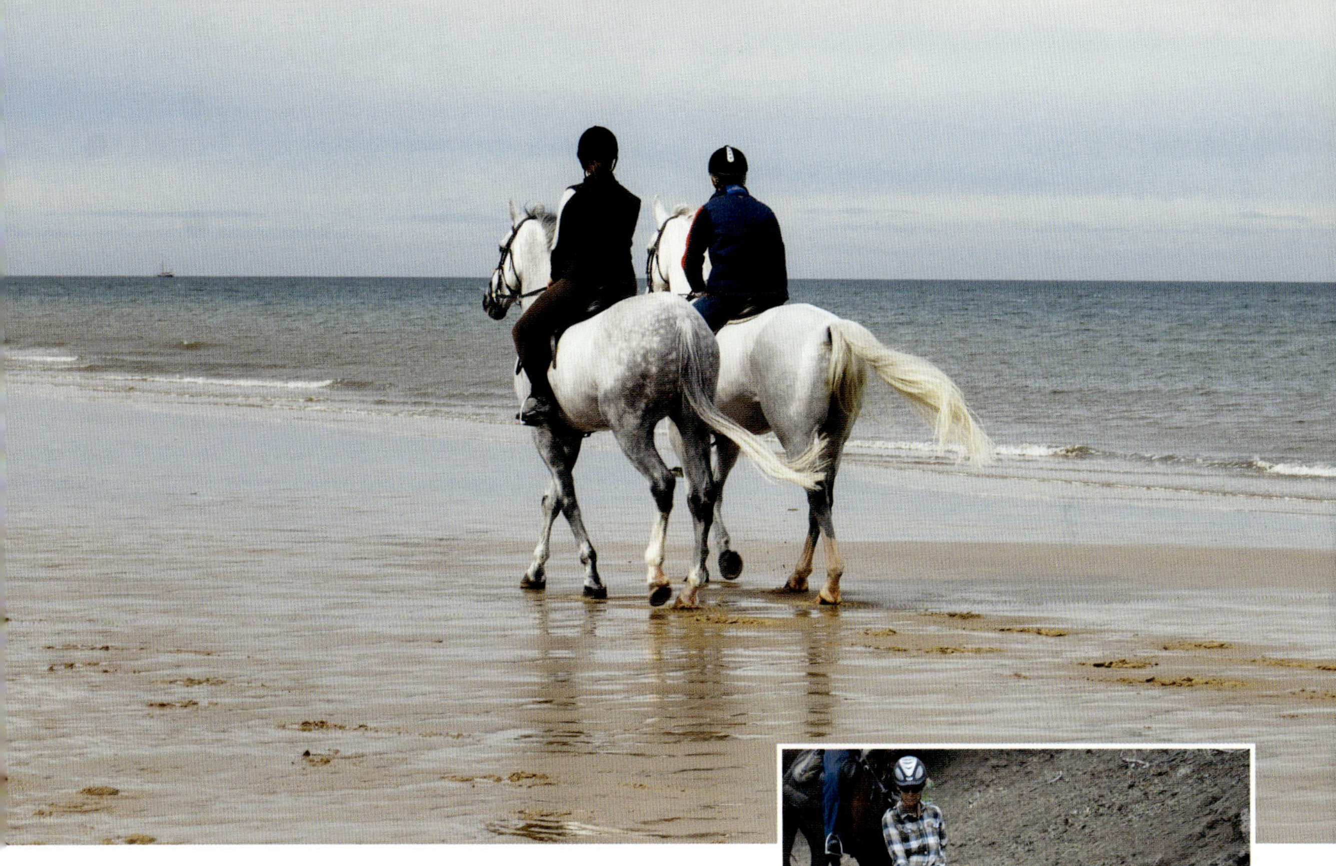

As personal trainers to our horses we need to know their 'gym' and expose them to a wide variety of experiences and surfaces. These can be natural such as fields, hills, tracks, turnout paddocks, the beach and sea or artificial which includes various manège and horse walker surfaces, concrete or tarmac, water and aqua-treadmills. Too hard a surface will expose the horse to the risk of concussion injury and too soft or deep will be tiring and expose the tendons and ligaments to strain. Horses worked only on one type of surface will be less resilient and more prone to injury when faced with an alien surface or situation.

**RIGHT** *Horses that are exposed to varied terrain are more surefooted, have improved proprioception, neuromuscular and motor control.*

## Hard ground

Hard ground, such as sun-baked earth or concrete, absorbs little energy, magnifies concussion forces and reduces stride length and swing. Horses can gallop faster on harder ground but there could be an increased risk of injury to bones, cartilage and joints. Horses often move less freely on hard ground. However, walking and short bursts of trot on hard surfaces improves bone density.

## Soft ground

Although a loose deep surface, such as a dry sandy beach, dunes or some sandy arenas, will reduce concussive forces to a negligible level it will dampen recoil, make the muscles work harder, require more energy and, particularly if very deep, increase the risk of soreness, injury, microdamage to muscles and strain to tendons and ligaments.

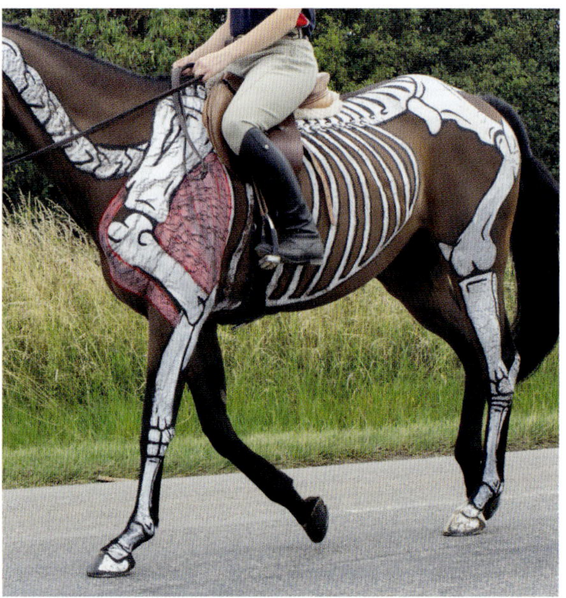

*Hard ground magnifies concussion forces.*

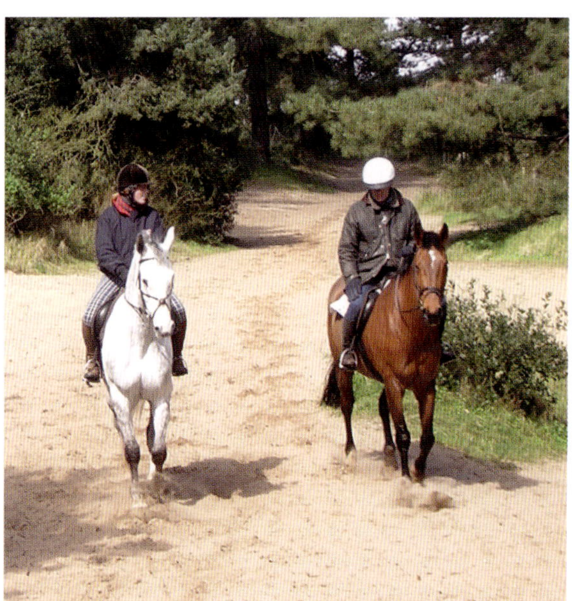

*Dry sandy surfaces will reduce concussive forces.*

### ARENAS

There is a wide variety of arena surfaces available, all with different properties, effects and benefits. Ideally a surface should allow slight penetration during impact and loading, absorb energy and provide stability and spring as the horse pushes off. For those who build their own arenas there are many non-slip, cushioning surfaces designed to reduce the risk of injury and make the most of the horse's ability and performance. For most riders, however, surface is dictated by location, home facilities, local equestrian centre, cost and availability.

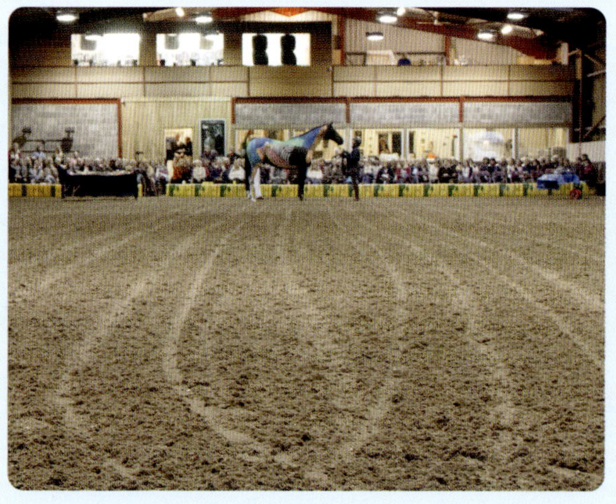

# Hills

Hill work is an ideal foundation for cardiovascular fitness, endurance and the strength required for all equestrian sports. Horses raised or turned out on hills tend to have stronger hindquarters, better balance and increased proprioception compared to those kept on flatter pasture. A consistent programme of hill work provides a full body workout, improving topline, balance, coordination and lower leg strength.

## Uphill

Walking or trotting uphill strengthens and conditions hamstring, gluteal and back muscles, of provide more pushing power for flatwork and jumping. Trotting encourages opening of the shoulders in preparation for medium and extended trot and is good for improving straightness and symmetrical muscle development. When cantering uphill, the thrust from both hind legs together develops jump and elastic recoil. To allow effective conditioning of the cardiovascular system, muscles, tendons, ligaments and joints to take place without strain, intensity of workout, steepness of incline, speed and frequency should be increased gradually.

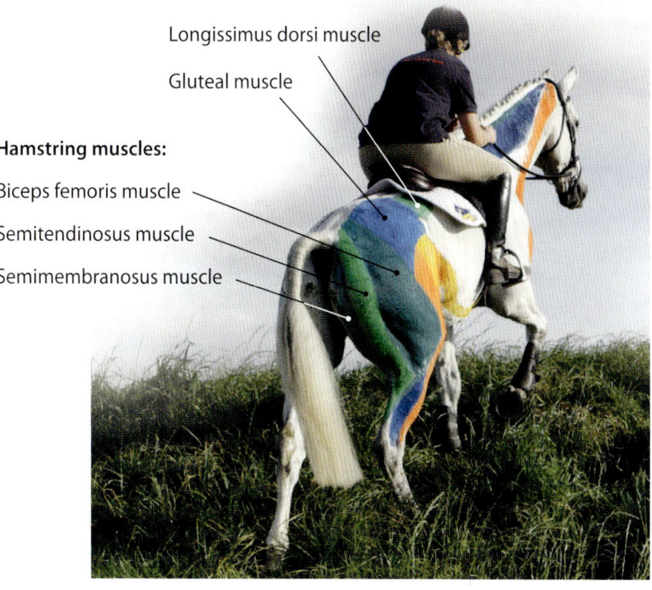


## Traversing slopes

Traversing Traversing a slope contributes to coordination and confidence and is an effective workout for the thoracic sling, abductor and adductor muscles. Riding curves and performing lateral work across, up and down slopes will encourage greater eccentric muscular contraction, develop lateral expression, control stability, balance and proprioception whilst still maintaining balance.

Too steep an angle can put the lower limb collateral ligaments under strain as they have to deal with torsional and sheer forces. Slope work should be avoided if the horse has a history of lower limb ligament conditions.

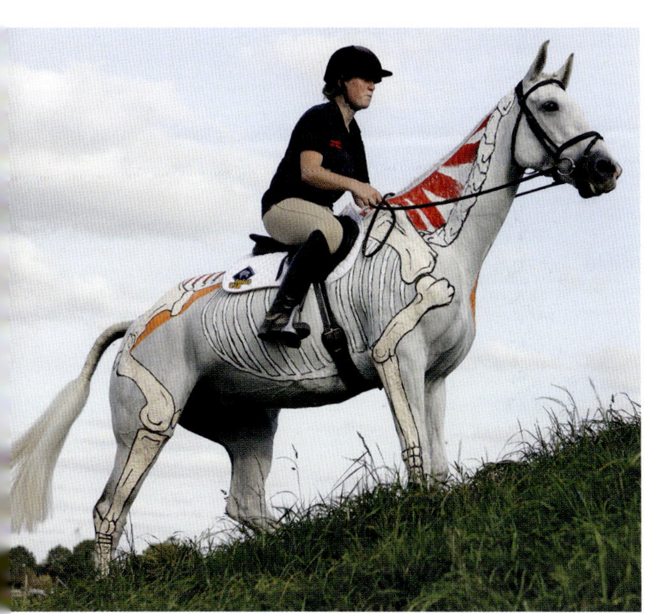

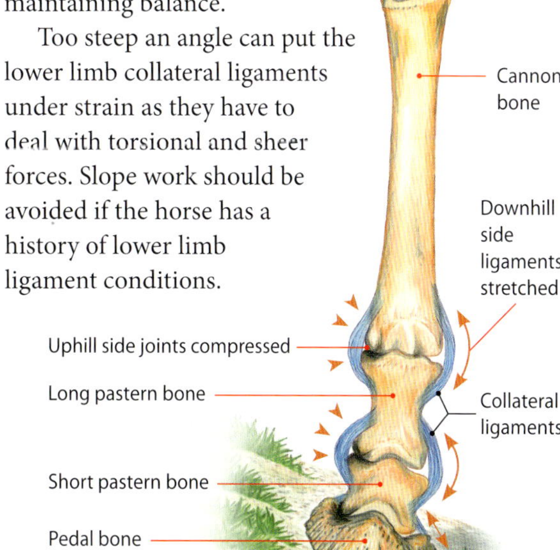

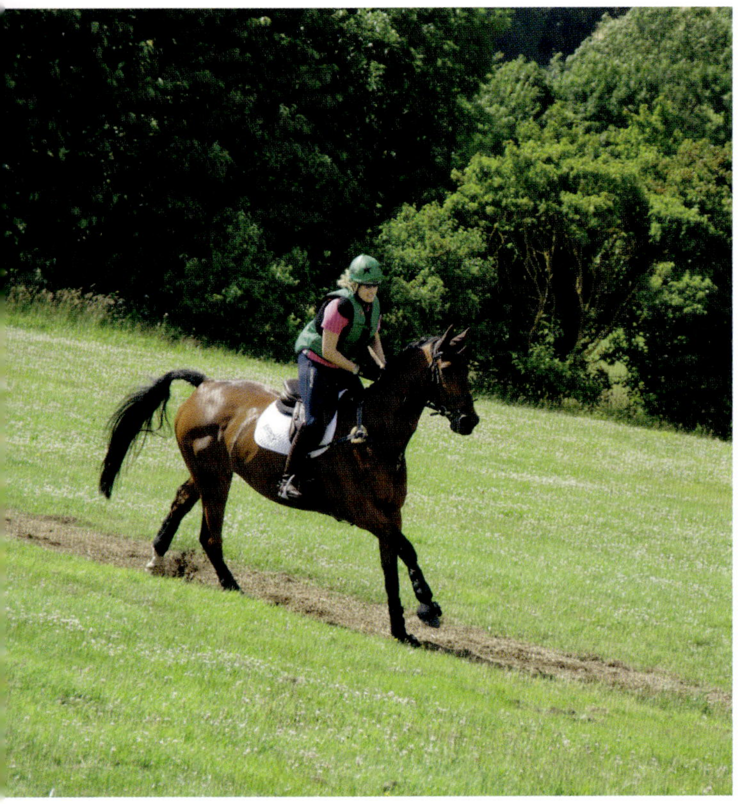

## Downhill

Downhill work also has its benefits. During descent greater eccentric and concentric muscle contraction is required to control braking power. The thoracic sling muscles must work hard to support the thorax between the forelegs and control the weight of both horse and rider bearing down the slope. The increase in muscle strength developed contributes to lightness of the forehand and forelimb expression. It also effectively strengthens the hindlimbs as they flex more and come further under the body for braking, balance and stability.

Performing downward transitions from trot to walk and halt whilst going downhill is an effective balance and core stability exercise. The aim is to ride a smooth downward transition whilst maintaining a consistent outline, contact, balance, control and self-carriage. Trotting slowly downhill builds hind end strength and condition required for jumping and hind expression.

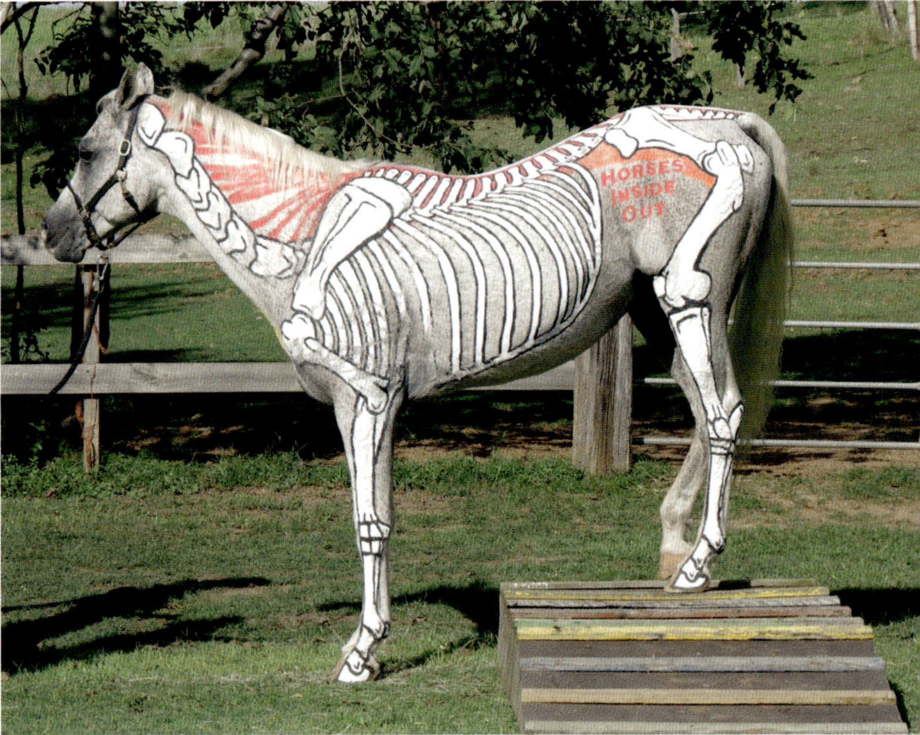



**RIGHT** *This picture has been included to illustrate how, when the horse is going down a steep hill, there is additional strain on the forelimbs and stress on the vertebrae, their spinous processes and vertebral discs. There is also increased extension through the cervicothoracic region. Horses with discomfort in their forelimbs or forefeet will take shorter, more cautious steps whilst those with weakness or discomfort in the hindlimbs may walk downhill reluctantly; drag the hind toes, or circumduct the limb. To mitigate all these effects and to help balance in descent it is important either to dismount or to allow complete freedom of the head and neck.*

# Water

Exercising in water has a number of benefits. It gives horses a completely different feel and experience and often promotes energy and enthusiasm. It is good for proprioception, training for event horses and provides therapeutic cooling for the legs.

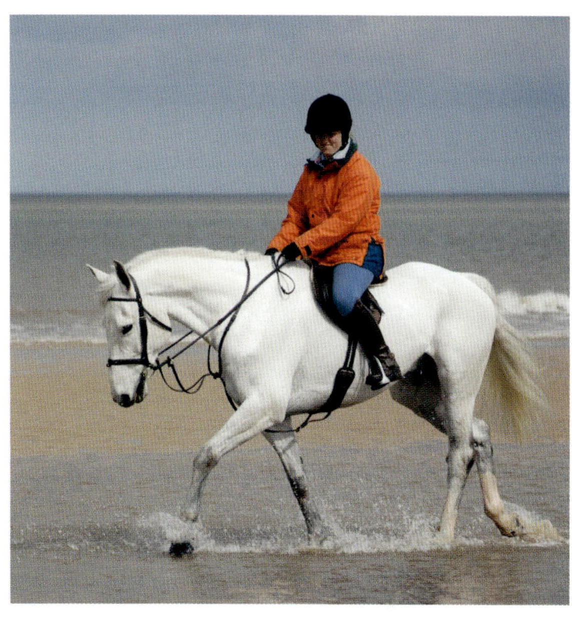

**RIGHT** *Walking in shallow water encourages the horse to lift and flex the limb joints. This strengthens the muscles during the swing phase and has a similar effect to walking over a series of raised poles. When walking in water it is important to be aware that the surface beneath the waterline can be inconsistent!*

**BELOW** *When trotting, additional lift conditions the muscles that are important in developing expression, power and cadence. Horses often lower their heads to look at the water. The splash and extra effort required benefits posture by encouraging recruitment of the abdominal and core muscles.*

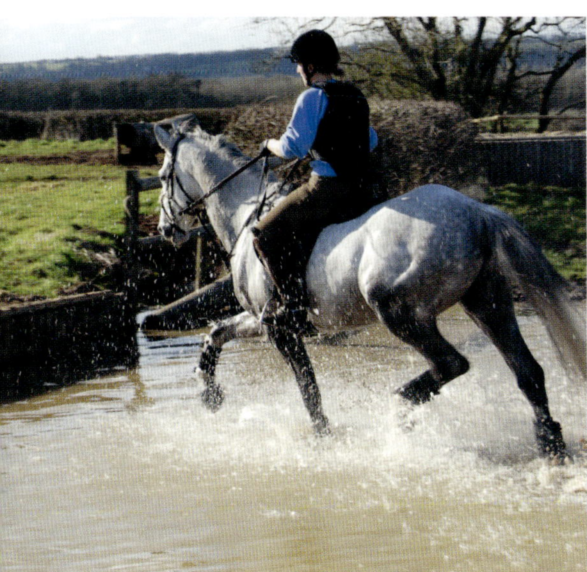

**RIGHT** *Moving through deeper water increases the resistance and therefore muscular strength training. The limb protraction muscles, (see page 120) involved in creating expression of movement, have to work particularly hard in deep water.*

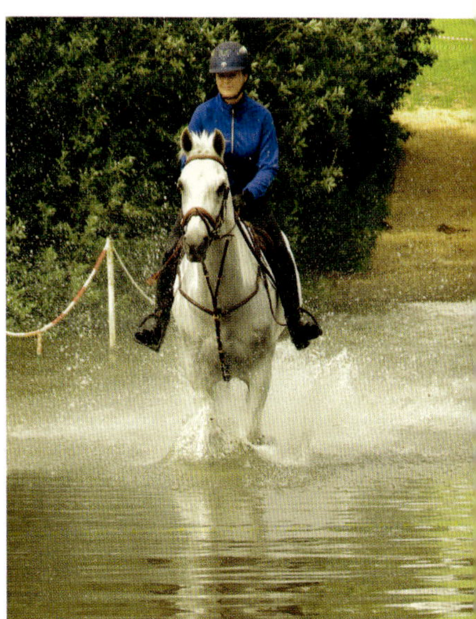

## SUMMARY

- Horses benefit from being exposed to a variety of surfaces.
- Hard ground magnifies concussive forces and reduces stride length and swing.
- Hill work is good for cardiovascular fitness, endurance and strength.
- Working in water cools the legs and, as the horse tends to lift his feet, is good for strengthening the abdominal muscles and core control.

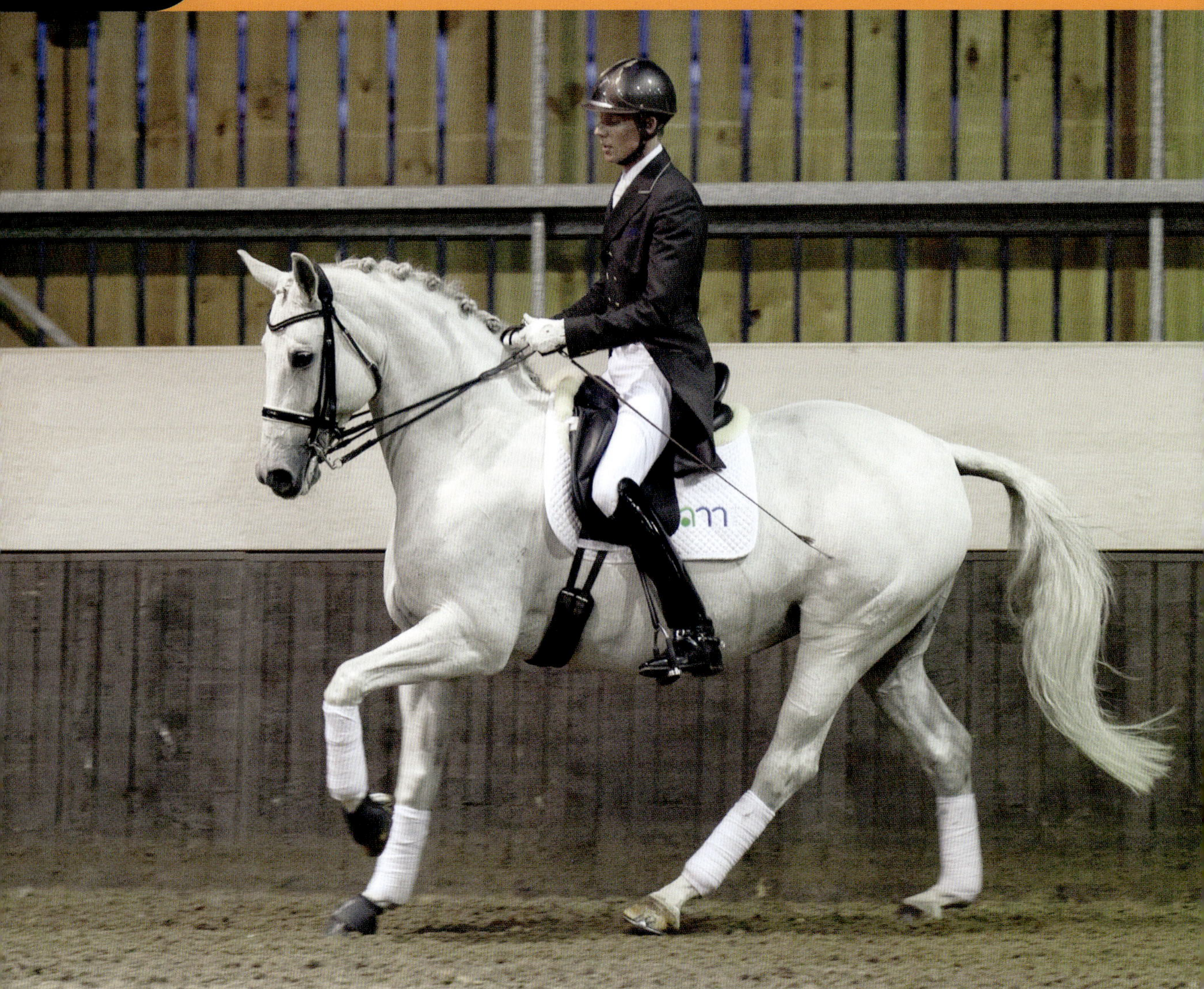

## The Journey to Collection

The journey to collection begins as soon as we start to handle a horse. True collection requires balance, energy, impulsion, skeletal maturity, correct posture and well-conditioned muscles. It is the culmination of the training principles of rhythm, engagement, relaxation, contact, impulsion and straightness. It requires the horse to flex the joints, lower and take more weight on the hindquarters whilst simultaneously shortening the frame and raising the forehand. This is a gradual process which takes time, patience and many years of musculoskeletal conditioning. As both horse and rider constantly change, evolve, improve, learn and develop it is a journey that never ends. At each milestone as the horse matures, mentally and physically, the requirements to reach the next stage alter and there is always room for improvement. The further along the road we travel the more demanding the tasks become and the longer it takes to reach them.

# How Horses Collect

Developing collection is progressive relative to age, stage, level of training and musculoskeletal strength. These photographs show two horses working towards collection – a novice on the right and a more advanced below.

During collection, as the centre of mass moves backwards, steps shorten as there is a reduction in the retraction of the hindlimbs. The quarters lower to carry more weight as flexion in the joints, and ideally in the back and lumbosacral junction increases. It is this flexion in the haunches which provides upward thrust and spring.

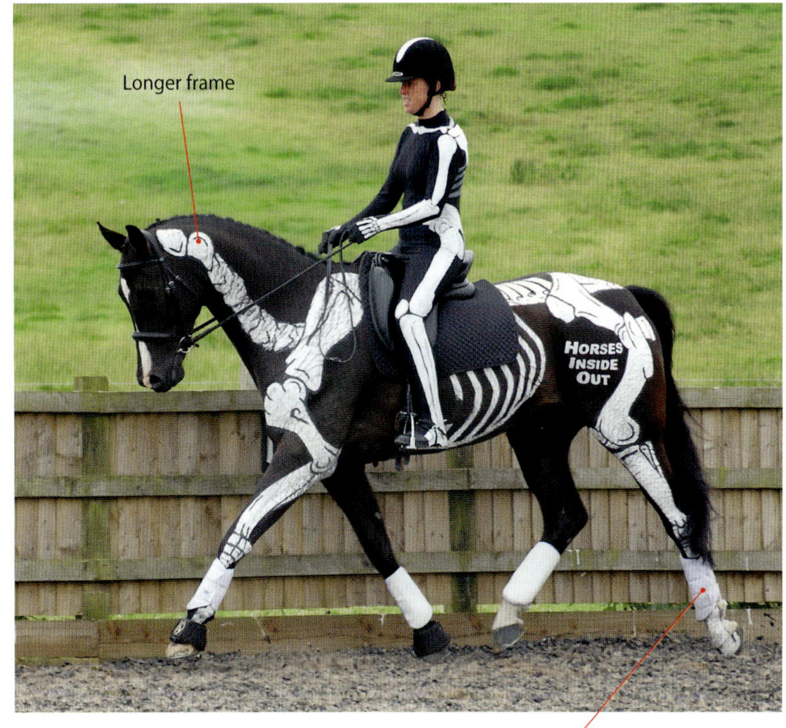

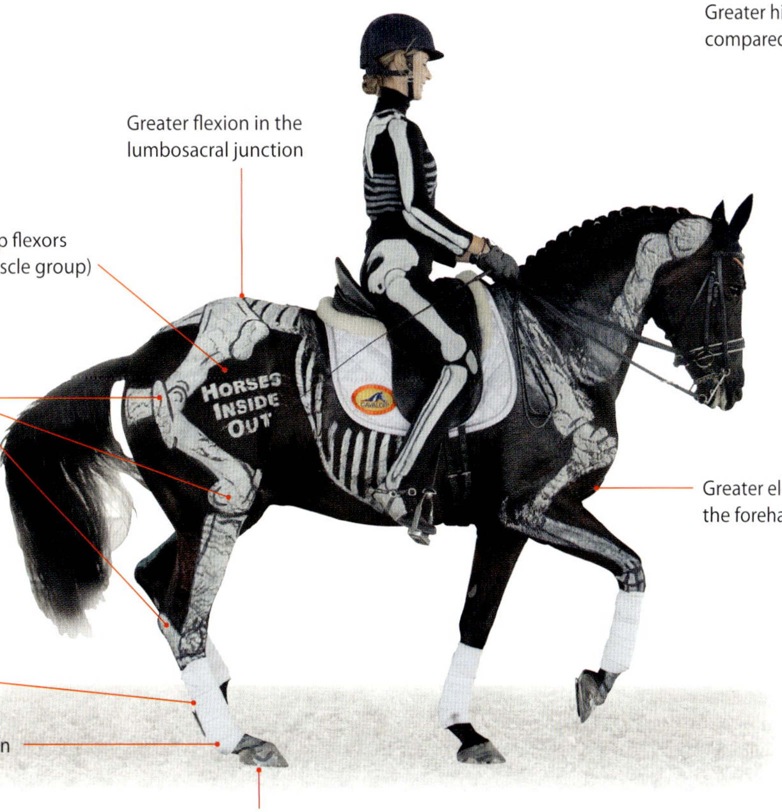

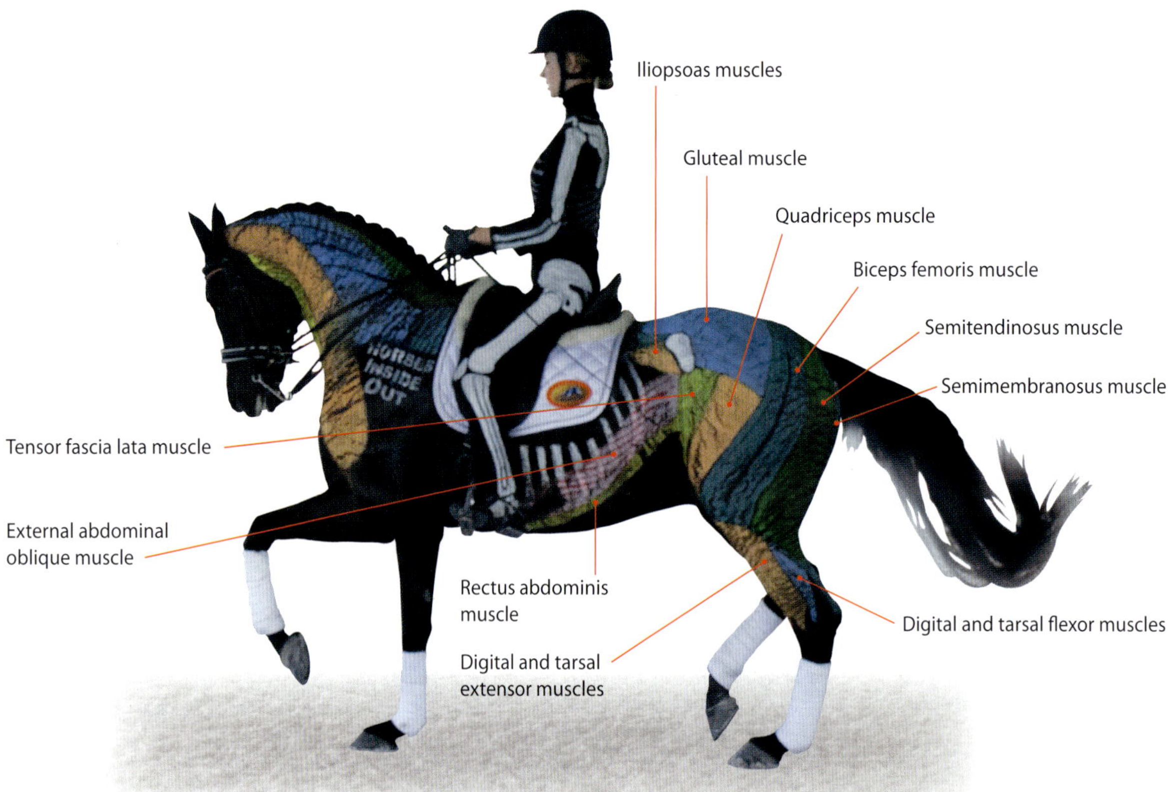


Flexion in the haunches requires muscular strength and a high degree of eccentric and isometric muscular contraction, particularly in the extensor chain. The back is supported by well-conditioned core muscles with the abdominal muscles, particularly the rectus and external oblique, pressing upon the visceral contents of the abdomen. This contributes to the horse working with good posture.

As more weight is carried behind, the forelimb is lightened, the base of the neck retracts and the head and neck come up. This lightens the forehand, makes the horse look and feel more 'uphill' and gives more freedom and expression to the forelegs. The 12-year-old horse in this picture has the muscular strength to perform collected movements and develop more engagement behind.

> **Note:** It is impossible to achieve collection by 'pulling' from the front. A horse that has insufficient strength to support a collected frame will be more prone to muscular and ligamentary damage. He may show resistance through swishing his tail, hollowing, evading the bit or displaying resistance in the head or neck.

This drawing illustrates a correctly conditioned horse, working well over the back, with a good posture and correct hind leg action.

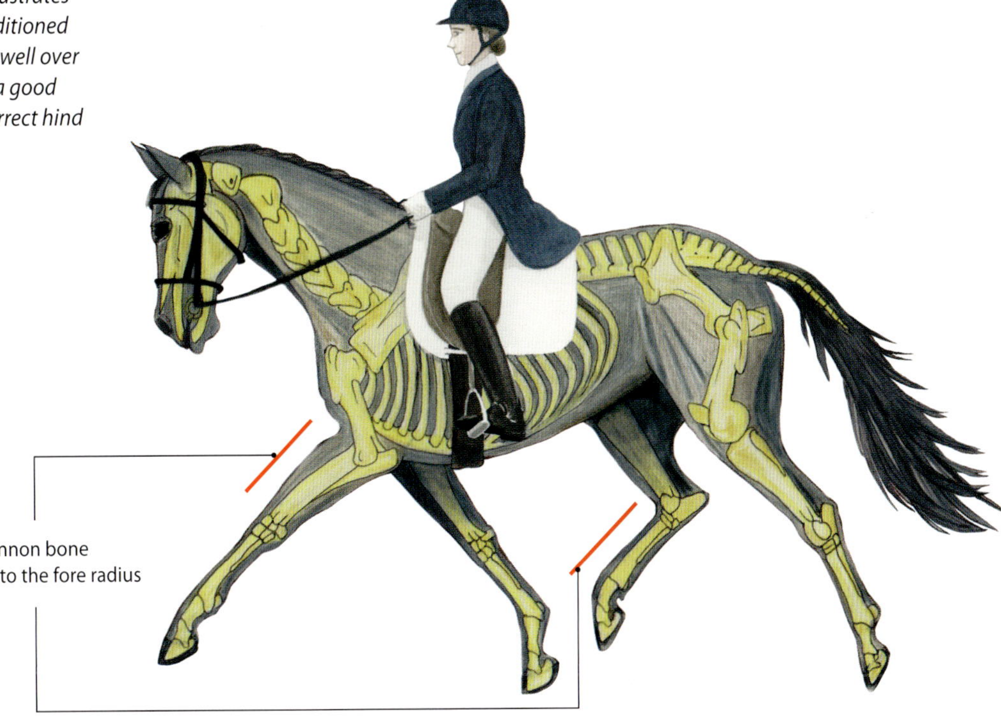

Hind cannon bone parallel to the fore radius

This drawing illustrates a horse with insufficient strength to lower his haunches and flex his hind legs sufficiently. He is unable to support his back correctly and will be more prone to injury.

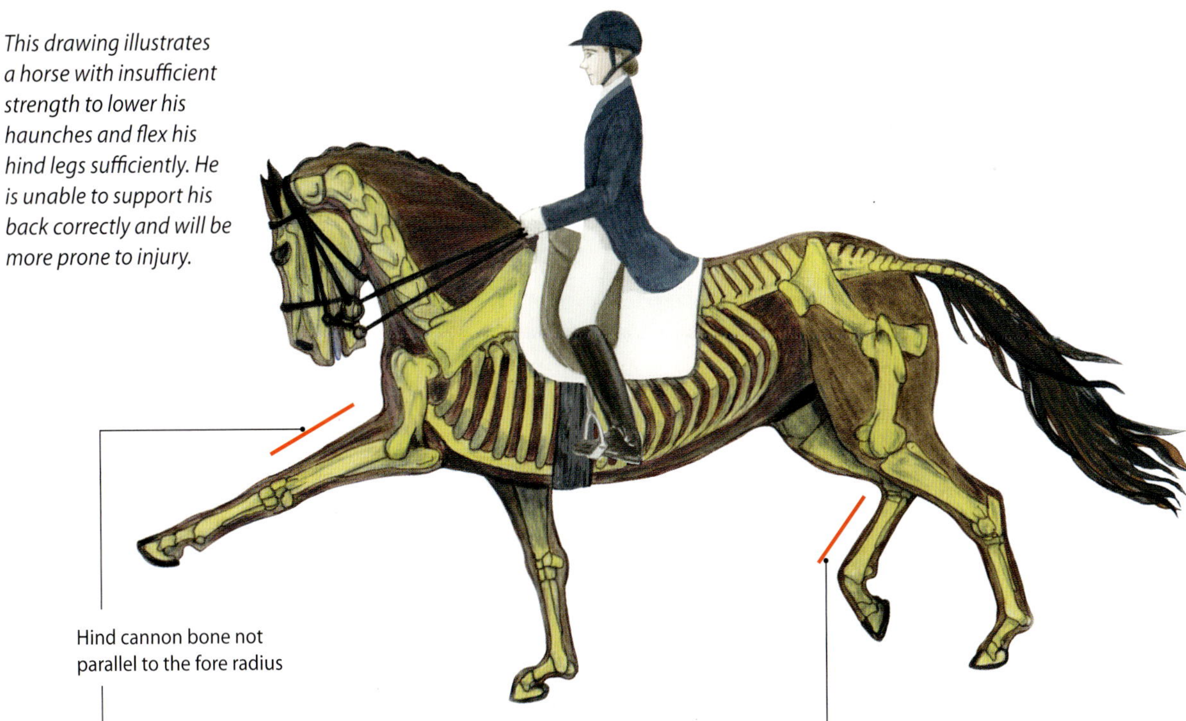

Hind cannon bone not parallel to the fore radius

# Developing collection

This novice horse is demonstrating how, when the hind leg comes well underneath the body and he is pushing evenly from behind, positive traction is created through the gluteal muscles, thoracolumbar fascia and latissimus dorsi. This raises the corresponding forelimb on that side. This correct action will pave the way for good forelimb expression as he progresses in his training.

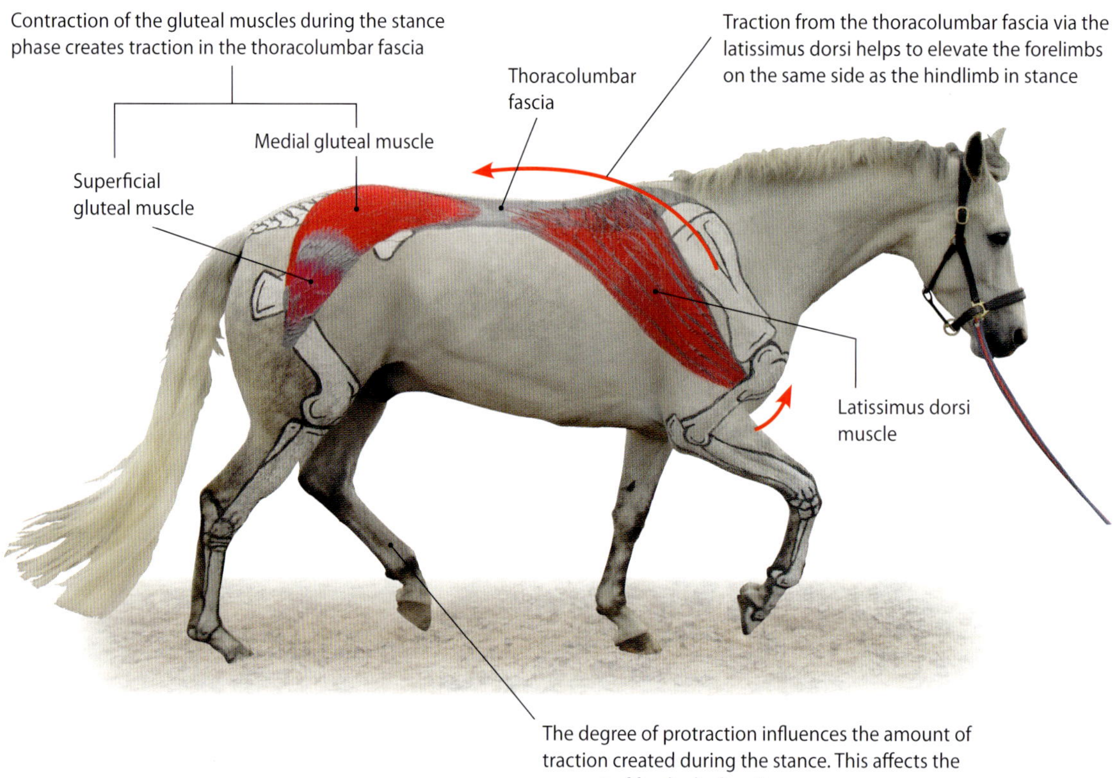


## APPLYING THE SCIENCE

Collection is a journey which begins as soon as we start to train the horse. To improve performance, reduce the risk of injury, derive maximum satisfaction and allow both horses and riders to reach their full potential, it is essential to fully understand and apply the basic principles of anatomy as outlined in Part 1. Achieving collection involves rounding the frame, developing impulsion, engaging the hindquarters, lightening the forehand and encouraging the horse to carry more weight behind. To do this the rider must sit tall to bring the weight back, develop a lightness of hand and minimise leg contact. This will bring a feeling of riding 'uphill'. A good trainer will help set realistic, achievable goals working in harmony with the horse. For maximum results, it is important to accept that true collection is the result of time, patience and many years of musculoskeletal conditioning. By working on backing up, transitions, riding corners and counter-canter the rider will be setting out on the road to true collection. The secret of success is to consolidate and enjoy each stage before moving on to the next.

## Piaffe

Piaffe is an advanced collected movement in which flexion of the haunches is combined with thoracolumbar and pelvic rotation as the croup lifts alternately on the side of the weight-bearing limb. The joints in the forelegs flex with the horse remaining light, mobile, free and calm. The back should round and the horse should retain an even, consistent rhythm, as he demonstrates a small moment of suspension between the footfalls. Good piaffe requires strength, control, patience and years of preparation on the part of both the horse and rider.

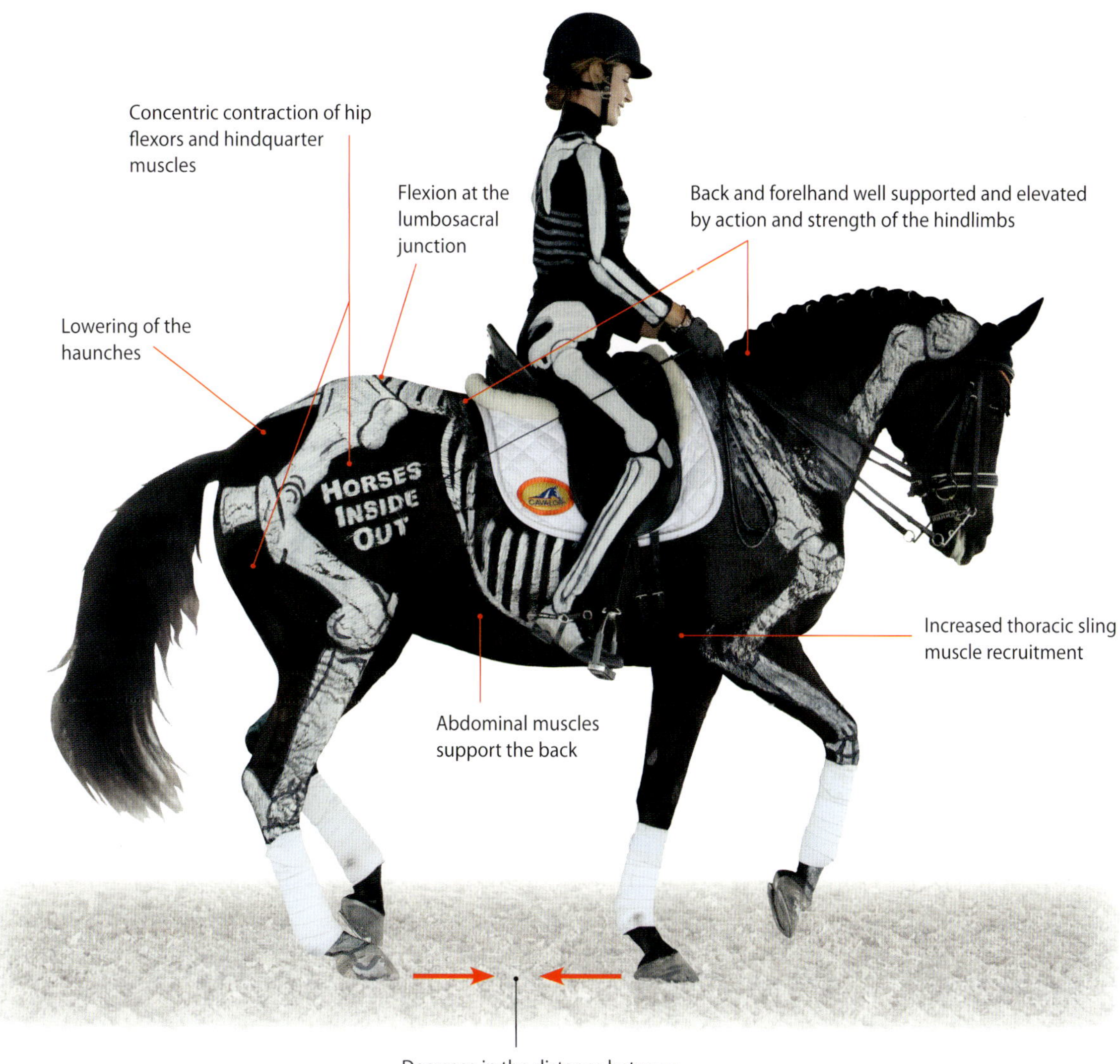

## Collection Exercises from an Anatomical Perspective

Anatomically working towards collection is good for:

- Developing back posture and strength
- Strengthening the hindquarter muscles
- Strengthening the core, abdominal, hip flexor and thoracic sling muscles
- Toning the muscles that carry the weight of the rider
- Enabling improved forelimb expression
- Developing the ability of the hind legs to carry weight behind
- Improving balance and muscular control.

From a training perspective collection exercises are good for:

- Developing power and strength
- Flexibility
- Improving responses
- Controlling speed
- Improving focus and concentration
- Adding impulsion, engagement and energy
- Increasing quality of the gaits.

## Backing up

Although it is not a natural movement for the horse, the anatomical and biomechanical benefits of backing up cannot be overemphasised. The exercise, which can be introduced in hand before the horse is ridden, should begin with one or two steps and progress to 20 plus. It should be performed with long marching steps with the head lowered. This increases thoracolumbar rotation, conditions the core muscles, raises, rounds and strengthens the back and contributes to good posture and the horse's ability to collect. Although in a formal dressage test the horse is required to step back in diagonal pairs with no moment of suspension in the same two-beat configuration as in trot, some horses find this difficult and tend to back up in a four-time sequence as in walk. In some horses this can be an indication of a spinal movement restriction or resistance but in others it is just preference. Whether performed in two- or four-beat time, this invaluable anatomical exercise has the best results if performed on a daily basis.

Backing up in hand is particularly beneficial for strengthening the flexor chain of muscles, particularly the hip and lumbosacral junction flexors, iliopsoas and the thoracic sling.

**SEQUENCE BELOW** *The anatomical and biomechanical benefits of backing up cannot be overemphasised.*

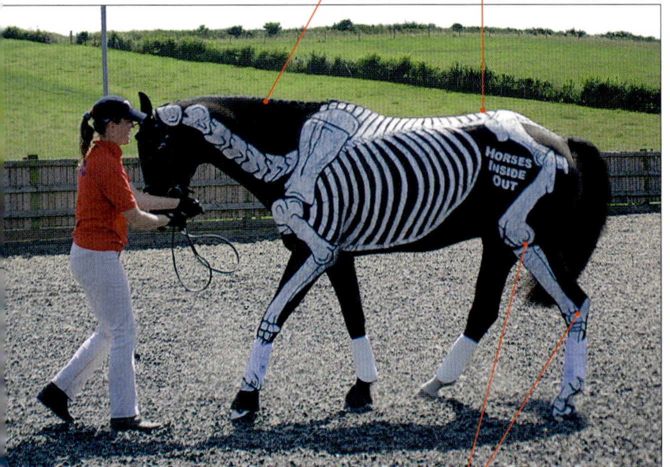


Topline muscles stretched

Increased hindlimb joint flexion

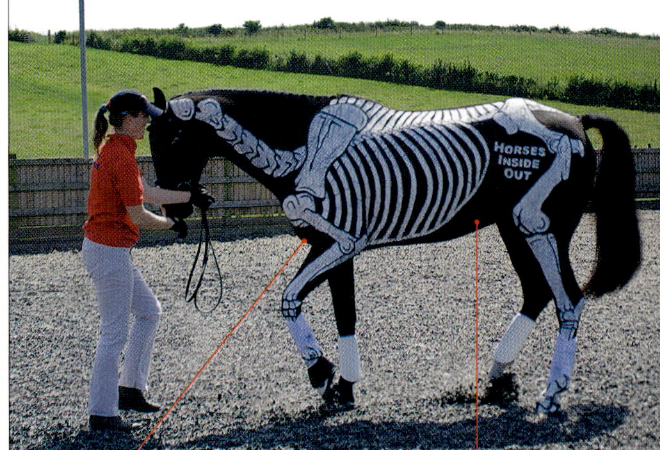


Thoracic sling recruited          Abdominal muscles shorten

Backing up is a low-impact exercise with no moment of suspension as the horse walks back with the diagonal pairs ideally moving together. For maximum benefit this exercise should be performed daily with the head kept as low as possible to encourage the back to raise. The aim should be twenty good quality, long, marching backward steps. Once achieved in hand this can also be performed as a ridden exercise.

**RIGHT, ABOVE AND BELOW**
*As it changes their action and develops muscular control, proprioception, coordination and balance, backing up or down a slope provides an alternative yet effective way of strengthening the thoracic sling, biceps femoris and gluteal muscles of the fore and hindlimbs.*

**Muscles which normally push the horse forwards must control the reach and placement of the hind foot.**

Biceps femoris

Semitendinosus

Semimembranosus

## Backing up a slope

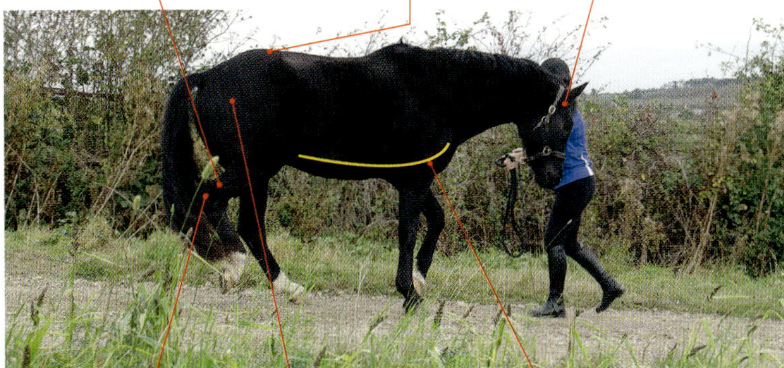


## Backing down a slope

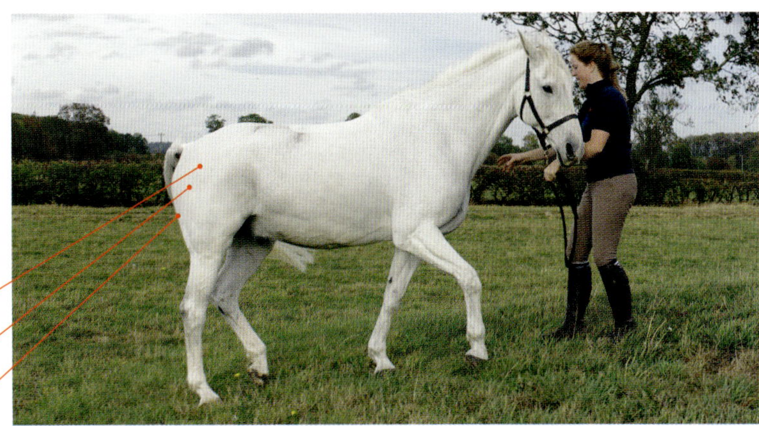

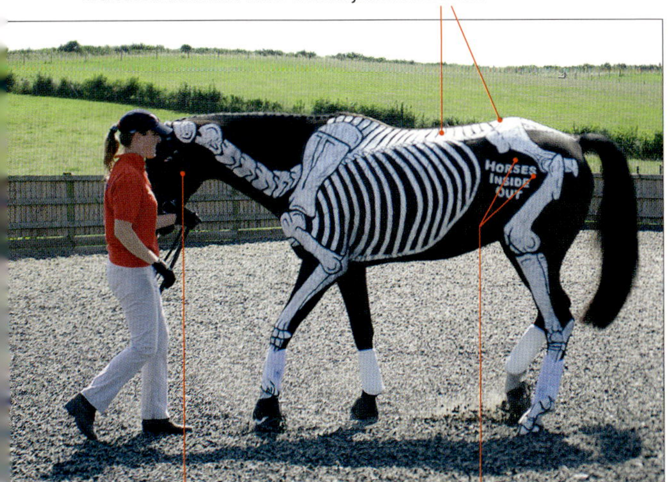


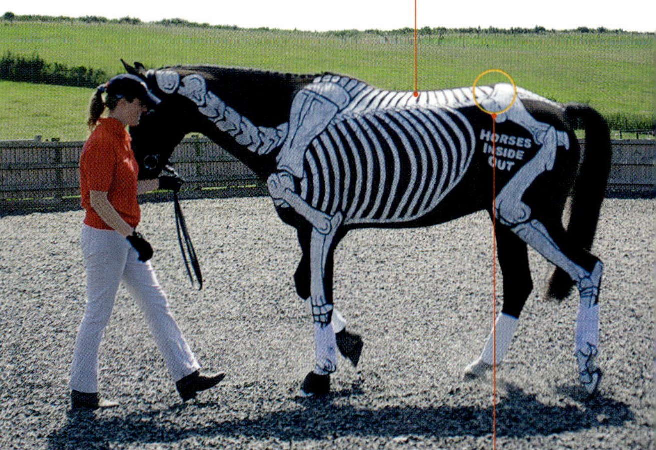

# Transitions

Transitions form the basis of all training, from young horses learning to go forward from walk to trot to horses performing high levels of advanced lateral and collected work. They take time, patience, repetition and careful preparation. An ideal smooth transition which involves a change of speed, gait, stride length or direction, requires balance, suppleness and a willing response to the aids and takes place without any loss of stability, rhythm or undesired change in posture.

## Trot–walk–trot transitions

This trot–walk–trot exercise, which gradually decreases the number of walk steps in the corners of the arena, improves both the engagement of the hindquarters and the quality of the trot immediately before and after the corner. They are also useful for calming and curbing speed in an over-enthusiastic horse.

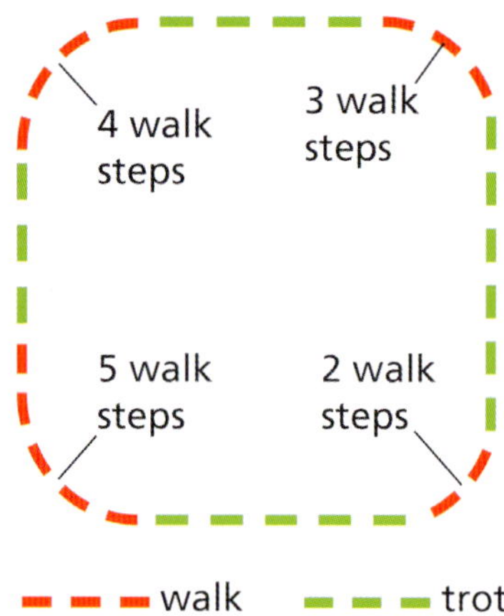


## Trot – canter, and canter – trot transitions

Because back function alternates between acting as a stabilising rod with only passive flexion and extension in trot to actively creating flexion and extension in canter, these progressive trot–canter and canter–trot transitions condition the abdominal muscles, improve stability and suppleness in the back, lumbosacral and sacroiliac regions and are an effective way of alleviating back tension and stiffness.

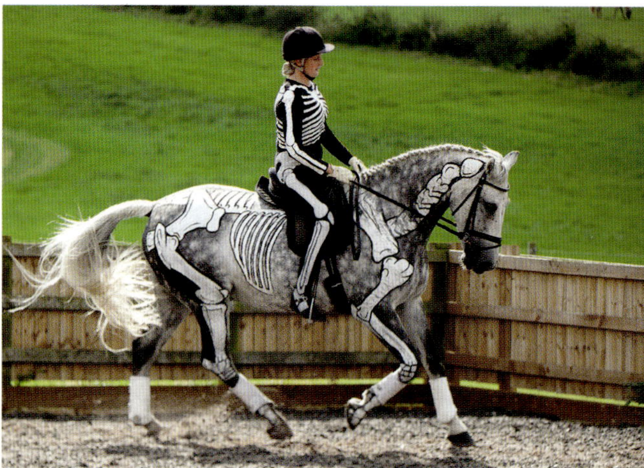

*Trot – canter, and canter – trot transitions.*

## Half-halt

The half-halt or 'nearly' transition is an essential collection exercise in which the horse's body comes back over the hind leg. This backward shifting of mass lightens the forehand and makes a considerable contribution to balance. Performed within the gait, it is good preparation for downward, and provides a surge of energy for upward transitions.

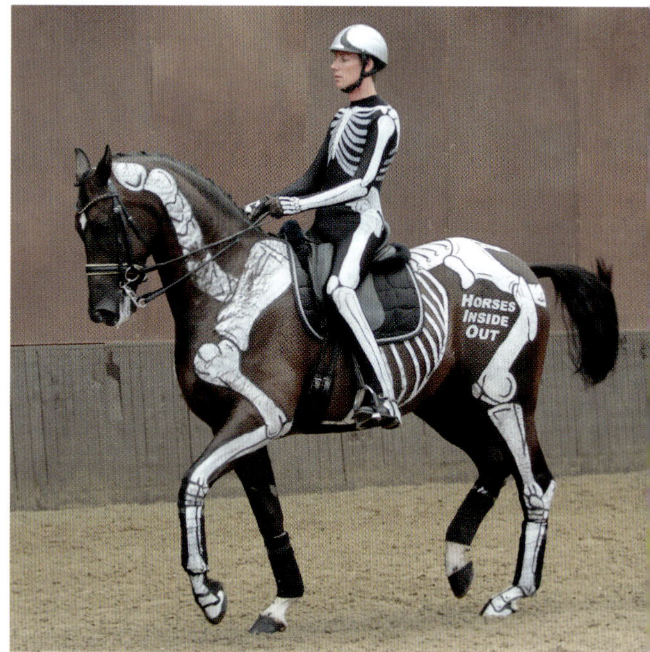


*The half-halt.*

A well executed half-halt is fundamental for developing hindlimb strength and recruits and shortens the iliopsoas muscle group as the lumbosacral junction flexes and the hindquarters carry more weight.

## Transitions within the gait

Transitions within the gait include altering speed, stride length or the degree of collection. They are useful for conditioning the gluteal and biceps femoris muscles, developing expression and power and sharpening the horse's response to the aids. Varying tempo and stride length within canter is a good exercise for improving manoeuvrability and achieving the required distances for showjumpers.

## Corners

Riding a corner, which is in essence a quarter of a circle, in perfect equilibrium, is an essential but difficult manoeuvre performed within the pace.

Any movement is only as good as the corner that precedes it. The corner requires the horse to master a combination of skills including the half-halt for preparation, balance, collection, lateral flexion and bend. It is particularly difficult for a young horse when he is learning to balance whilst carrying the rider. A corner is a good test of and developmental exercise for core strength, posture and athletic ability.

As training progresses, the principles of leg-yield, shoulder-in and turn about the forehand and haunches (see Chapter 12) can all be incorporated into riding the corner which, if ridden consistently, will become 'automatic'.

Once mastered, balance and self-carriage can be enhanced by riding a square in the centre of the school and by varying the gait and pace between the corners.

If practising corners other than in an arena, using dressage boards or equivalent is useful for focus and balance and to improve the accuracy and quality of the turn.

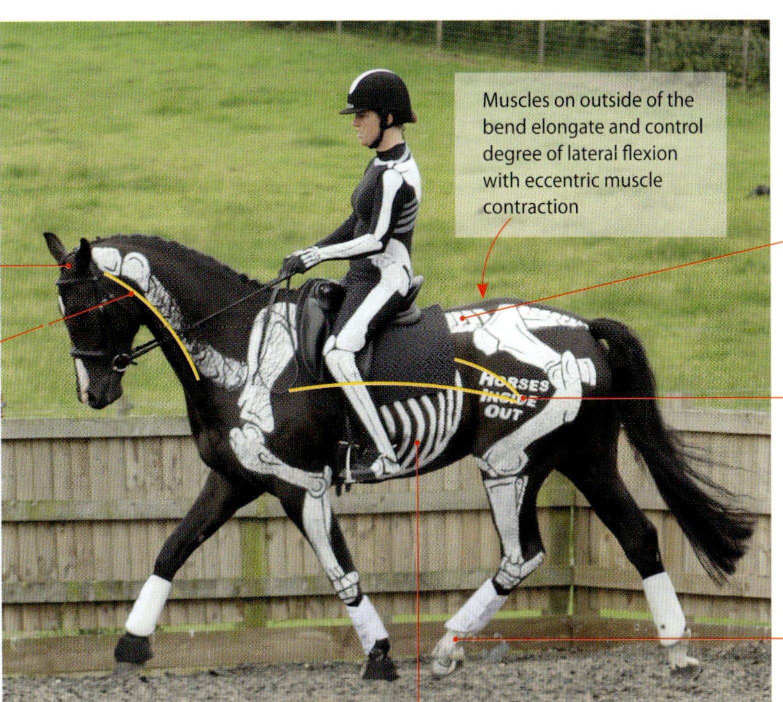


*Riding a corner.*

# Counter-canter

Riding counter-canter with the neck straight or flexed slighted to the side of the leading limb is an advanced movement requiring and training the horse to be straight. To maintain the correct outline and posture requires balance, muscular strength, core stability, coordination, skill and musculoskeletal control. For dressage horses, counter-canter develops collection, hock flexion and engagement. It is also is a good precursor for flying changes and canter pirouettes. For jumping horses it contributes to overall balance, improves agility and the ability to change leads and direction.

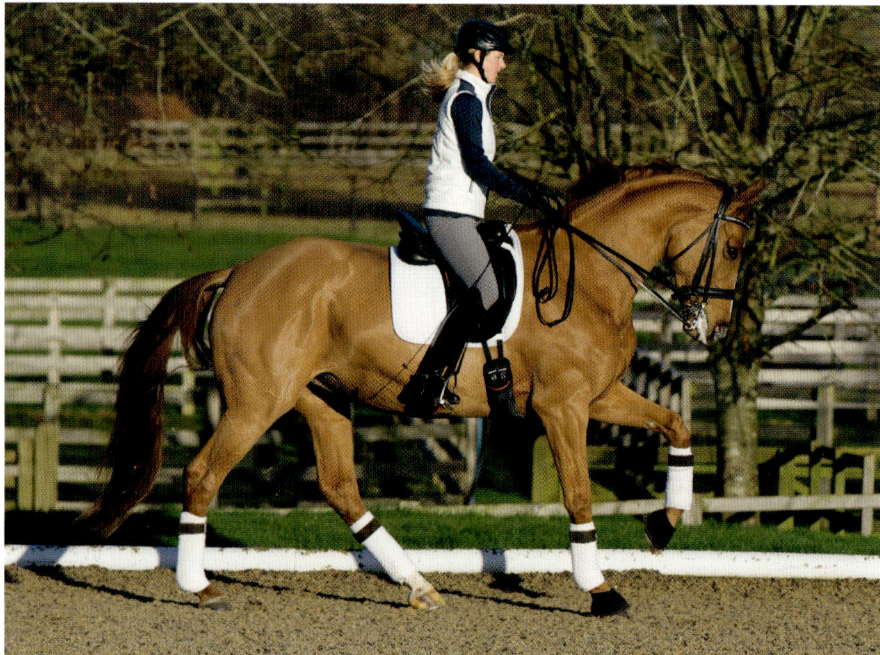

*For dressage horses, counter-canter develops collection, hock flexion and engagement.*

Counter-canter straightens the horse. Biomechanically when the neck is flexed to the inside (see right) and the outside leading leg has to push harder to reach further, the brachiocephalic and omotransversarius muscles on the outside of the bend are stretched. This will also help free the shoulder and improve forelimb expression.

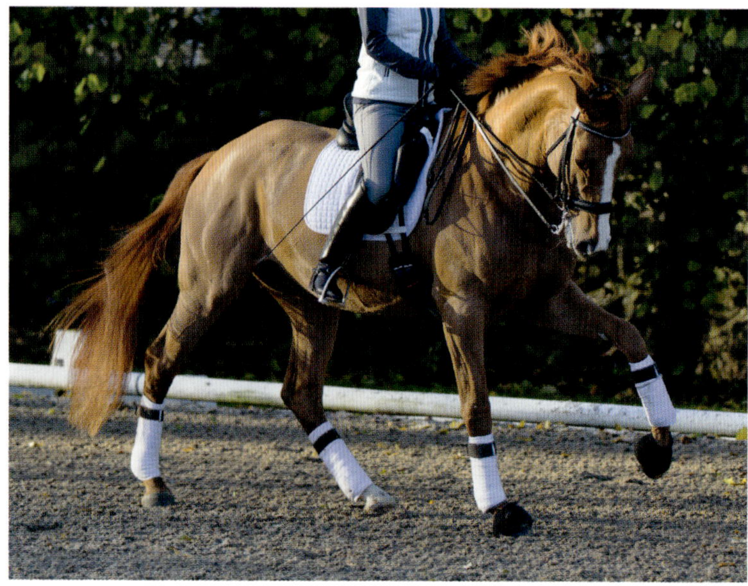

# 11 Bending Exercises

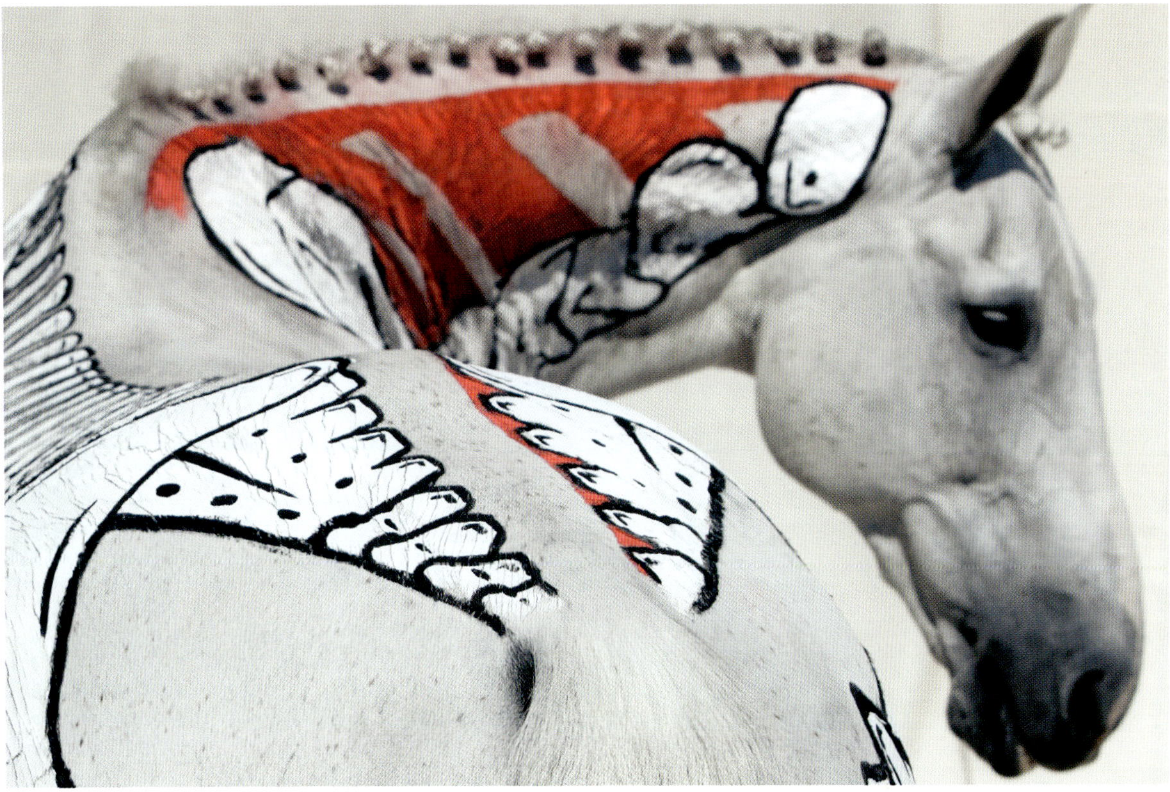

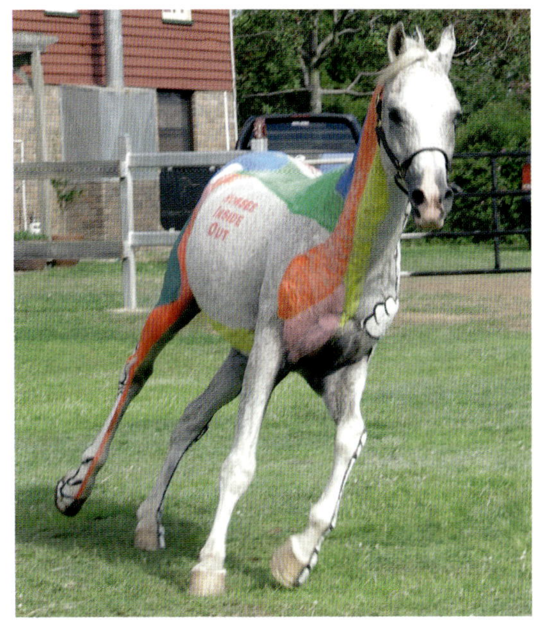

Correct bend is essential for maintaining balance and smooth movement. Because of the rigidity of the spine it is not possible for horses to bend uniformly from nose to tail. This is a concept often misunderstood by both riders and trainers who frequently refer to the horse bending evenly through the body.

## Neck Contribution to Bend

Horses use the head and neck as a counterbalance to help with turning and stability. This explains why young and untrained horses tend to lean in and move with their heads to the outside on the lunge. As this is discouraged in the ridden horse, he must find alternative ways to balance and turn whilst holding his head still and bending his neck to the inside. This requires strength, suppleness and coordination.

## Superficial neck muscles

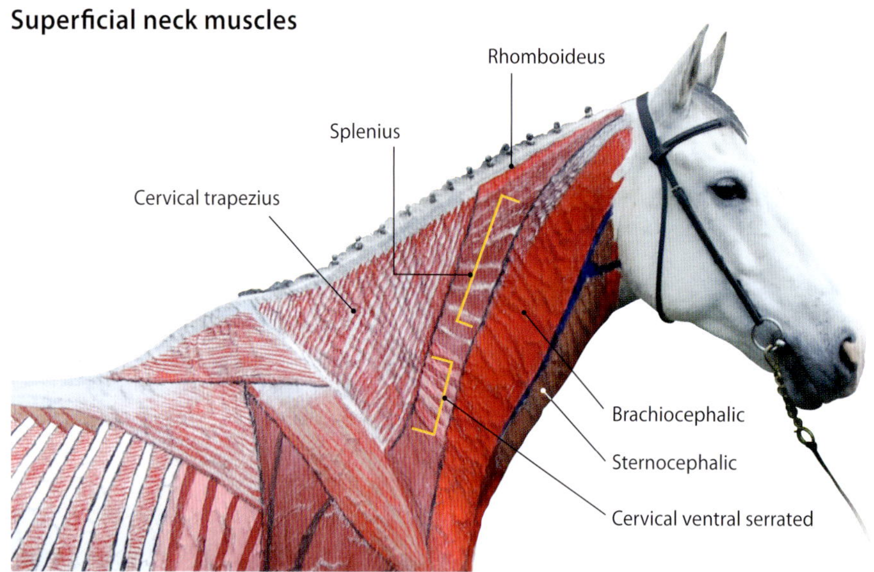


## Deep neck muscles

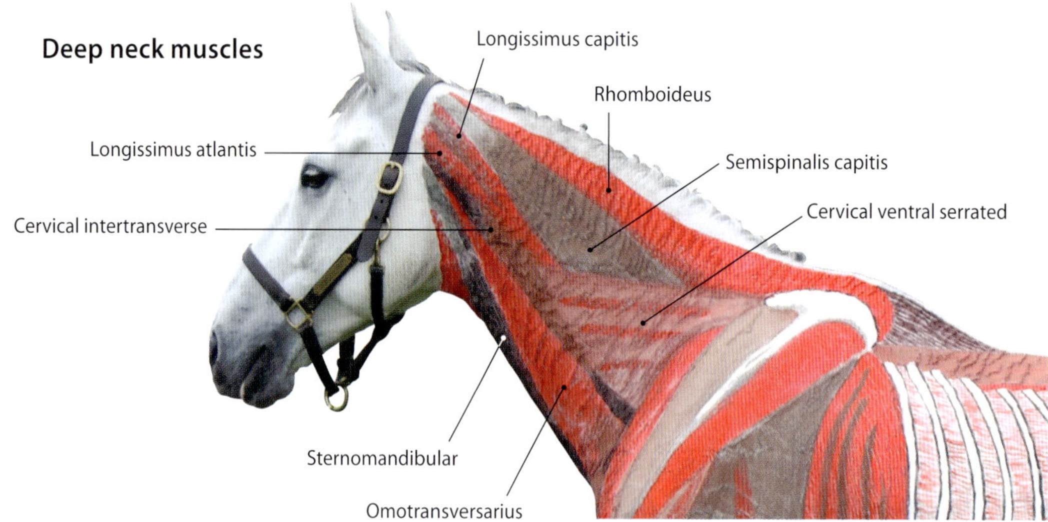


# Lateral flexion within the neck

Any stiffness in the neck not only limits suppleness and the degree of bend but, as the neck muscles (particularly brachiocephalic and omotransversarius) attach into the humerus and scapula this can also inhibit forelimb movement. Tension in the neck muscles that attach into the back extensor chain, for example the splenius, longissimus capitis, longissimus atlantis and multifidus, can also increase back stiffness and extension which will, in turn, affect posture.

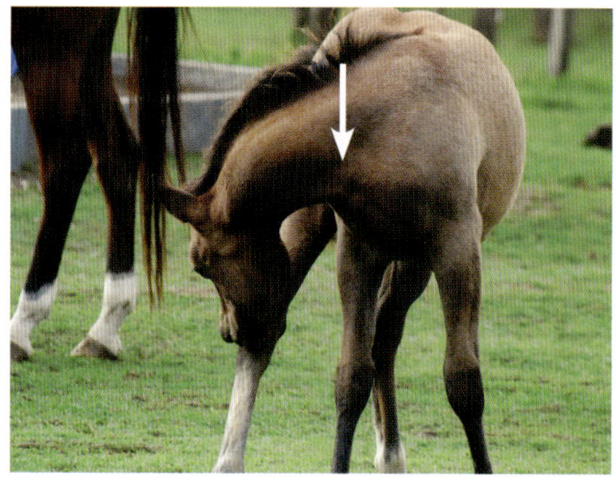

**RIGHT** *Most lateral flexion occurs at the base of the neck.*

## Riding with lateral flexion in the neck

Encouraging the horse to hold his head slightly to the inside or outside for several steps is an effective exercise for stretching the neck muscles. The bend should only be introduced and the number of steps increased gradually with the neck only being flexed as far as the horse can comfortably maintain rhythm, balance and impulsion. Performing this exercise in a faster gait or on a slope further strengthens the thoracic sling and neck muscles. Lateral flexion in the neck is good for:

- Core stability and balance
- Coordination and proprioception
- Developing straightness and symmetry
- Forelimb movement and expression
- Reducing tension and restriction in the neck muscles
- Muscular strength, control and suppleness
- Neck joint flexibility.

## Lateral flexion at the poll

Lateral flexion at the poll refers to the slight bend to the left or right created at the atlanto-occipital joint, which is located between the first cervical vertebra and the skull. It is important in the ridden horse because it indicates acceptance of the bit and allows the horse to develop correct posture, alignment and straightness. It also contributes to relaxation of the jaw, topline muscles of the neck and longitudinal suppleness. Both lateral flexion and rotation here are limited by the bony processes and shape of the joint itself and any further bend in the neck actually comes from much lower down. When riding with lateral flexion, there should be just enough flexion to see the inside eye or the inside cheekpiece

The horse will find it difficult to demonstrate lateral flexion at the poll if he:

- Is over-extended or hyperflexed at the atlanto-occipital joint
- Has tension, injury or scar tissue within the small muscles or tendinous attachments in that area
- Is tense through the temporomandibular joint
- Clamps his jaw shut
- Is stiff, resists the rider, has psychological tension or is nervous.

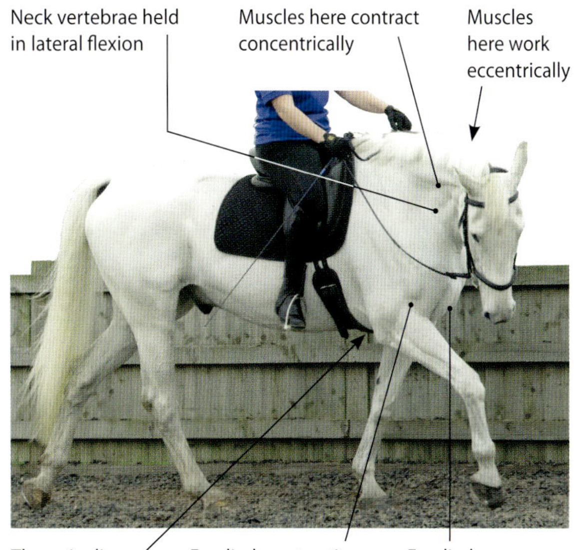


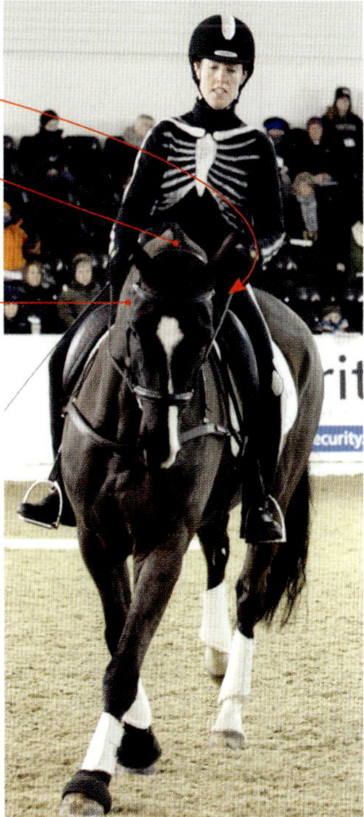


**RIGHT** *Riding with lateral flexion keeps the atlanto-occipital and atlanto-axial joints flexible, improves lateral suppleness through the poll and neck and improves bend in response to the bit aids.*

To compensate for lack of lateral flexion at the poll, the horse may rotate from the atlanto-axial joint; the joint between the first and second cervical vertebrae. This will result in the nose twisting.

# Back Contribution to Bend

Although contraction of the longissimus dorsi and the internal abdominal oblique muscles does contribute to bend, it is ultimately the negligible degree of flexion between each the thoracic and lumbar vertebrae that limits the overall amount of lateral flexion. This is further restricted by the saddle.

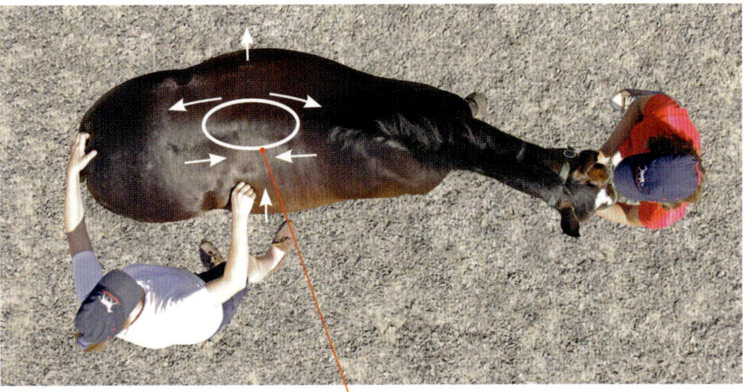

Most lateral flexion in the back occurs here

# Rib Contribution to Bend

Rib movement makes a significant contribution to lateral flexibility and gives the rider the feeling of the horse 'bending' around the inside leg. The photograph on the right shows that most rib movement occurs in the caudal ribs and the whole barrel of ribs swings to the outside.

**BELOW** *Each rib attaches into two adjacent thoracic vertebral bodies at the costovertebral joints. Movement of the ribs stimulates the production of synovial fluid, lubricating the surrounding joints and keeping the back supple.*

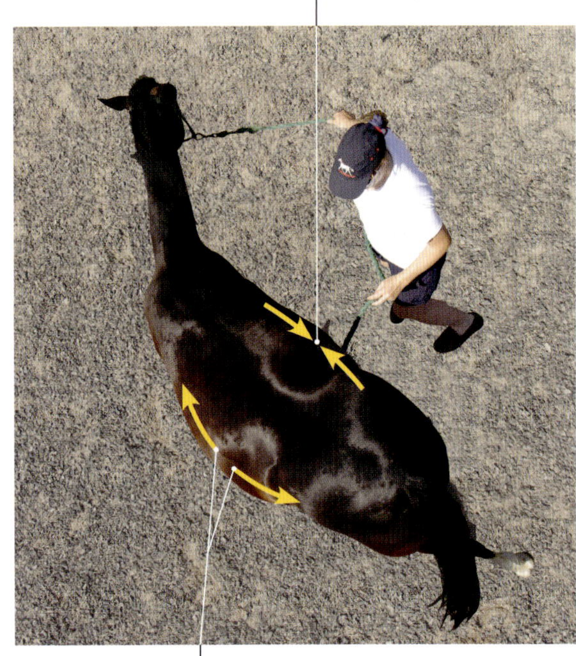


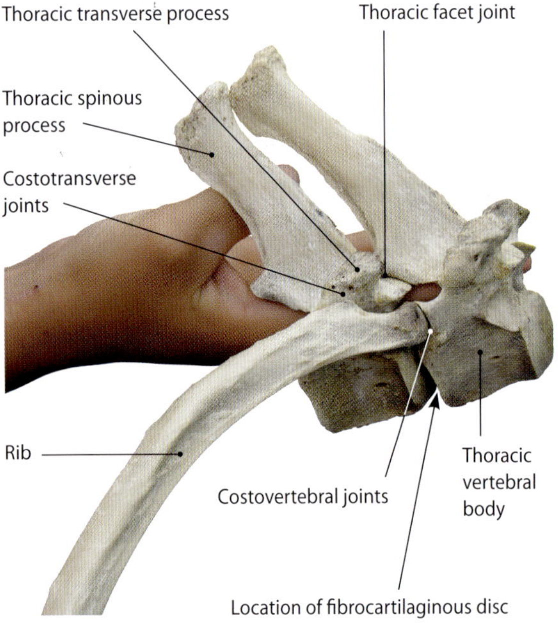


# Forelimb Contribution to Bend

The muscular attachment of the forelimbs to the axial skeleton contributes to range of movement. When turning, the outside forelimb reaches further across the thorax. The thoracic sling also allows the thorax to rotate between the front limbs, further contributing to bend.

## Hindlimb Contribution to Bend

The hindlimb contributes to bend through adduction and abduction. Although the inside hindlimb carries more weight, more force is transmitted through the outside hindlimb as it has to push harder in propulsion. This is more pronounced and has a greater influence on back and rib movement on a smaller circle.

## Muscular Contribution to Bend

On a small circle the lateral flexor muscle chain, responsible for creating bend through the body, shortens concentrically on the inside (Picture 1) whilst the outside chain (Picture 2) elongates eccentrically to allow the bend to occur. It is not possible to achieve optimum lateral flexion in an over-flexed or over-extended spinal posture.

### The lateral flexor muscle chain

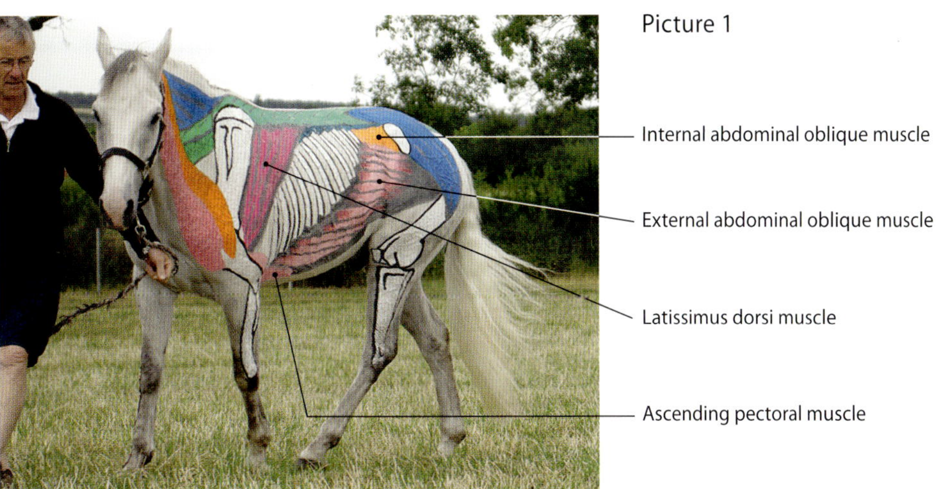


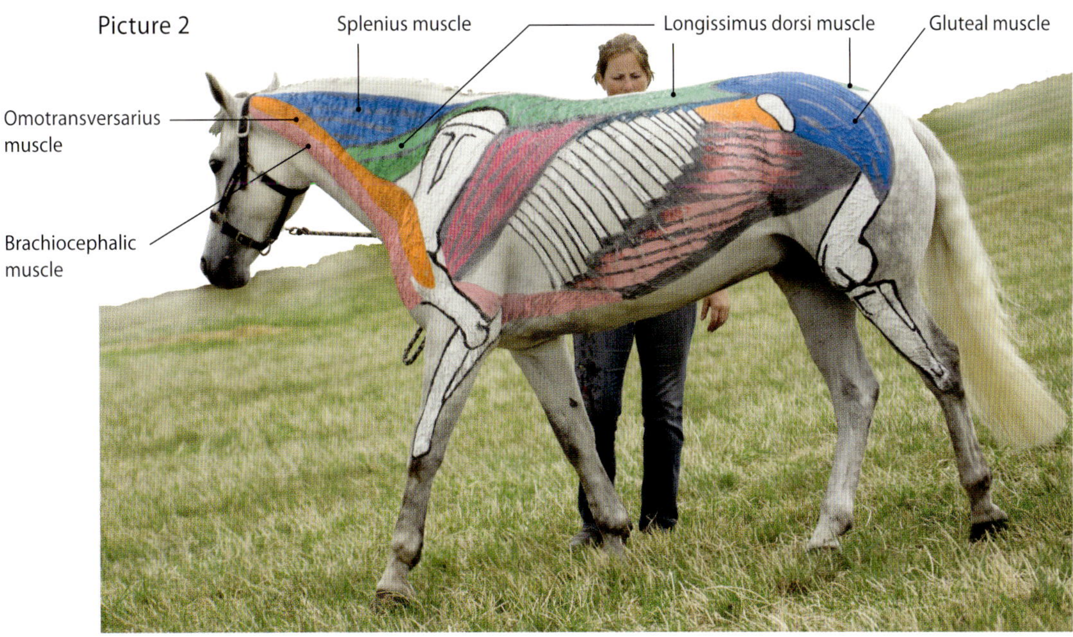

# Bending Exercises from an Anatomical Perspective

Understanding how horses bend, and performing bending exercises, is useful for suppling, providing feedback for weaknesses and for checking and establishing correct posture and way of going.

Turns, loops, circles, figures of eight and serpentines can all be combined to produce an infinite number of bending exercises. These form a sound basis for training. Begin with shallow loops and large circles to promote balance, suppleness and accuracy before progressing to tighter turns, smaller diameters and exercises requiring more changes of bend as the horse becomes skeletally mature, strong and more flexible. The intensity of all the bending exercises can be increased by varying the gait, degree of collection, speed and tempo.

Anatomically all bending exercises are good for:

- Mobilising the vertebral and costovertebral joints
- Suppling the ribs and back
- Recruiting the abdominal oblique muscles
- Strengthening the core
- Improving the reach of the outside fore and hindlimbs.

From a training perspective they are good for:

- Enhancing bend and flexibility
- Developing balance and straightness
- Preparing for a transition
- Preparing for lateral work
- Initiating engagement and collection
- Improving body awareness, coordination, control and balance
- Improving expression
- Reducing psychological and physiological tension.

## Loops

Loops and shallow turns, which require uniformity and a gradual change of direction, are a good introductory bending exercise for young and inexperienced horses. Most of the bend should come from the poll with only a small amount through the neck and body. This exercise is also good preparation for counter-canter.

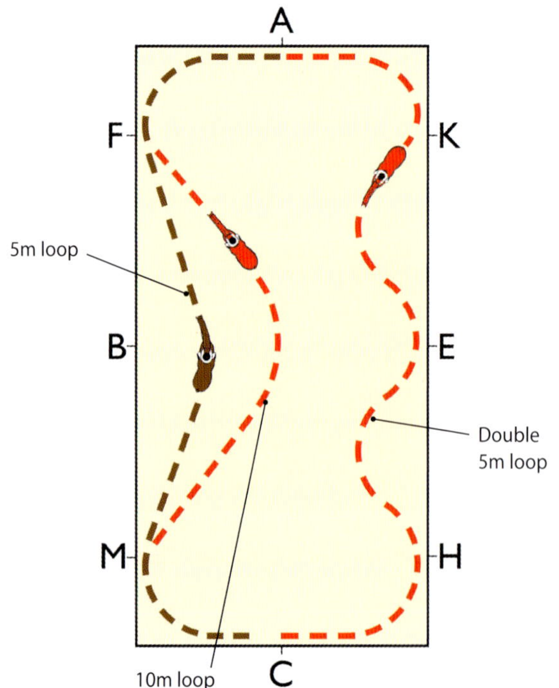

## Circles

Riding a circle accurately in walk, trot or canter is one of the most difficult movements for horse and rider to achieve. It requires well established lateral suppleness, balance, control, core strength, collection, accuracy and perseverance.

Circles require the inside hind leg to come under the body whilst tracking up, keeping the head level, maintaining balance, suppleness, uniformity of bend, impulsion and rhythm. The smaller the circle the greater the degree of collection, balance and impulsion required.

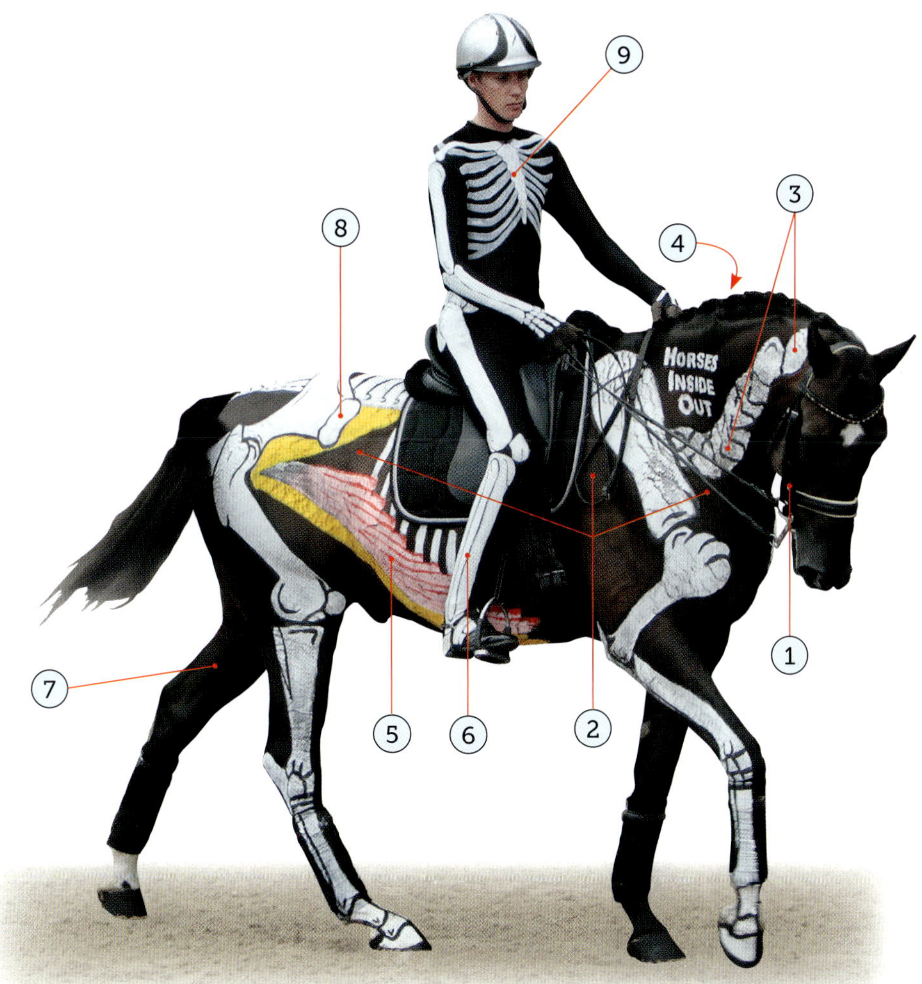


1. A relaxed jaw encourages softness at the poll

2. Muscles on the inside of the circle work in a shortened form

3. Lateral flexion through the cervical vertebrae

4. Muscles on the outside elongate to allow bend

5. Abdominal oblique muscles contribute to rib movement as well as bend

6. Influencing rib position with leg aids directly affects lateral suppleness

7. Outside fore and hind legs reach further across the body

8. Inside tuber coxae leads

9. Rotation through the body enables correct positioning of the seat bones, legs and arms.

## Changing the bend

Exercises that involve a change of bend are beneficial for horse and rider. A smooth change of bend can only be achieved if the horse is straight for one or two steps. Changing the bend requires balance, flexibility and accuracy and releases any build-up of tension within the muscles on the inside of the bend. For jumping riders, circling around fences and repeatedly changing the rein can help with manoeuvrability and quick reflexes.

Riding a series of 10m half-circles across or down the centre of the school requires the horse to be attentive, calm and responsive. This is an advanced suppling exercise which necessitates accuracy, collection, muscular strength, good balance and an increased degree of bend. Once the horse can maintain balance and collection the exercise can be extended to riding figures of eights or linked complete circles down the centre line. Riding more than one 10m circle in each position allows time to establish the bend before changing the rein and progressing to the next circle.

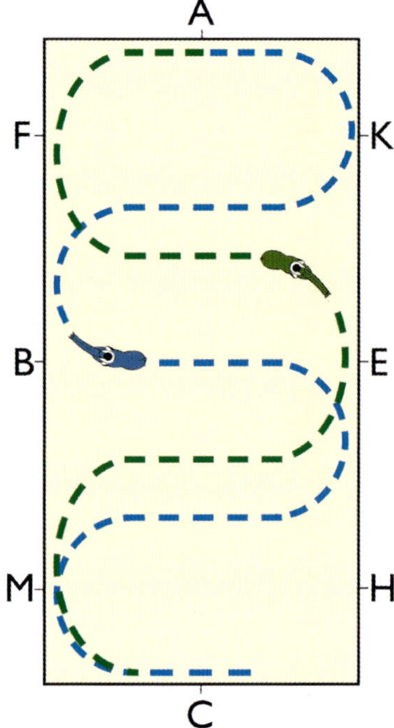



*BELOW Serpentines are good for developing fluency, rhythm, outline, accuracy and creating a smooth and even bend. They also contribute to symmetrical muscle development and straightness.*

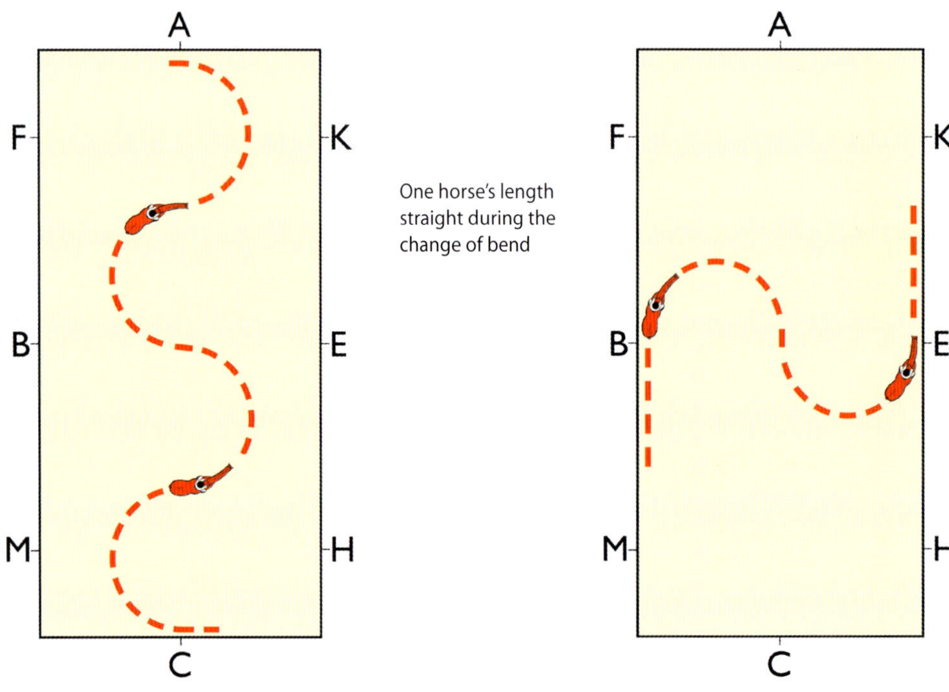



One horse's length straight during the change of bend

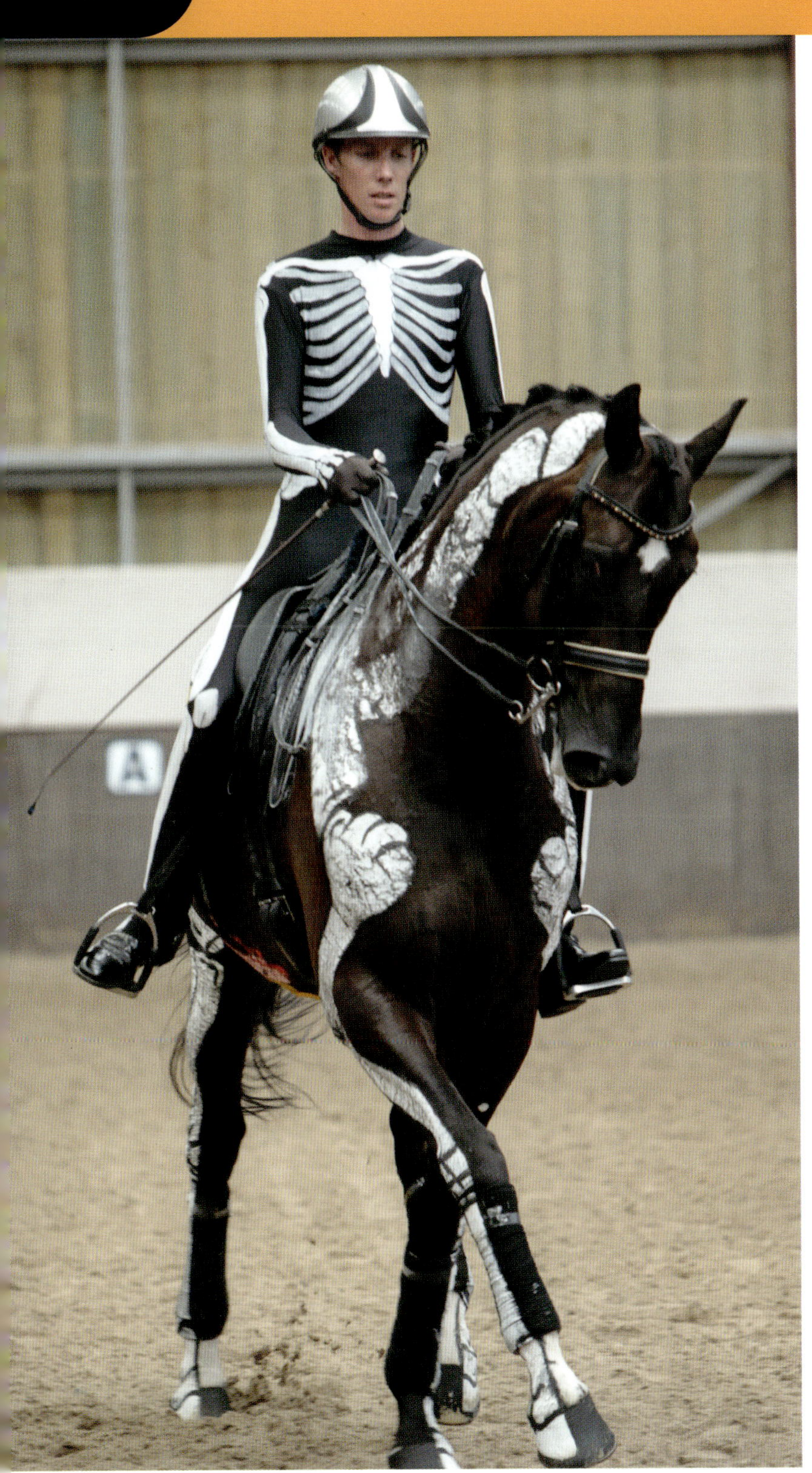

Lateral movements require the horse to move sideways with fluidity and grace. He does this by:

- Moving his legs across the midline of his body in *adduction*
- Moving his legs out and away from his body in *abduction*.

Moving laterally is introduced to a youngster as he is nudged over in field or stable. Regardless of age type or discipline it can be thought of as gymnastic exercise which creates a supple athlete who is loose, flexible and in balance. It has therapeutic benefits and contributes to manoeuvrability, lateral strength, stability, coordination and confidence.

The most basic lateral exercise is leg yield. Lateral exercises should be introduced in walk before progressing to trot and canter.

# Forelimb Contribution to Lateral Movement

The shoulder is the only joint in the forelimb that can actively create lateral movements. This joint is limited by the fact that it is located within the body, the muscles that control it and the position of the first few ribs.

**RIGHT** *This photograph, which shows both forelimbs in abduction, illustrates how greater demands are placed on the muscles of the right forelimb, which is in retraction, rather than the left, which is in protraction.*

## The forelimb abductor muscles

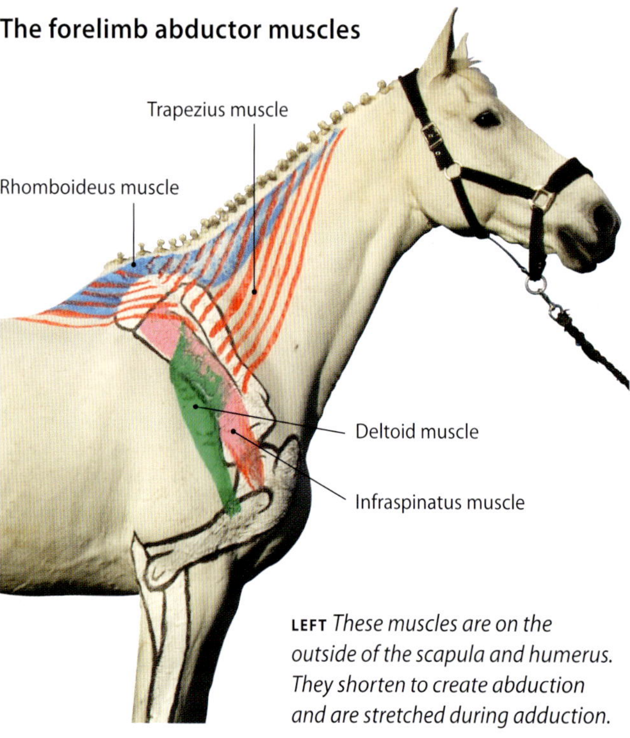


**LEFT** *These muscles are on the outside of the scapula and humerus. They shorten to create abduction and are stretched during adduction.*

## Abduction

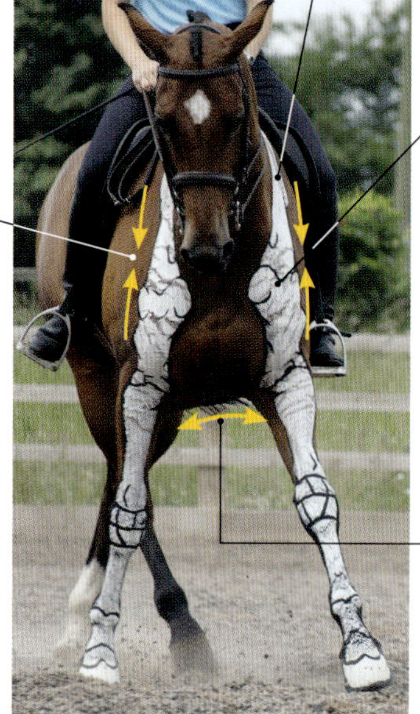


**BELOW** *The trapezius and rhomboideus muscles lift the scapula towards the withers when the limb protracts and abducts (yellow arrow) and pull the withers towards the weight-bearing scapula (black arrow) when the limb retracts and abducts. This positions and stabilises the scapula and withers during lateral work and contributes to forelimb reach and elevation in abduction and protraction as the limb moves forwards and away from the body. This is particularly exaggerated in shoulder-in. It also makes it a useful exercise for jumpers as these muscles, conditioned by shoulder-in, help to raise the scapula. This in turn improves forelimb technique over a fence.*

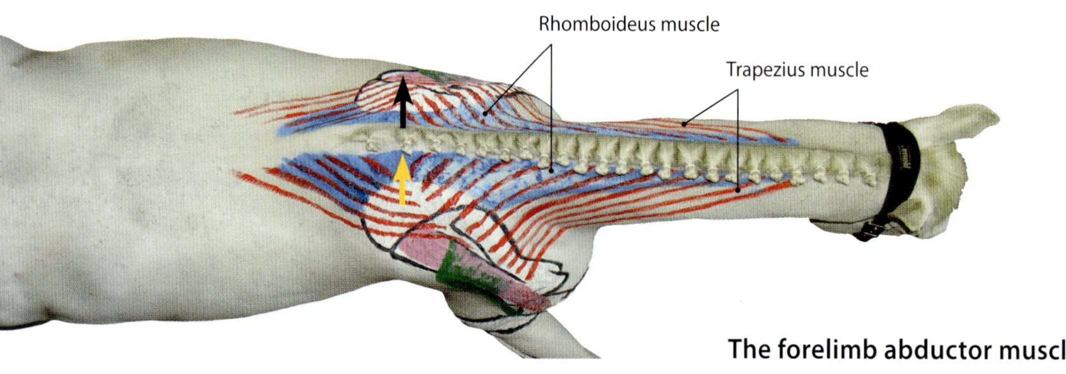


## The forelimb abductor muscles

## Adduction



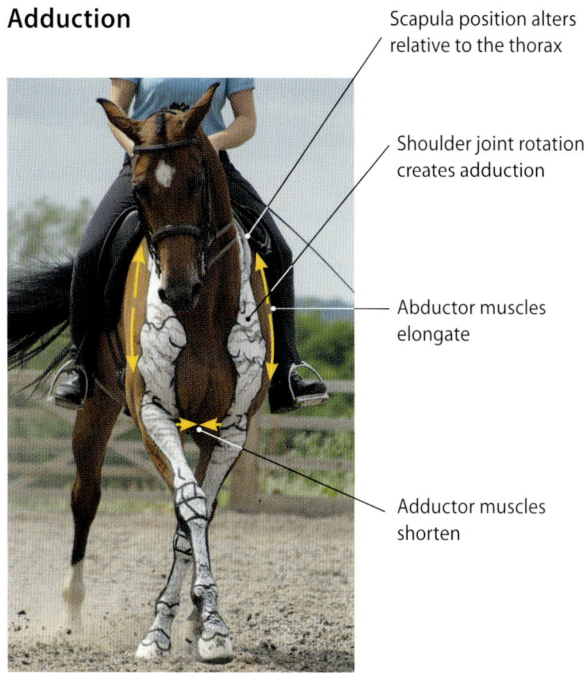

**RIGHT** *In this photograph, although both forelimbs are in adduction, the left is in retraction and the right is in protraction.*

## The forelimb adductor muscles

These muscles are on the inside of the scapula and humerus. They shorten to create adduction and are stretched during abduction. Owing to the muscular connection of the forelimb to the rest of the axial skeleton, forelimb adduction and abduction can affect the position of the thorax and spine.

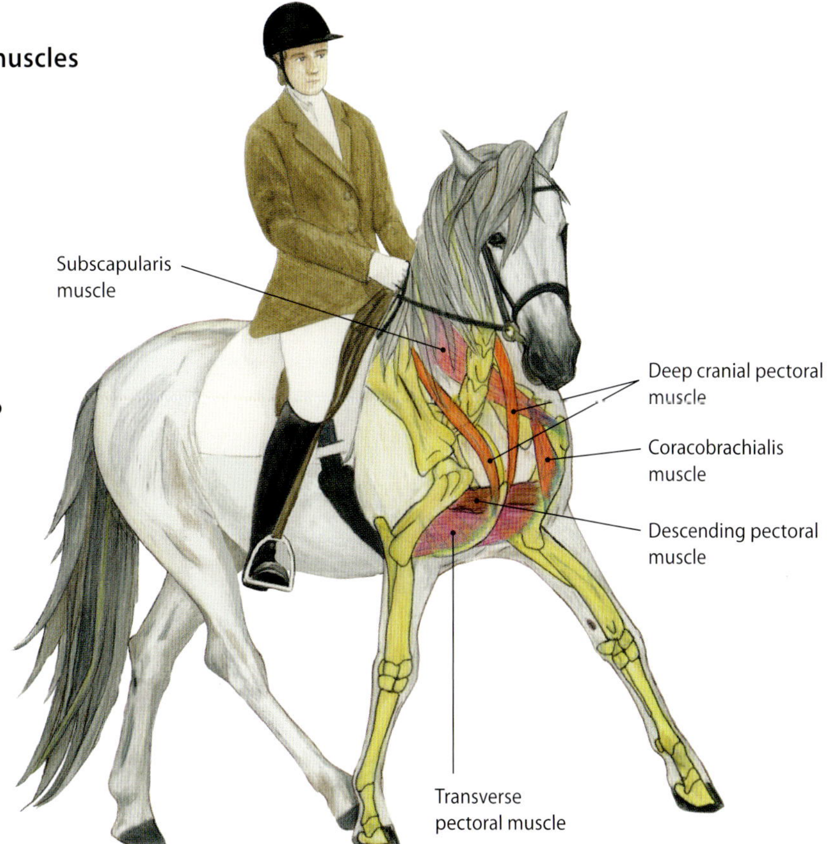

## THE ROLE OF THE LOWER LIMBS DURING LATERAL EXERCISES

The joints below the elbow and stifle can only flex and extend, although there is a small amount of passive lateral and rotational movement in the most distal joints. This enables the horse to cope with sideways loading of the limbs during lateral work or on an uneven surface.

**RIGHT** During lateral work the hoof impacts on the medial side and breaks over on the lateral side on one limb and vice versa on the other. This puts strain through the lower limb joints. For this reason it is important to:

- Warm up appropriately before performing high-intensity lateral work

- Work on a consistent surface

- Avoid lateral work if the horse has had any sort of collateral ligament injury.

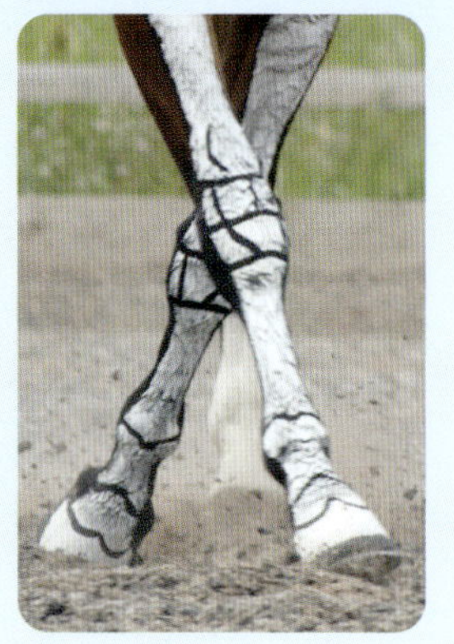

# Hindlimb Contribution to Lateral Movement

The hip is the only joint in the hindlimb that can actively create lateral movements. Although this ball and socket joint allows rotation, the ligament that control it limit sideways movement.

**BELOW RIGHT** *In this photograph, although both hindlimbs are in abduction, the right is in retraction and the left is in protraction.*

**BELOW LEFT** *In this photograph, although both hindlimbs are in adduction, the right hind is in protraction and the left is in retraction. The ribs, which always swing away from the protracted limb, are swinging to the left.*

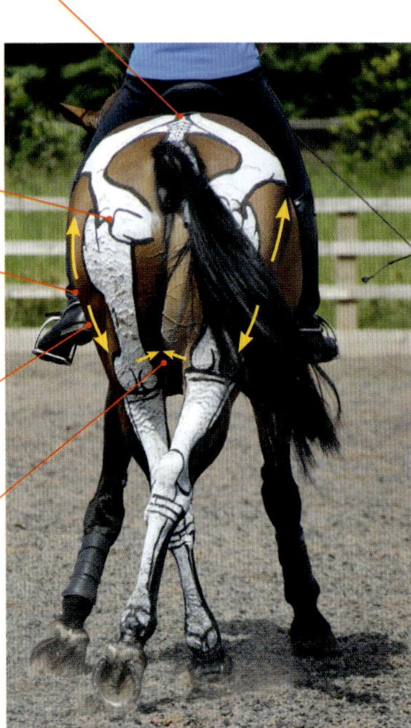


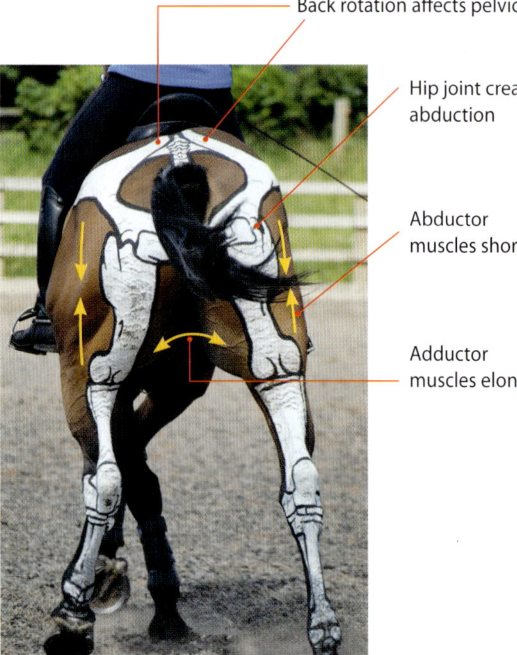

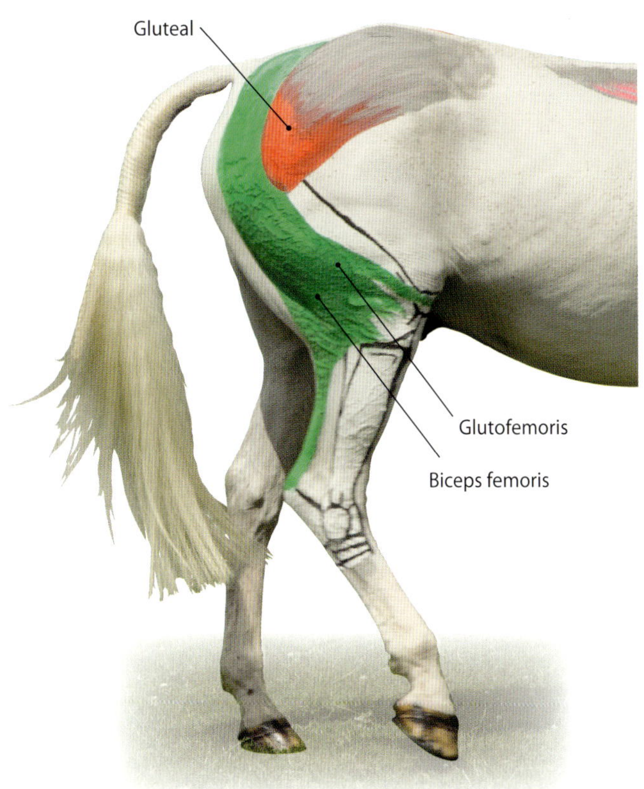



## The hindlimb abductor muscles

*These muscles are on the outside of the pelvis and femur. They shorten to create abduction and are stretched during adduction.*

## Abduction

**BELOW** *Contraction of the gluteal group, the most powerful of which is the middle gluteal muscle, results in extension and rotation of the hip joint. This has a very strong tendinous attachment to the greater trochanter, an extension lever on the top of the femur and above the level of the hip, which is pulled forwards and inwards to bring the limb away from the body during abduction. Lateral work strengthens the gluteals and stronger gluteals lead to more expressive lateral work.*

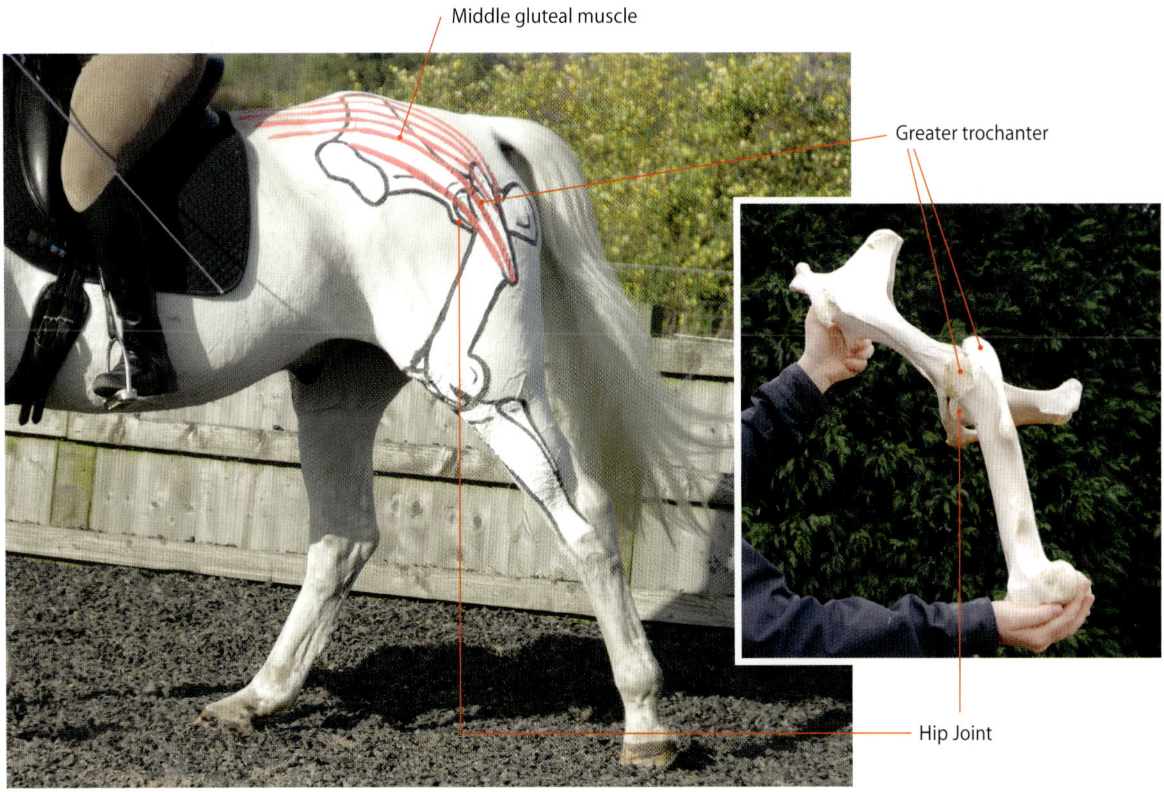

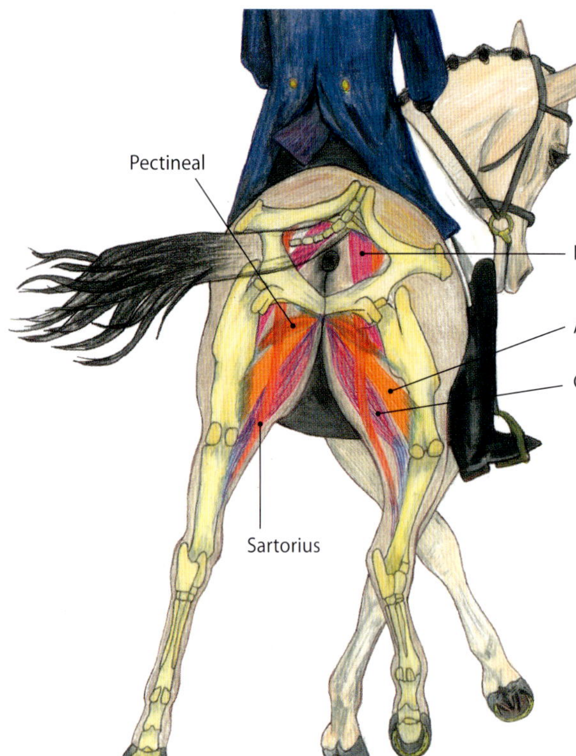


## The hindlimb adductor muscles

*These muscles are located underneath the pelvis and inside the femur. Their primary function is to support and stabilise the limbs. They shorten to create adduction and stretch during abduction.*

## Adduction

**BELOW** *During protraction and adduction, as the hindlimb is taken forwards and across the body, the middle gluteal muscle elongates as the greater trochanter moves back and away from the midline. This further stretches the middle gluteal muscle and encourages relaxation of the extensor chain which, in turn improves posture and promotes relaxation in a tense horse.*

Owing to the skeletal and muscular attachments of the hindlimb to the spine, lateral work will increase spinal flexibility, posture and rotation particularly in the caudal thoracic region. This results in an upward spiral of increased spinal flexibility and greater range of sideways movement.

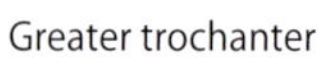

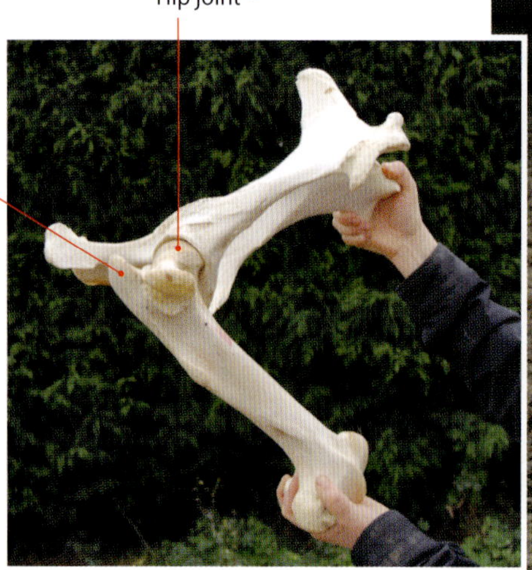


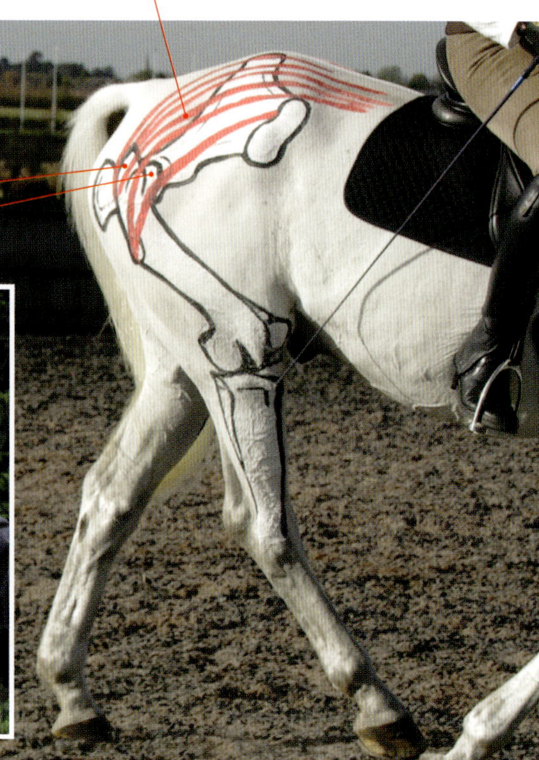

# Lateral Exercises from an Anatomical Perspective

Understanding how horses move sideways, and performing lateral work exercises is useful for suppling, assessing and establishing correct posture and way of going.

Anatomically all lateral exercises, the intensity of which can be increased by varying the gait, angle and degree of collection, are good for:

- Mobilising the structures of the shoulder and hip
- Strengthening and stretching the upper forelimb, hindlimb and trunk muscles
- Developing topline musculature
- Strengthening the core
- Toning abdominal oblique muscles which further support the back
- Encouraging relaxation of the extensor chain
- Improving spinal lateral suppleness and flexibility
- Improving body awareness, coordination, proprioception, control and balance.

From a training perspective they are good for:

- Reducing psychological and physiological tension
- Improving bend and agility
- Developing balance, straightness, stability and hindquarter engagement
- Preparing for and developing collection work
- Improving hindlimb protraction
- Improving posture and expression.

## APPLYING THE SCIENCE

Sitting tall and still whilst riding lateral exercises and keeping the basic anatomical principles in mind, gives combinations the best possible chance to reach their full potential. Applying the aids correctly and in harmony with the horse's rib movement will allow the rider to enjoy a feeling of harmony and ease. To achieve maximum potential it is important to warm up correctly and work on a consistent surface. Understanding adduction and abduction and strengthening the gluteal muscles leads to more expressive lateral work and enables the rider to produce lateral movements more efficiently and competently. Developing balance, straightness, stability and hindquarter engagement by performing lateral exercises also contributes to and is a good preparation for collection work. True enjoyment and satisfaction are only achieved through patience and persistence.

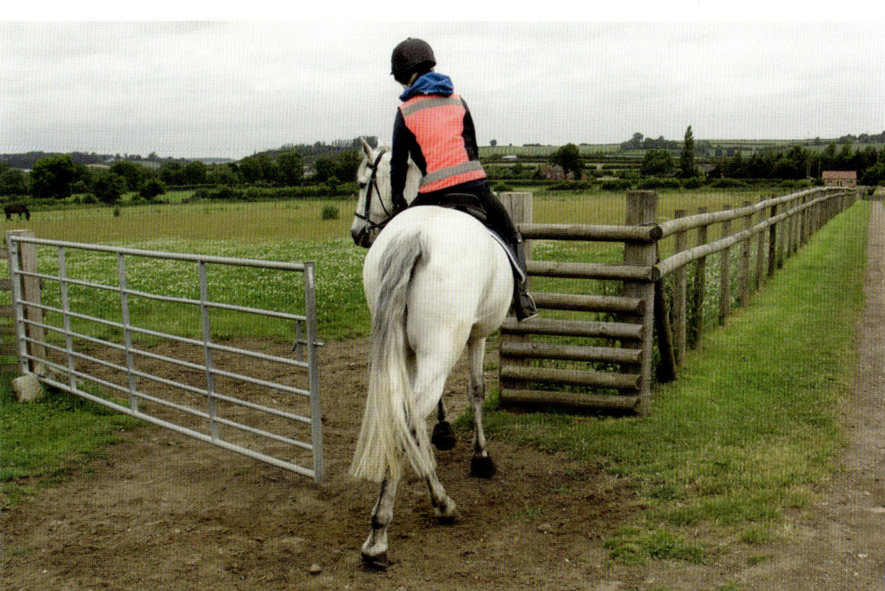

*Opening a gate is a useful practical application of when lateral work.*

# Turn About the Forehand

Turn about the forehand is a four-beat lateral turning exercise performed in walk. As the forelimbs turn on a small circle the hindlimbs adduct and abduct to step around in a 180 degree arc on a larger circle until the horse is facing the opposite direction.

Turn about the forehand requires and teaches the horse to be relaxed. It is good for encouraging young horses to move sideways away from leg pressure, provides a good way of releasing stiffness and tension from the muscles and is an excellent introduction for dressage riders progressing to further lateral work.

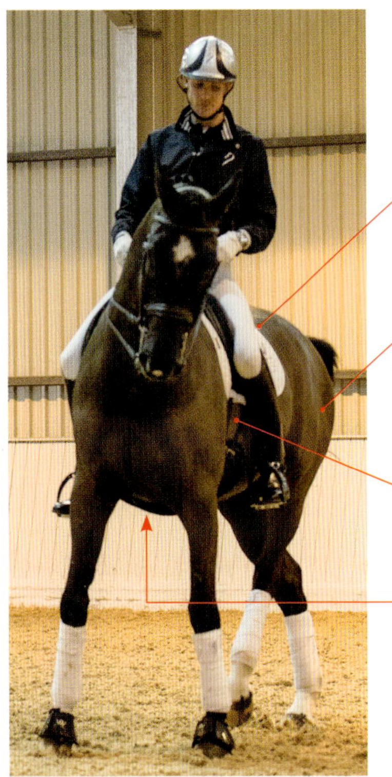


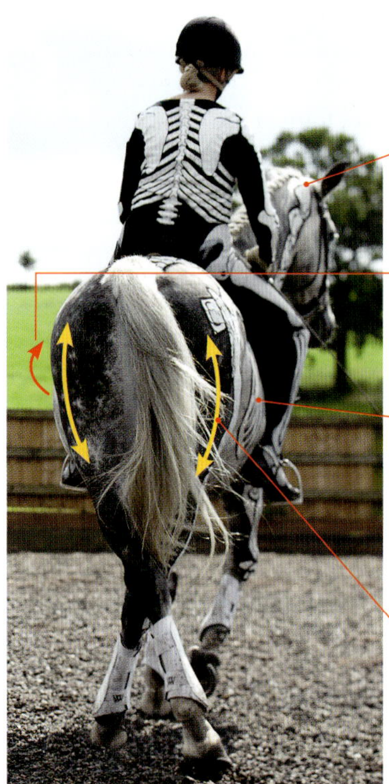


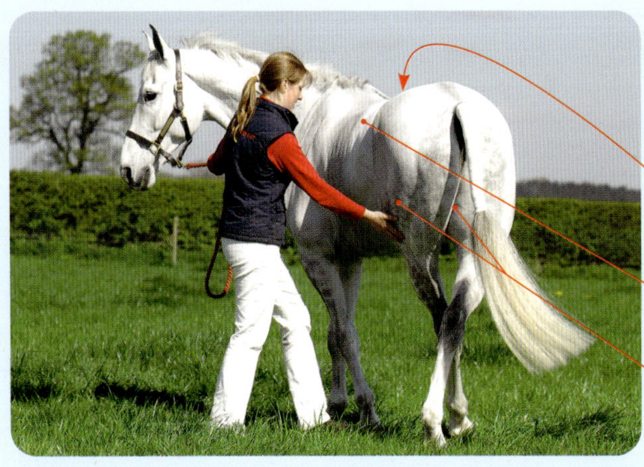


Performing this exercise in hand requires skill and practice. Three circles each way each day will improve ridden suppleness, bend and hindlimb adduction.

# Leg-yield

Performed on two tracks, leg-yield is a fundamental, versatile, suppling exercise in which the fore and hindlimbs adduct and abduct to move the horse sideways whilst the spine is laterally flexed away from the direction of travel. This mobilises the ribs, back and hips, activates the deep vertebral muscles and is a useful contributory factor in developing longitudinal and lateral flexibility. Leg-yield forms a solid foundation for all lateral work and should be mastered before progressing to more advanced lateral movements.

RIGHT *This horse is leg-yielding evenly across the diagonal with slight lateral flexion through the head, neck and body. The degree of shoulder joint and scapula movement in relation to the thorax determines the degree of lateral reach of the forelimbs.*

BELOW LEFT *Leg-yielding can also be performed head to the wall.*

BELOW RIGHT *Increased lateral flexion through the neck and spine can be seen in this horse leg-yielding out from a 10m to a 20m circle.*

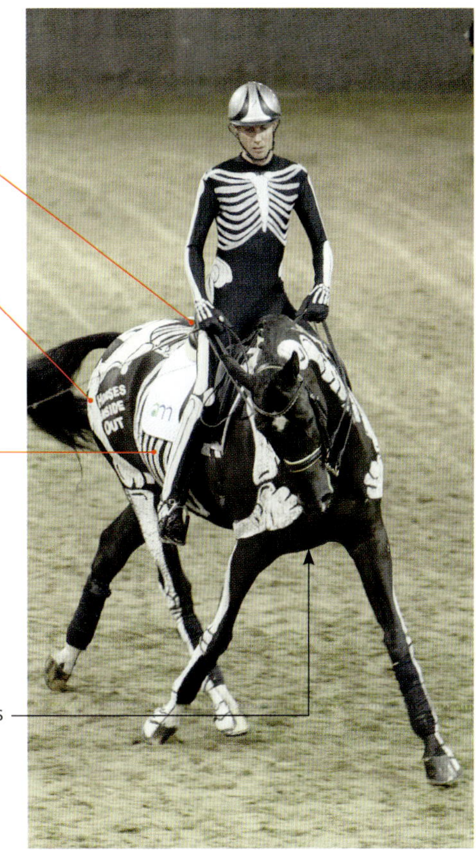


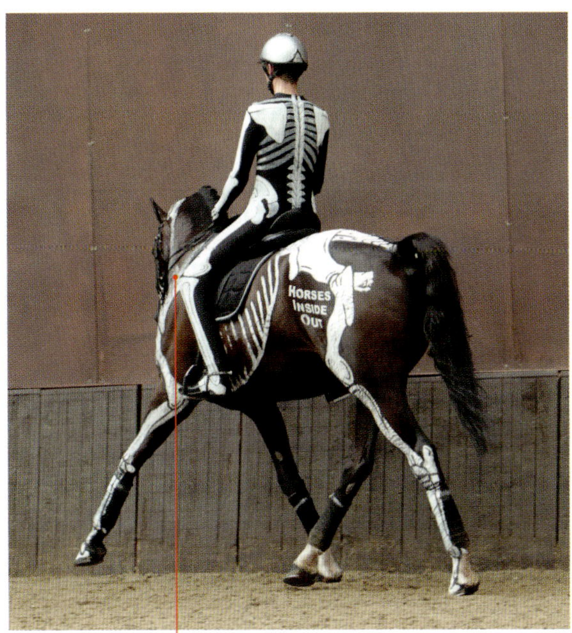

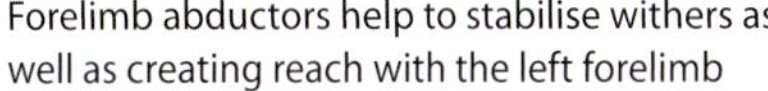

Forelimb abductors help to stabilise withers as well as creating reach with the left forelimb

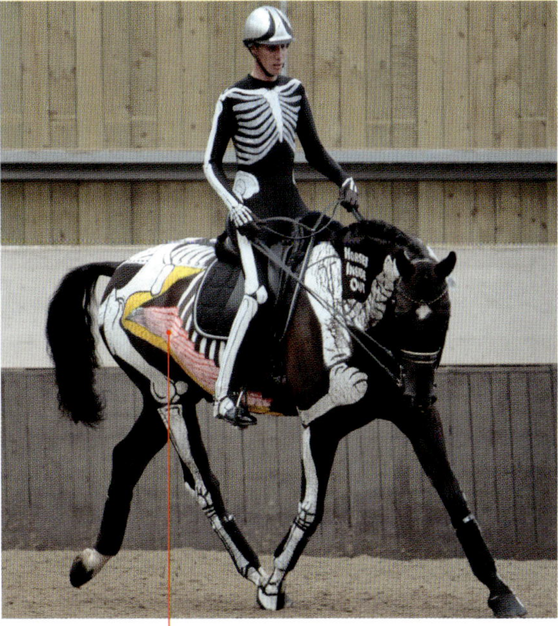

Abdominal oblique muscles contribute to bend, rib movement and adduction of the hindlimb during protraction

# Shoulder-in

Shoulder-in and shoulder-fore, which requires about half the angle of shoulder-in, are natural progressions from leg-yield and are good exercises for suppling and developing straightness, symmetry and strength. Shoulder-in, which improves forelimb expression and shoulder mobility, improves engagement of the inside hindlimb and is an excellent preparatory exercise for collection. It strengthens the forehand adductor and abductor muscles and improves suppleness by inducing spinal rotation and lateral flexion within the back, particularly the cranial thoracic region.

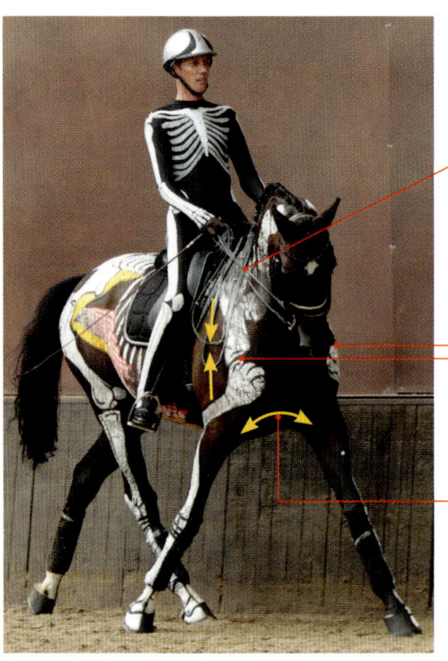


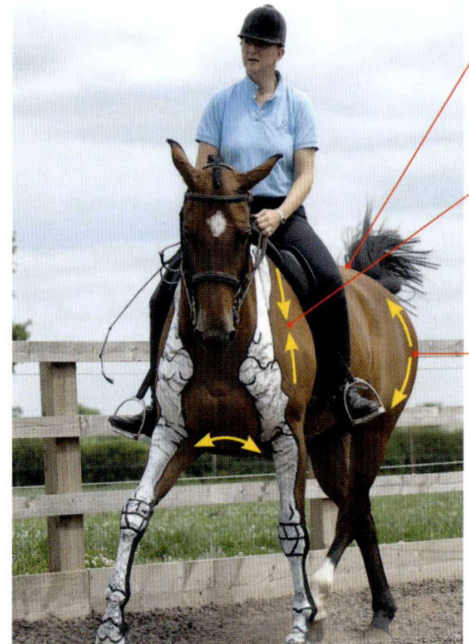


*These photographs illustrate forelimb abduction in shoulder-in.*

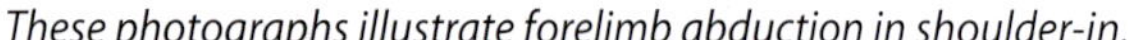

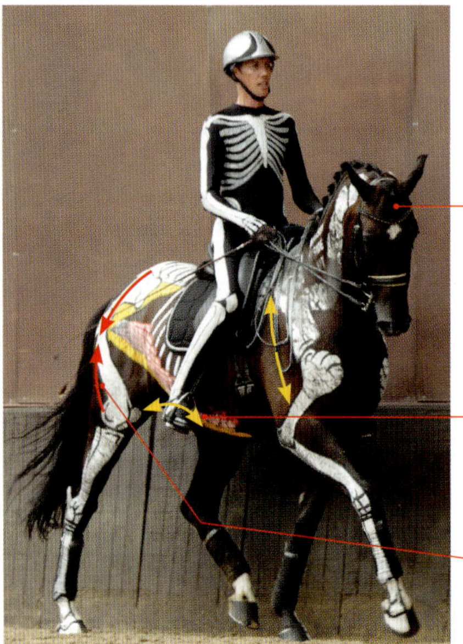


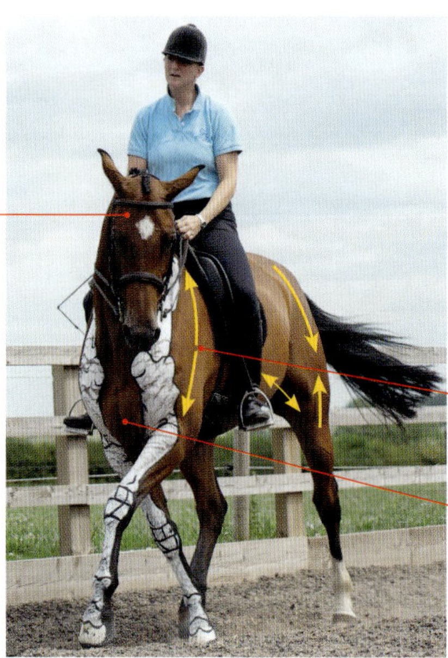


*These photographs illustrate hindlimb abduction and forelimb adduction.*

# Travers

Travers is a lateral exercise in which the horse travels on four tracks with the body bent towards the direction of travel and the quarters on the inner track. The movement, which comes mainly from adduction and abduction of the hindlimb and lateral flexion and rotation within the caudal thoracic and lumbar regions of the spine, is good for overall suppleness, strengthening and engagement of the hindquarters. Travers is particularly good for developing elasticity, reach and freedom of hindlimb movement, lateral bend, suppleness and as a preparatory exercise for collection and progression to half-pass.

## Hind adduction during travers

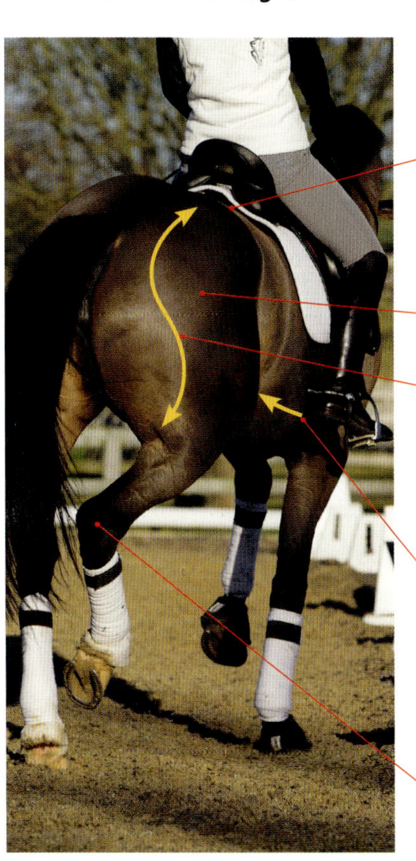


## Hind abduction during travers

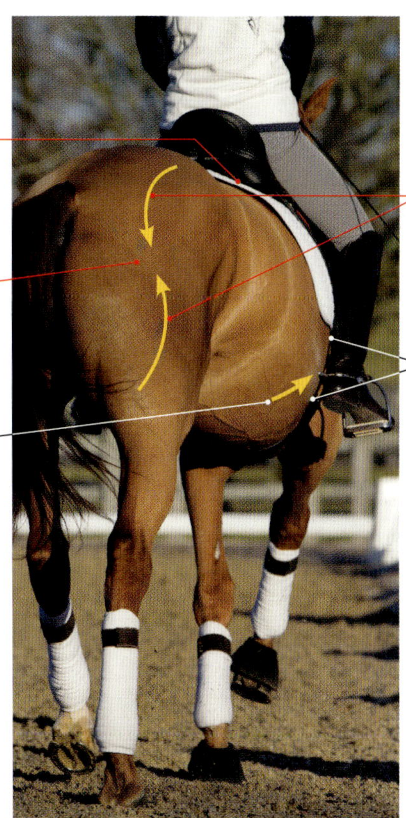


**ABOVE, LEFT AND RIGHT** *Here the horse is engaging the hindquarters as he steps forwards and sideways with the hind legs.*

# Half-pass

Half-pass is a progression from travers which can be ridden in walk, trot or canter. It is a movement in which the hind leg comes well under the body as the horse is ridden forwards and sideways on a diagonal line with body parallel to the arena wall. During this movement as both forelimbs abduct, both hindlimbs adduct or as both hindlimbs abduct the forelimbs adduct. Half-pass is the most demanding of all lateral movements; it requires the horse to maintain balance, rhythm and impulsion and differs from leg-yield in that the body is bent towards the direction of travel. A successful half-pass is dependent on the degree and control of elongation of the gluteal and longissimus muscle groups on the outside of the bend.

*These photographs show (1) and (2) hind leg abduction during half-pass and (3) and (4) hind leg adduction.*

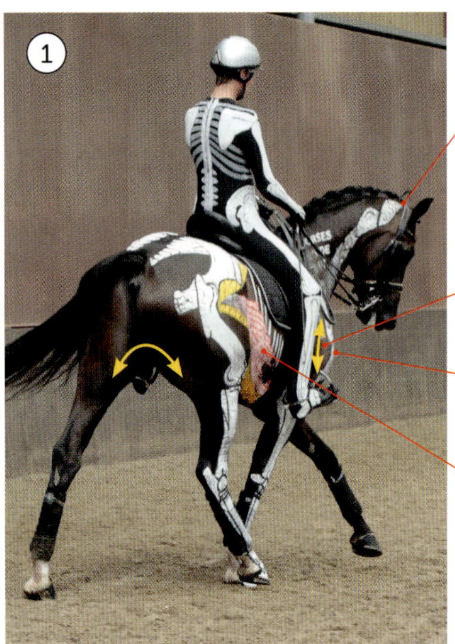


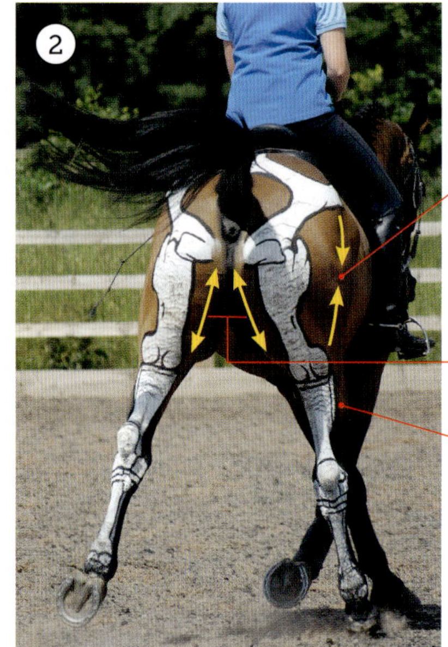


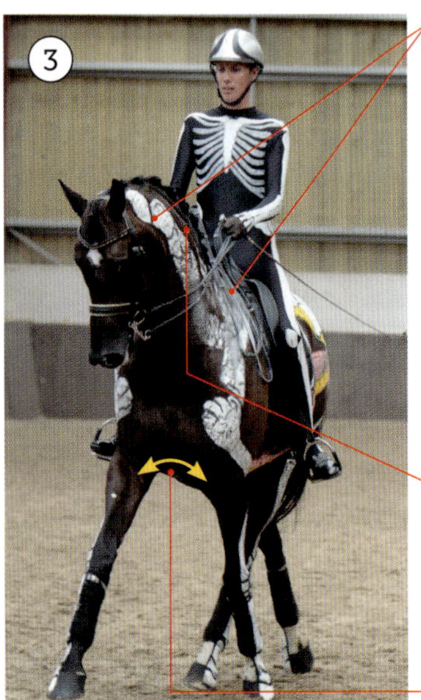


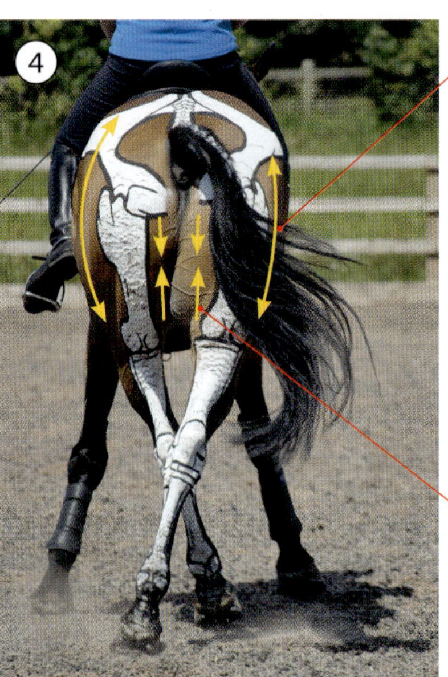

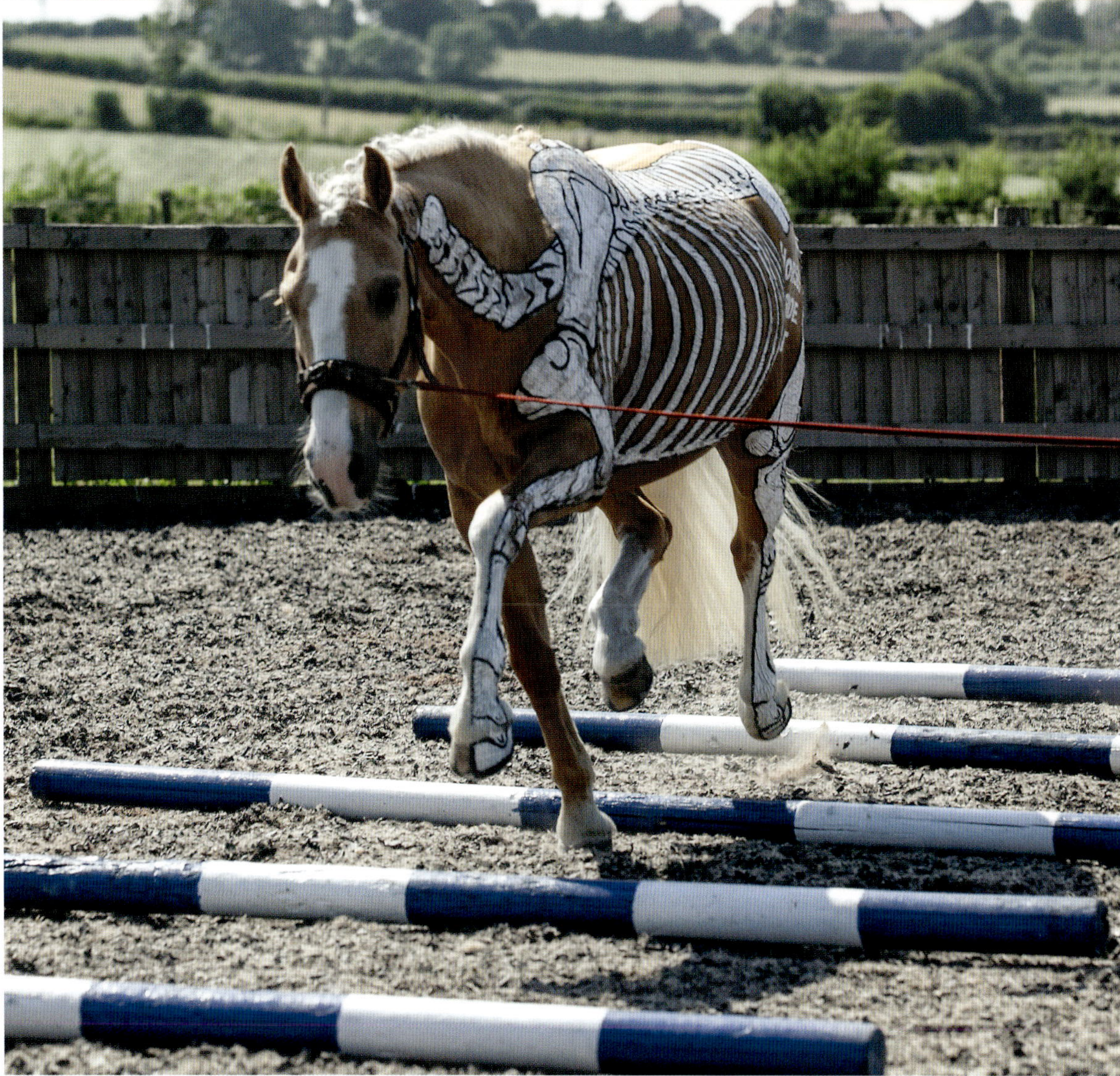

Pole work is useful for horses from all disciplines and its benefits should never be underestimated. It is good for maintaining balance, developing rhythm and energy, toning muscles, encouraging symmetrical movement, stimulating the production of synovial fluid within the joints, keeping the horse flexible and improving proprioception and hoof/brain coordination. It can also be used to rehabilitate horses from injury or neurological conditions. More specifically:

- **Walk poles** are good for developing back rotation, lateral flexion, strength and control
- **Trot poles** are good for developing core and abdominal strength, back stability, momentum, power and spring
- **Canter poles** are good for strengthening the back, raising the forehand and hindquarters, strengthening the thoracic sling and, as the horse rocks between the fore and hindquarters are good for back mobility flexion and extension.

# Pole Work Exercises from an Anatomical Perspective

For maximum benefit, pole work must be practised on a regular basis. Whether ridden or performed in hand the horse should have a long rein and freedom to lower his head. This enables him to assess how and where to place his limbs and, as lowering the head and neck raises the back and engages the abdominal muscles, it will help improve posture. Pole work exercises help straightness and symmetry as stride lengths are forced to be equal. With a little imagination and ingenuity poles and blocks can be configured in many ways to provide fun, variety and challenge whatever the gait.

**Distance guide**

| | |
|---|---|
| Walk poles | 0.7–1M |
| Trot poles | 1.2–1.7M |
| Canter poles | 2.6–3.2M |

When placed closer together poles encourage the horse to shorten and collect and if placed further apart to open out, lengthen the frame and develop extended gaits.

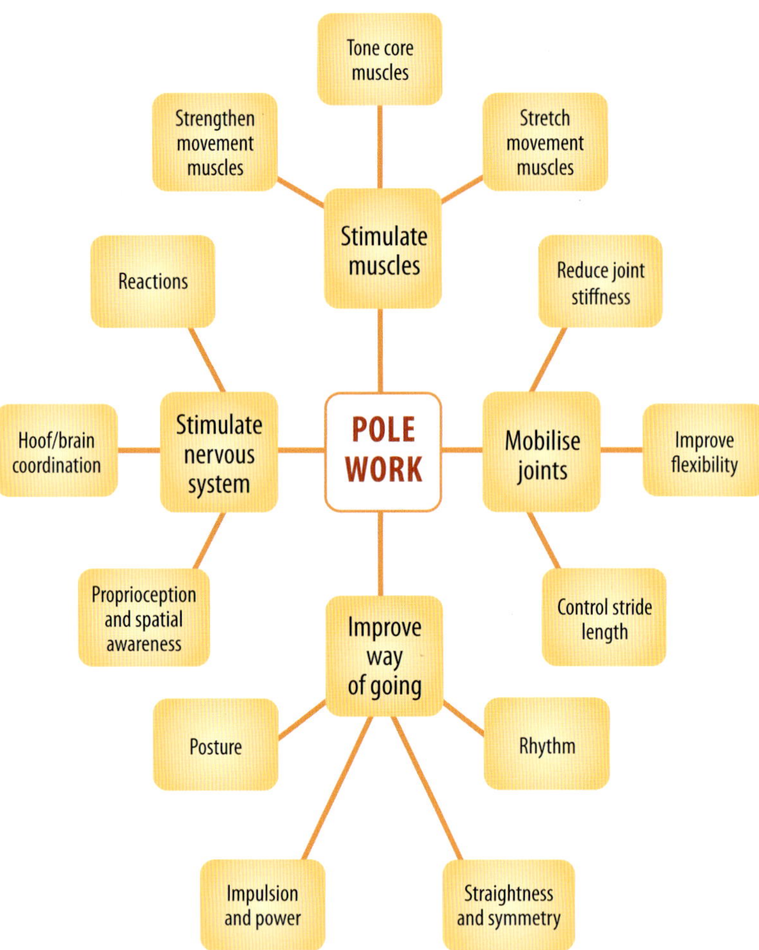


## APPLYING THE SCIENCE

Pole work is useful for horses and riders from all disciplines. Its benefits cannot be underestimated. As skills and accuracy advance through practice proprioception, hoof/brain coordination, balance and flexibility improve. As stride lengths are forced to be equal, pole work contributes to balance, straightness and symmetry, strengthens the core and mobilises the back of both horse and rider. As with all aspects of flatwork, a thorough understanding of the principles of anatomy together with the help of a skilled trainer will allow riders to apply those principles successfully. Pole work helps to sharpen riding skills as it is essential for the rider to maintain balance with the weight equally distributed in both stirrups whilst maintaining a steady rhythm in both trot and canter. With increased skill comes a feeling of confidence, pleasure and satisfaction which can be transferred to all areas of riding.

# Walking Over Individual Raised Obstacles

As the horse lowers his head to look at the obstacle, which should be at knee or hock height, the back is supported by the spinal ligament system. As there is no moment of suspension in walk he must clear the obstacle by stabilising his back, recruiting his core and by physically lifting his legs rather than by using momentum as he would in trot or canter. This action strengthens the muscles involved in carrying the weight of the rider, is good for horses recovering from sacroiliac, pelvic and back problems and those recovering from abdominal and back surgery.

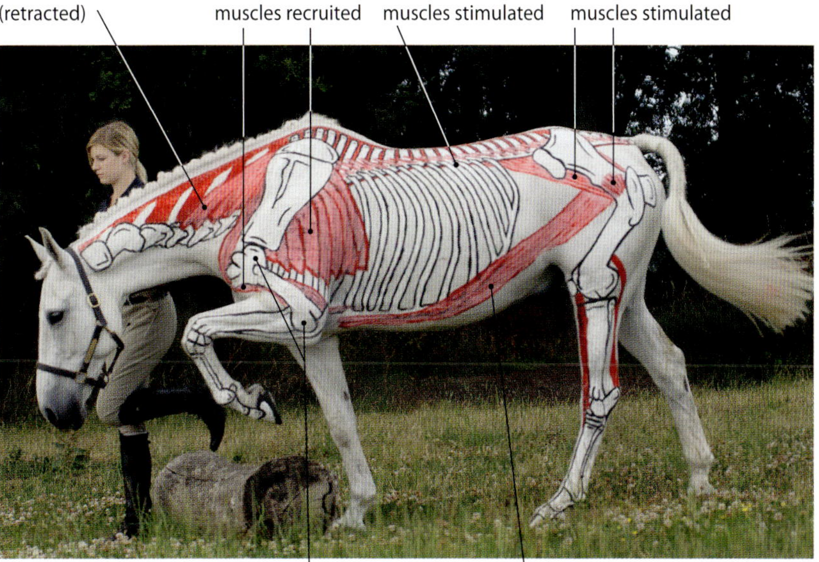


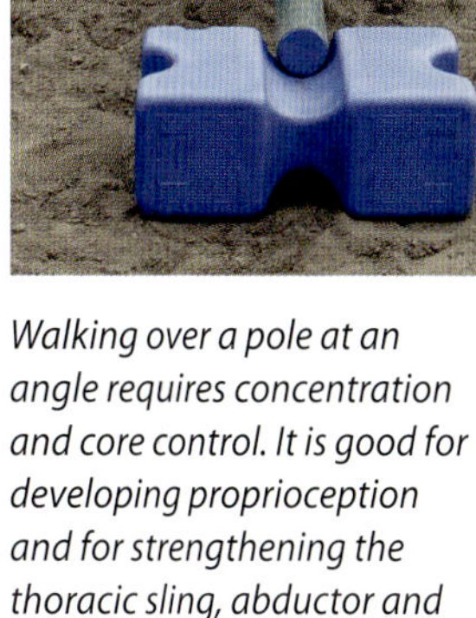

*Walking over a pole at an angle requires concentration and core control. It is good for developing proprioception and for strengthening the thoracic sling, abductor and adductor muscles.*

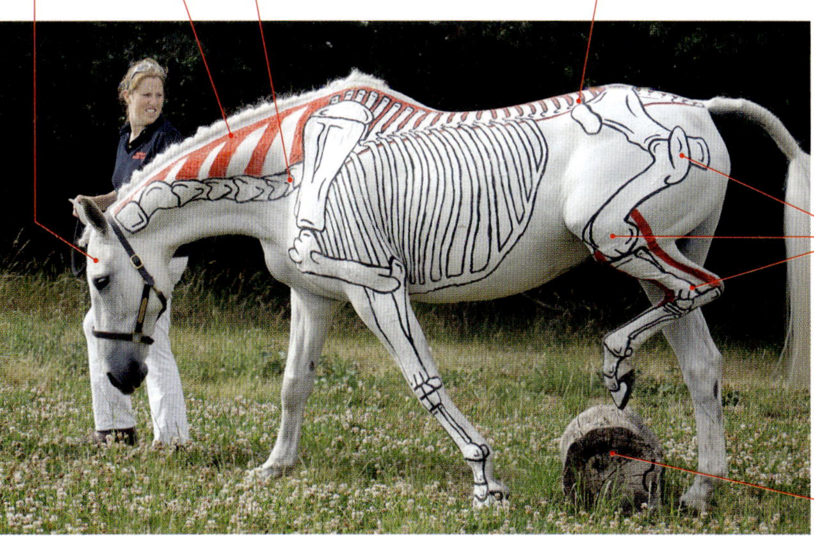

# Walk Poles

Walking over a series of poles improves rhythm and regularity of the footfalls. It is particularly useful for correcting jogging or an irregular or 'lateral' walk.

**BELOW** *Arranging the poles on a curve develops proprioception and enables the rider to easily vary the distance between them by riding to the inner or outer of the curve.*

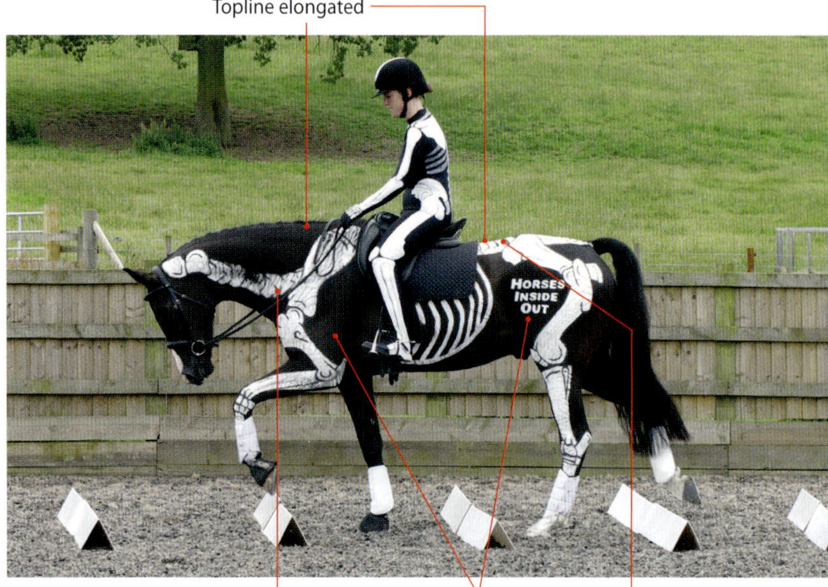


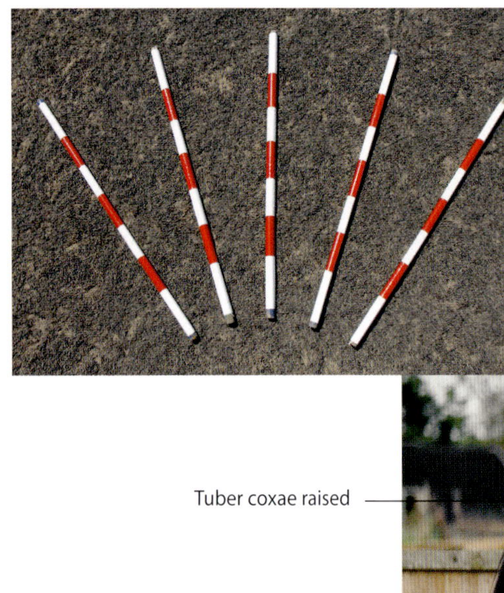

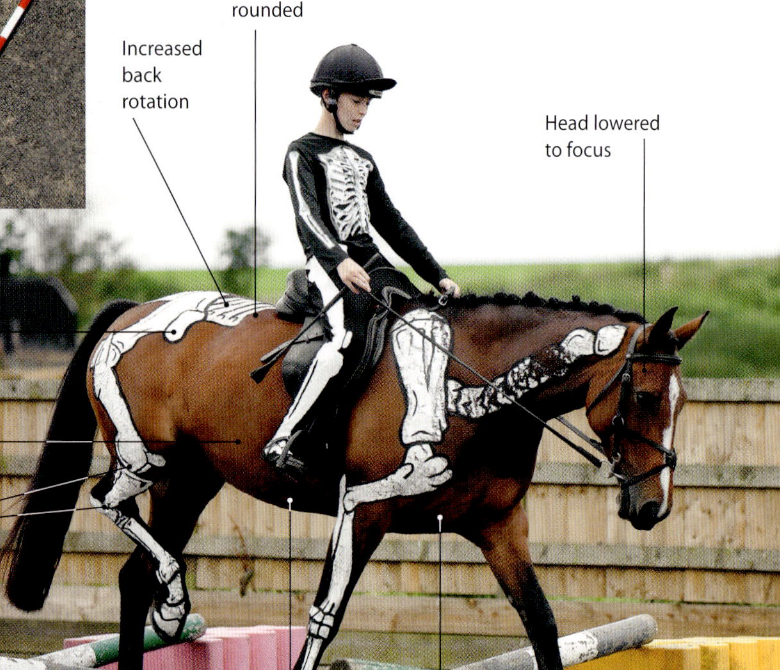


**RIGHT** *Raising poles at alternate ends improves focus, spatial awareness and hoof/brain coordination.*

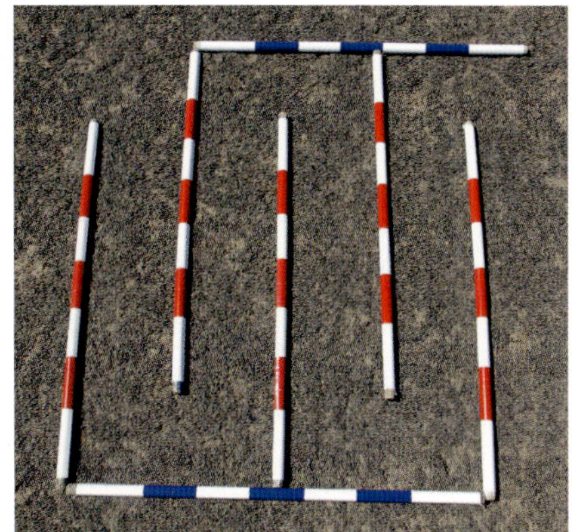

This in-hand exercise encourages and improves lateral suppleness, core control, coordination and proprioception. As the horse is led in a serpentine line between the poles he must bring his hind and forelimbs closer together to negotiate the grid, core muscles are recruited and the back is rounded.

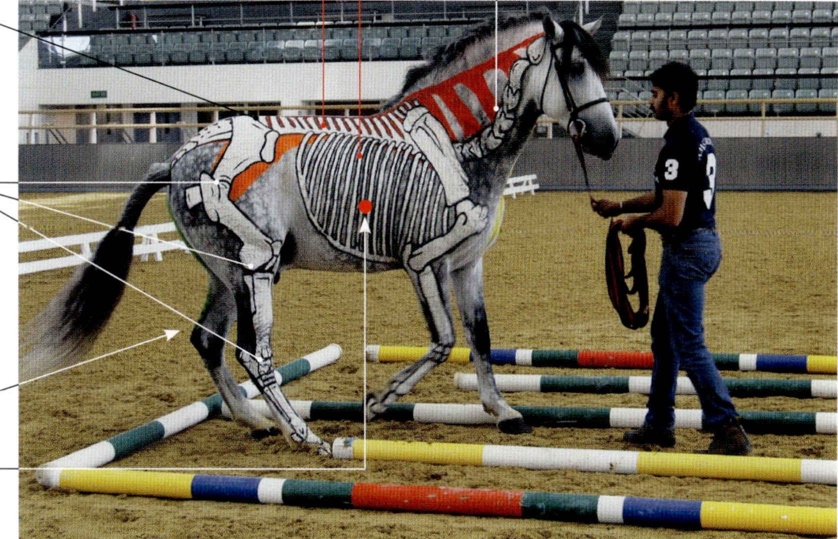


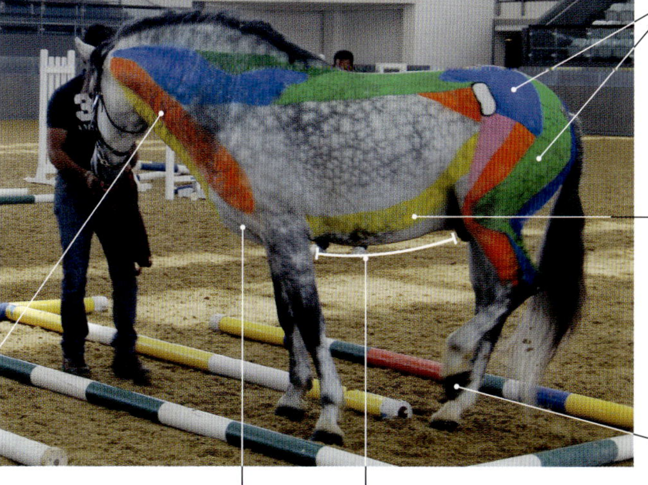

# Trot Poles

As trot has a moment of suspension and is a higher impact gait than walk, to negotiate poles successfully requires increased momentum, flexion in all the limb joints, power and spring.

As they encourage the horse to push equally from behind, trot poles are an excellent exercise for developing an equal stride length and for improving symmetry, straightness and coordination. They are particularly useful as a rehabilitation exercise following injury or lameness.

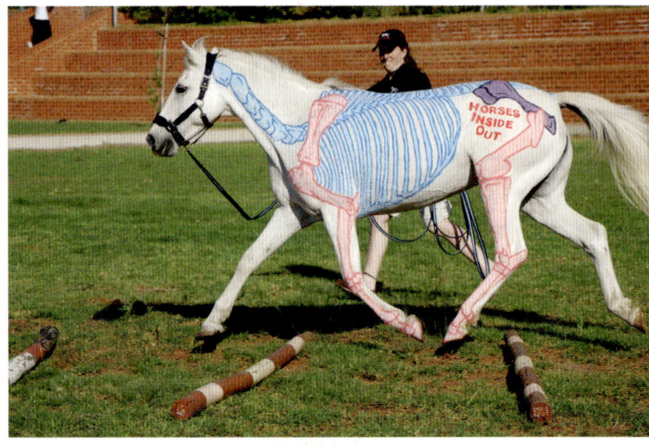


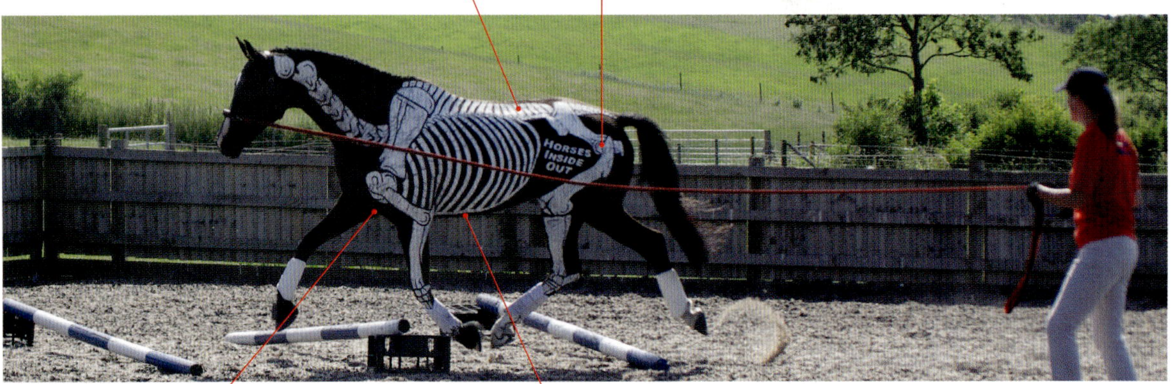


*ABOVE AND BELOW Raised trot poles require core strength to stabilise the back and facilitate increased lift and flexion of the limb joints.*

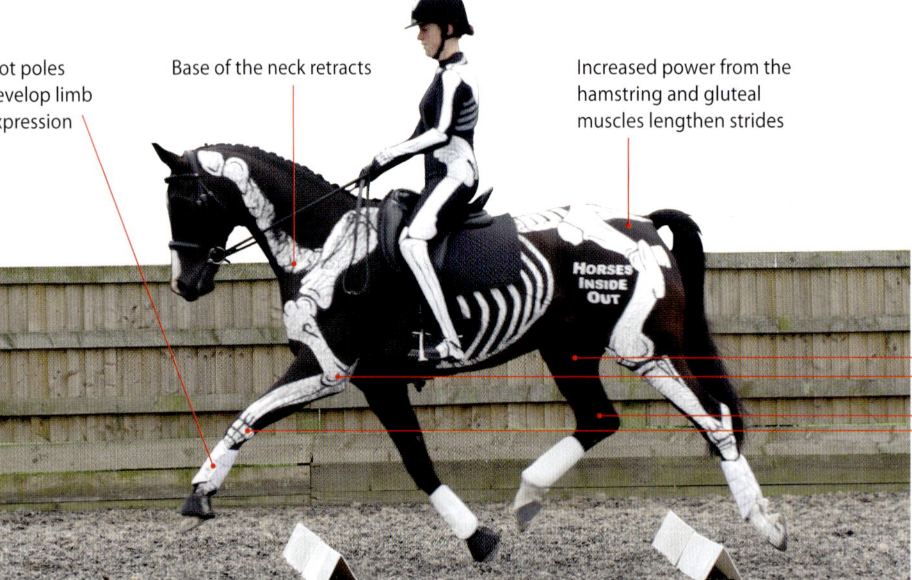

Raising the poles on the outside of a curve encourages reach and range of movement in the outside forelimb. This exercise stretches the latissimus dorsi and forelimb retractor muscles, increases the range of movement in the shoulder and elbow joints and is useful for helping straighten a horse with asymmetrical forelimb movement.

Raising poles on the inside of the curve encourages the horse to lift the inside shoulder, strengthens the rhomboideus and trapezius muscles and prevents him from 'falling in'.

Riding through trot poles arranged on a gentle uphill slope strengthens the gluteals and hamstrings as the horse must push harder from behind. Trotting downhill requires greater core control, balance and increased recruitment of the thoracic sling muscles.

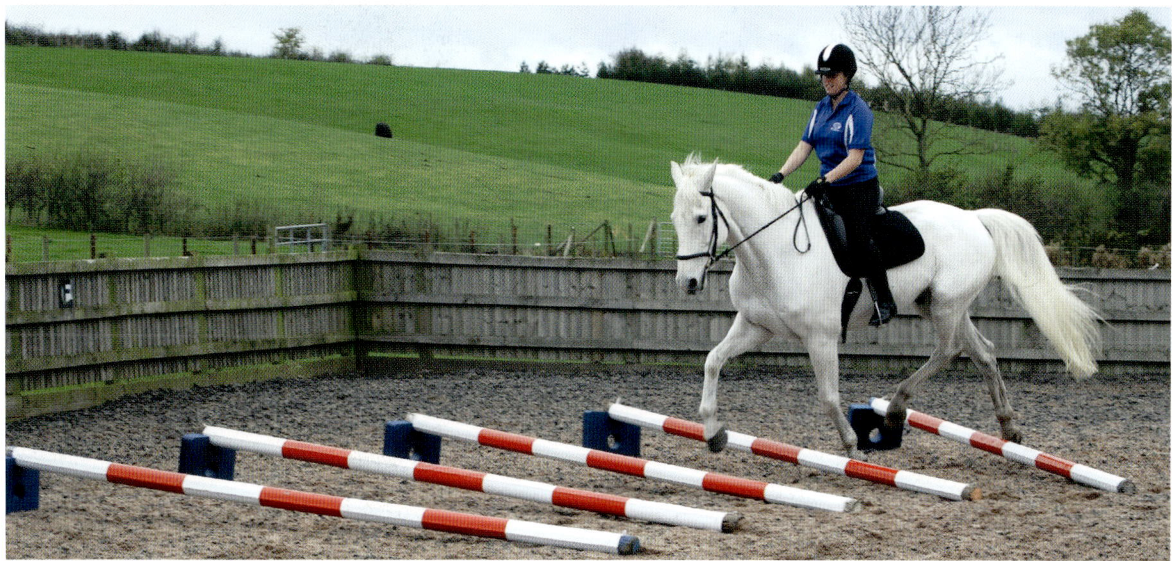

ABOVE *Raising the poles on the outside of a curve.* BELOW *Raising poles on the inside of the curve.*

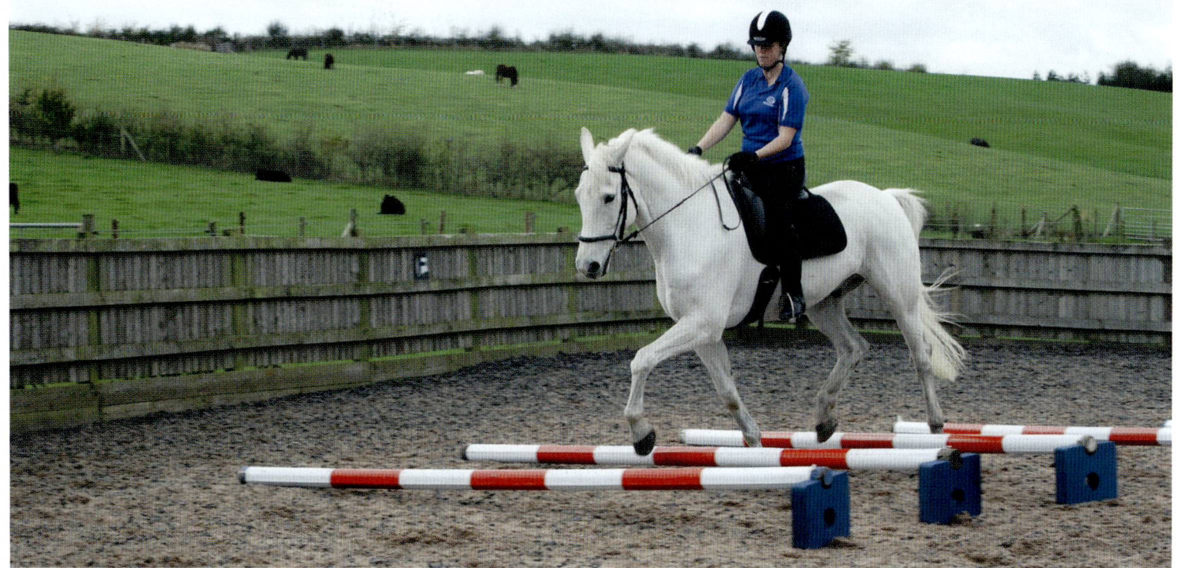

# Canter Poles

Canter poles encourage flexion and extension of the lumbosacral junction and improve rhythm and balance. They are particularly useful for suppling the back and as a rehabilitative exercise for horses recovering from back injury.

## Related distances

Cantering over two ground poles set at a 6–8 stride distance gives the scope to increase or decrease the number of strides between the poles. This is good preparatory exercise for collection and extension, adjusting the number of strides in preparation for jumping and improving rhythm and the regularity of steps.

## Raised canter poles

These are useful for:

- Encouraging rounding of the back, flexion and extension of the lumbosacral junction and hindlimb reach
- Strengthening the back and hindquarters
- Strengthening the muscles involved in supporting and raising the forehand
- Recruiting and toning the abdominal muscles, hip flexors and the spinal flexor muscle chain
- Agility and coordination
- Reducing back stiffness.

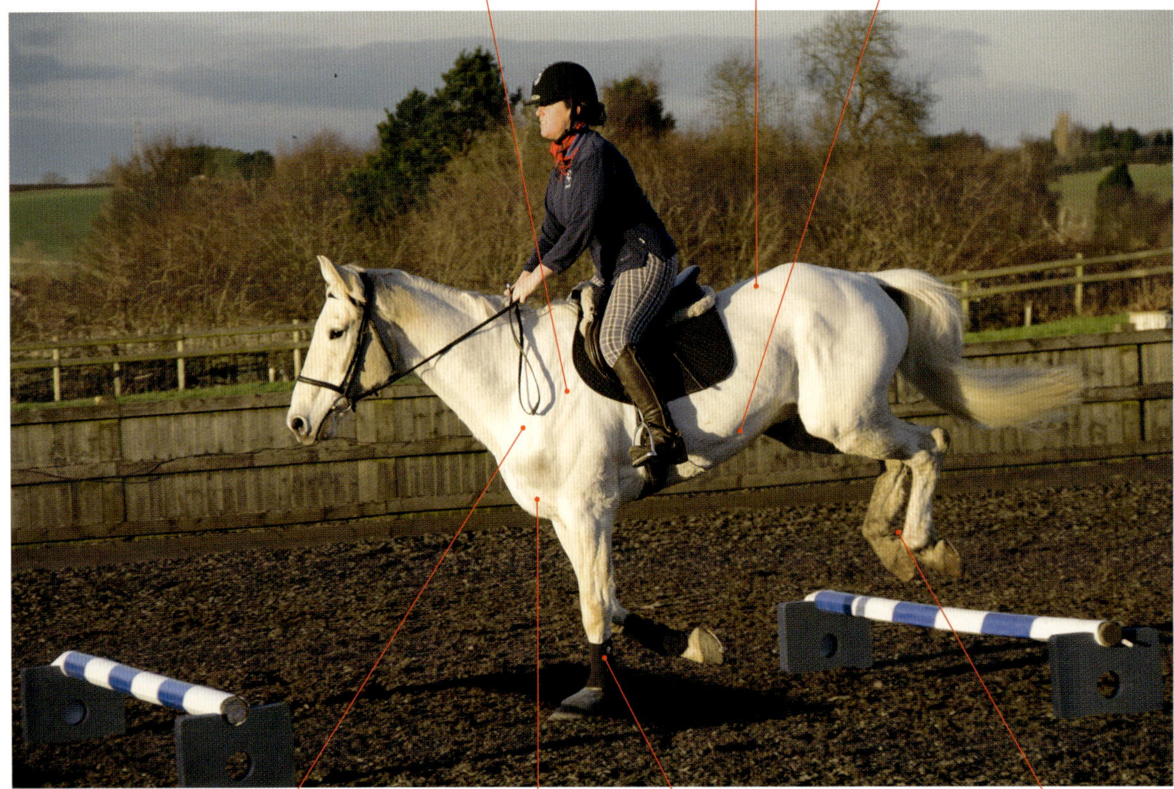

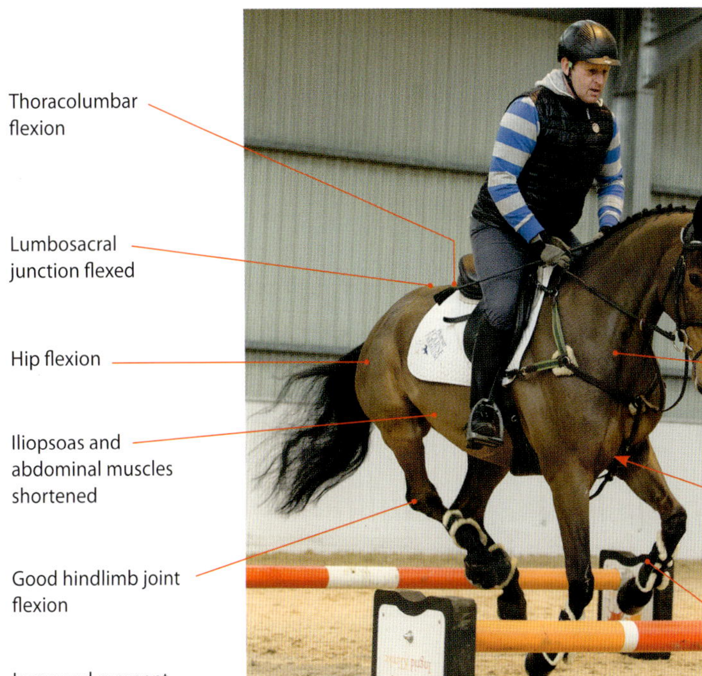





Raising the poles alters the footfalls of the canter, causing the diagonal pair to dissociate and resulting in the horse 'rocking' between the fore and hind limbs. This is a good core strengthening and back mobilising exercise can be considered as a precursor to and has the same anatomical benefits as the bounce (see page 162).

**Note:** Cantering through a line of raised poles, particularly when ridden, increases the load placed on the limbs. If the horse has a history of lower limb tendon and ligament injury this exercise should be avoided.

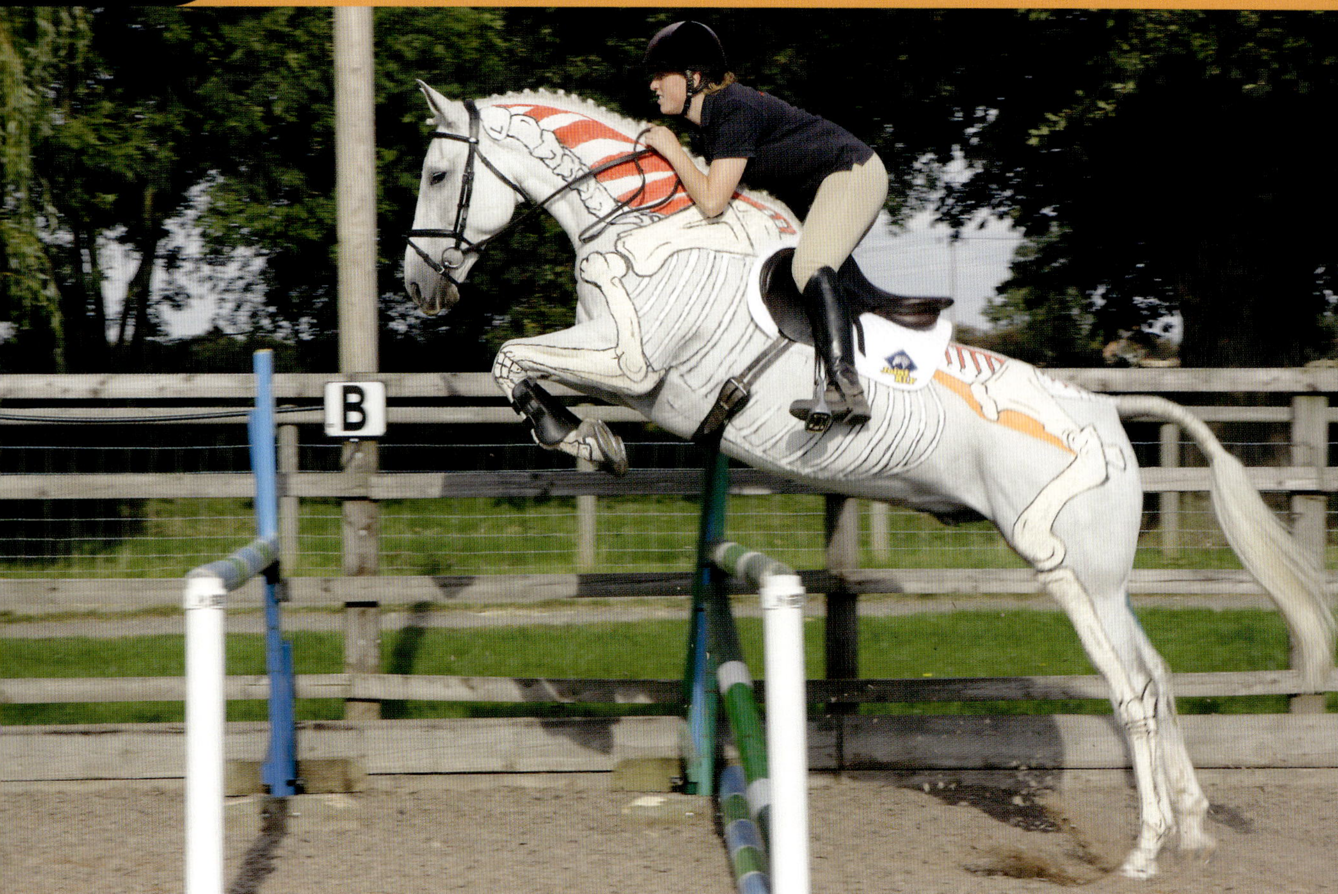

To jump successfully horses need physical strength, a good mental attitude and a balanced rider. The ability to jump comes from suitable conformation, a good power to weight ratio, technique, willingness, coordination and the ability to convert forward momentum to upward thrust.

Although horses do jump in the wild (they clear streams and obstacles that get in their way), they are not natural jumpers. A substantial hind gut, heavy forehand, long neck, heavy head and an inflexible spine increase the stress and risk of injury to skeletal, muscular, tendon, ligament and fascial structures. These do not correspond with the physical requirements for jumping. Jumping also increases stress on the cardiovascular, respiratory, nervous and endocrine systems.

## How the Horse Jumps

In approach, the horse lifts his head to assess the fence, gathers energy, power and impulsion by bringing his hind feet well under the body and compresses his frame rather like a coiled spring. He then brings his weight back and shortens the last stride to convert forward momentum to upward thrust. At the last moment he lowers his head and sinks through the thoracic sling. The fetlocks drop then the energy stored in muscles, tendons and ligaments is released as the forelegs straighten to push and lift the forehand. At this point the hindlimbs come through together, flex and compress before pushing powerfully upwards. A well-angled shoulder and elbow conformation allows good lift and tuck of the forelegs. The horse then lowers his head and rounds his back in bascule as his body follows the line of a parabola. As he comes in to land, he raises his head and the back extends once again as the forelimbs stretch out in front. He lands on the trailing forelimb. The fetlock sinks to the ground as the thorax also sinks and the structures of the lower limb bear the brunt of the concussive forces with the trailing limb taking considerably more force than the leading limb. The hindlimbs land together. The first stride after landing is short before the horse regains his rhythm.

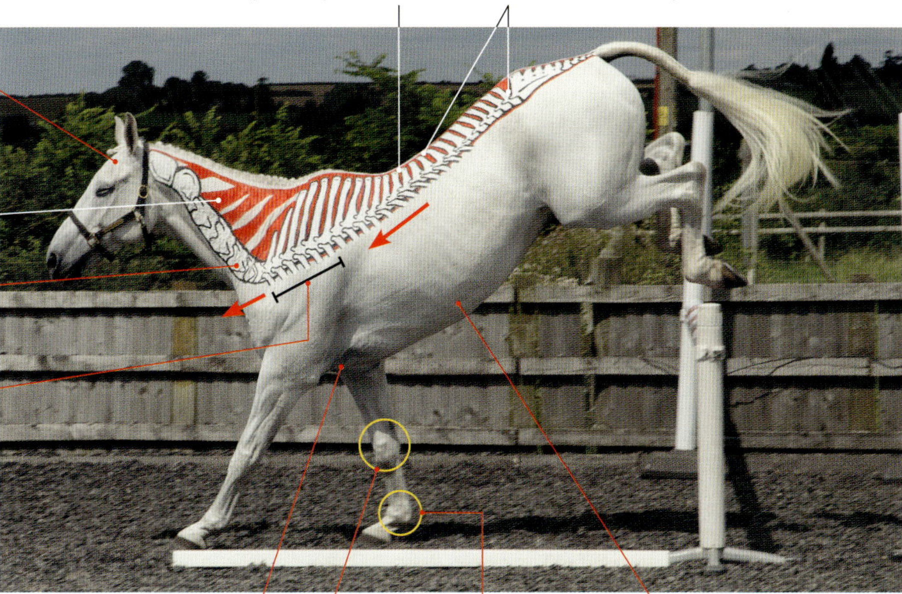


**ABOVE** *There is considerable stress through the vertebrae in the cranial thoracic region as the horse lands from a jump and the thoracic spinous processes take some of the weight. A rider and the restrictions of tack compound the strain.*

**RIGHT** *This horse is preparing to take off.*

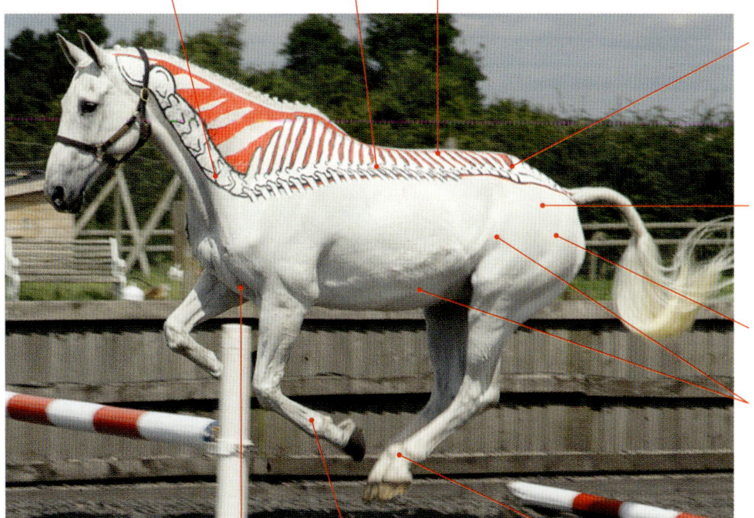

# Comparison of the Biomechanics of Jumping Upright versus Wide Fences

## Upright fences

Effect of placing poles on jump trajectory

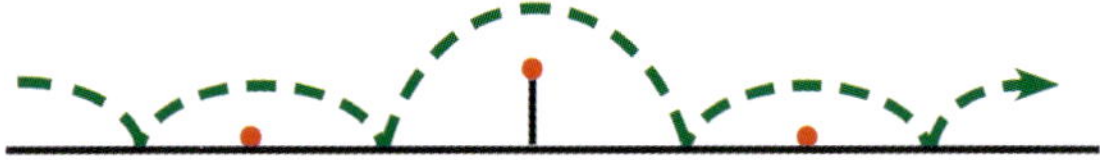

- When jumped well from a close take off spot the angle of ascent and descent is steep. This increases the vertical forces the horse must create at take off and absorb at landing. The higher the fence the more force created.

- Jumping high upright fences is good for encouraging the horse to compress his frame, develop spring, power and the ability to raise the forehand.

    When the horse lands steeply from a vertical fence the forelimbs are almost perpendicular to the ground, the head is up and the back is extended. This puts more strain on the tendons, ligaments and joints particularly those in the lower limb.

1. Head and neck movement contributes to forelimb flexion

2. Stretch of topline over neck and thoracic region

3. Retraction of the base of the neck

4. Good shoulder action

5. Back and gluteal muscles working to further raise the forehand

6. Powerful contraction of hindlimb muscles creates upward thrust

7. Hindlimb joints extending

8. Hind tendons recoiling, contributing to upward thrust.

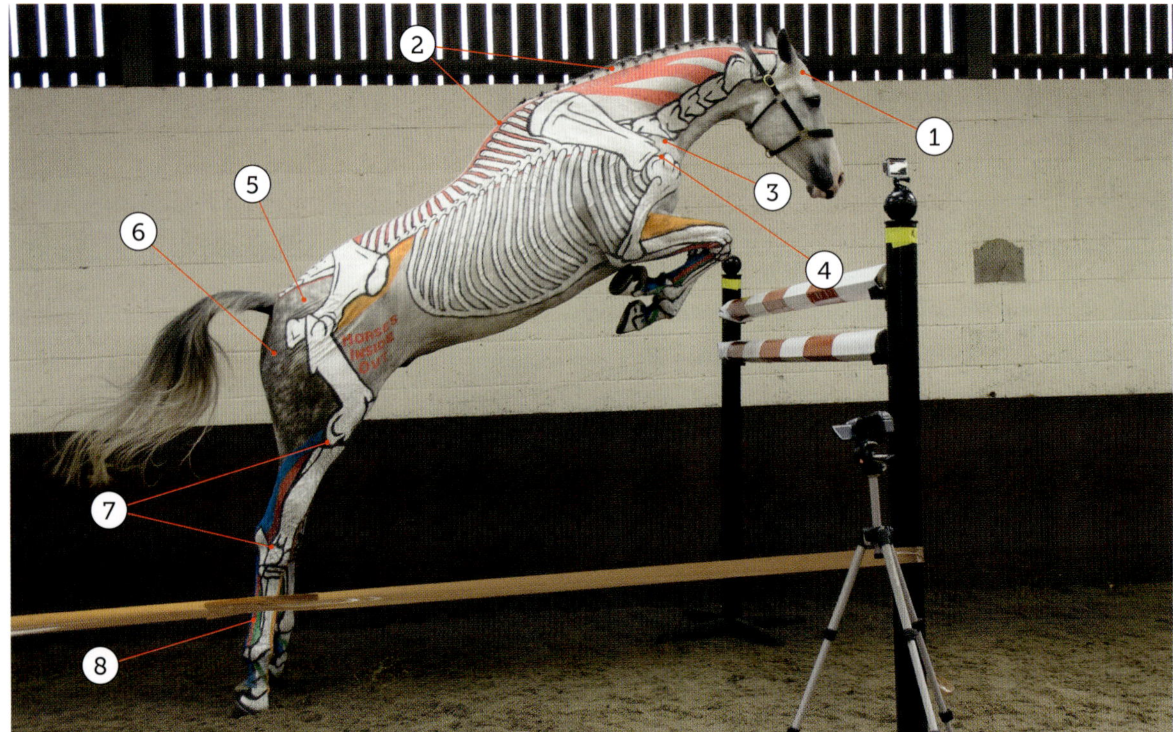

*High uprights strengthen the back, gluteal and thoracic sling muscles to bring the forehand up.*

# Wide fences

Jump trajectory over an ascending spread

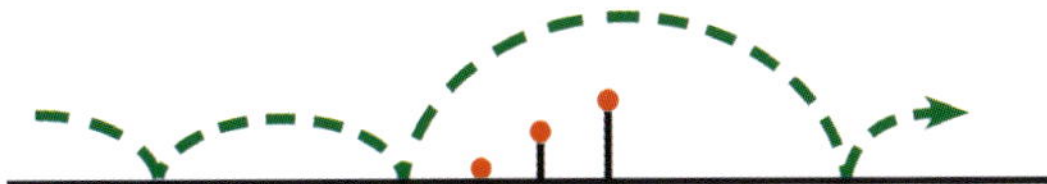

- Jumping a wide fence from a forward stride encourages a more sloping trajectory. A wide fence with a lower front rail or an ascending triple bar allows for a more gradual take off whilst a wide fence with both rails the same height requires a sharper take off and neat forelimb action.

- A wide fence encourages the horse to elongate in his frame, open up through the back and stretch the head, neck and topline. A flatter flight-path helps to develop reach, scope and stride length.

1. Head stretches forward

2. Neck elongates

3. Back elongates

4. Spinous spaces in the cranial thoracic region are opened

5. Extension of the lumbosacral junction

6. Good joint movement as back end flicks away

7. Muscles stretched.

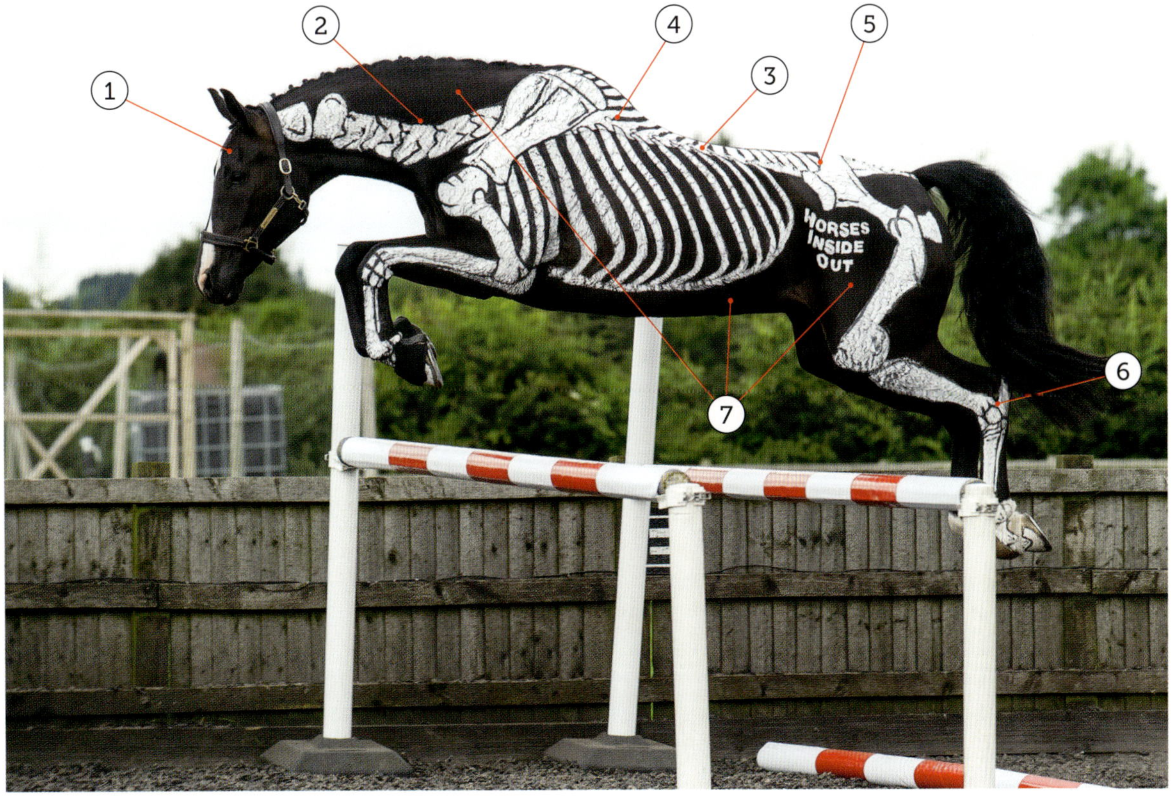

*Wide fences strengthen the gluteals and hamstring muscles to improve forward thrust.*

## Jumping Exercises from an Anatomical Perspective

Most horses can improve their jumping performance with correct training and conditioning. This involves targeting muscle strength, general fitness and jump training. For gymnastic jumping the horse requires:

- Well-conditioned gluteal, hamstring and biceps femoris muscles
- Well-toned thoracic sling and triceps muscles
- A flexible spine
- A strong sacroiliac area
- Sloping pasterns and strong limbs to absorb concussive forces
- A supple neck to use as a counterbalance.

If the horse is suitably agile and fit, jumping is good for:

- Improving the anatomical requirements outlined above
- Improving muscular strength, elasticity and speed of contractions
- Power, scope and expression
- Core stability, balance and rhythm
- Flexibility and range of movement
- Hoof/brain coordination, proprioception and surefootedness
- Quick neurological reactions, reflexes and athleticism.

## Factors Influencing back Movement when Jumping

Owing to the physical impact on the musculoskeletal system, jumping should form part of a structured exercise programme rather than being an everyday activity. The height, width, type and shape of the fences, the distance between obstacles, the line of approach and speed will all influence the shape the horse makes over the fence and the effect on the musculoskeletal system.

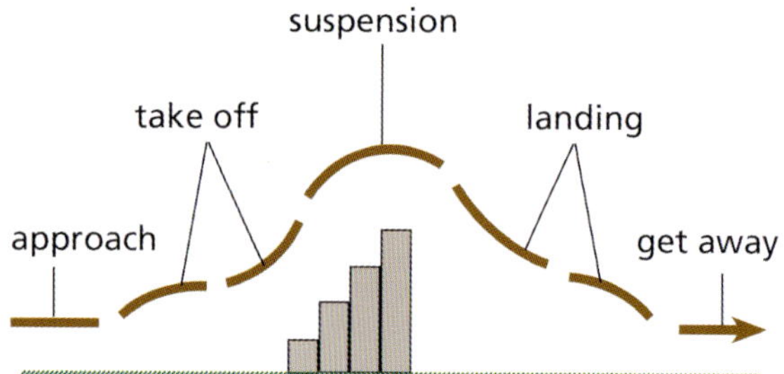


The line diagram above illustrates back movement over a fence. When jumping, the back flexes and extends dramatically. This means that, although jumping horses can be more supple and mobile through the back, they can also be more prone to back and sacroiliac problems than horses from other disciplines.

### APPLYING THE SCIENCE

Jumping is a fun activity. To jump safely and successfully it is essential the rider remains in perfect harmony with the horse. Developing the two-point position with the rider lifting the seat and taking the weight on the balls of the feet will develop independent balance. This, together with understanding the biomechanics of jumping, will allow the horse the freedom to use his head, neck and back correctly. A good trainer will be able to assess the capability of both horse and rider; suggest an appropriate, enjoyable, achievable training programme; maintain enthusiasm and ensure the rider is in the correct position to give the horse the best possible chance of success whatever the age, stage or jumping discipline.

# Placing Poles

Placing poles on the approach influence rhythm, balance and take off point. They are useful for assessing distance and 'training the eye' of both horse and rider. A single take off pole, correctly positioned:

- Brings the horse to the correct take off point
- Encourages him to compress
- Brings his hind legs underneath the body together in the take off canter stride
- Propels him upwards and forwards
- Maximises the use of the gluteals to raise the forehand
- Extends the hip
- Increases flexion in the back and lumbosacral junction.

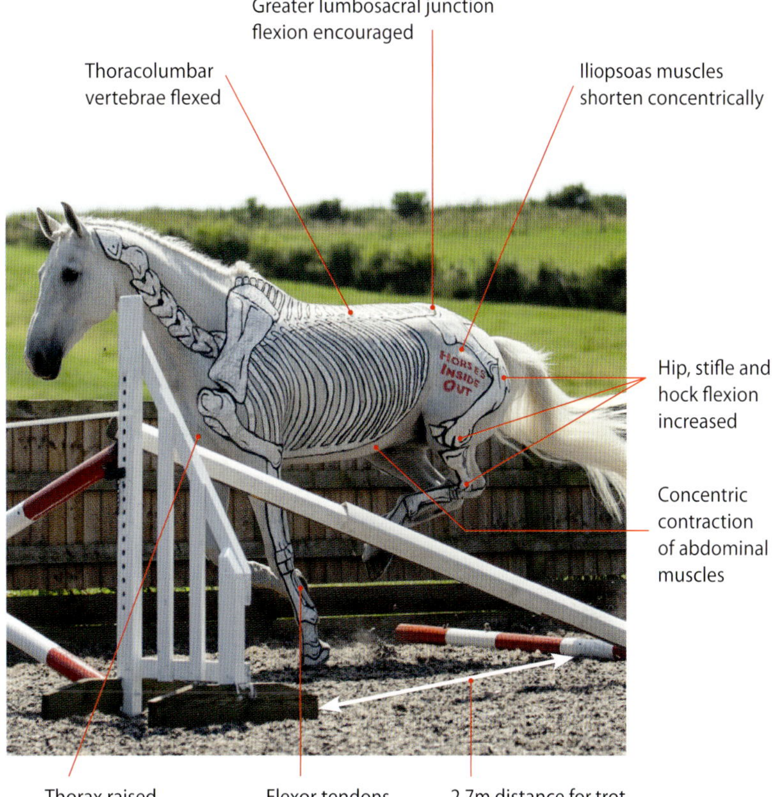



## Landing poles

Landing poles, which should always be at least 3.2m away from the fence, are useful to encourage the horse to slow down, lower his head and round his back over the fence as he looks at the pole. They are also useful for encouraging a steeper parabola if the horse tends to jump too long and flat over a fence. Correctly placed a landing pole will encourage the horse to compress his body during the landing stride, balance and bring his hind legs well under his body ready to push on after the fence.

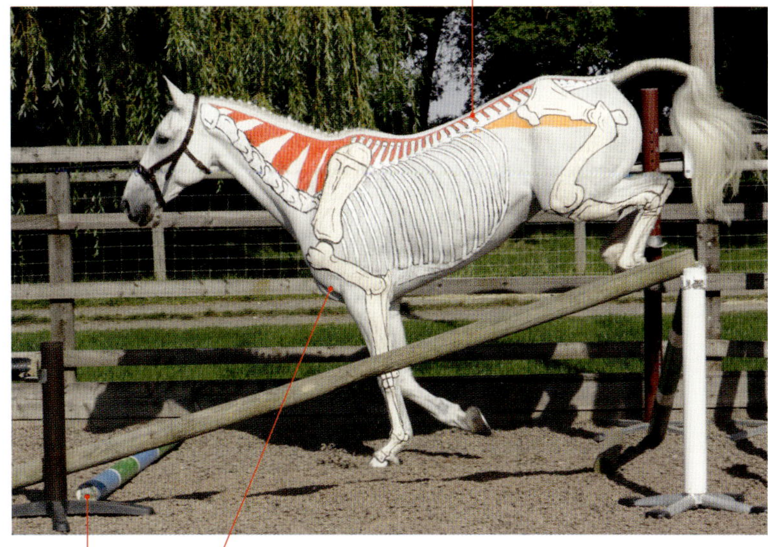

# The Skeletal System in Bounces

When cantering through a bounce (which, for an average-striding 16.2hh horse should be set at 3.5m), as the forelimbs leave the ground, they are immediately replaced by the hindlimbs. This initiates a dynamic rocking motion which requires power, athleticism, agility and quick reactions.

Bounces are good for joint mobility, suppling the back and lumbosacral junction, muscle strength and flexibility, developing technique and controlling speed. They should not be attempted if the horse is suffering from back pain, is recovering from injury or has known tendon or ligament problems.

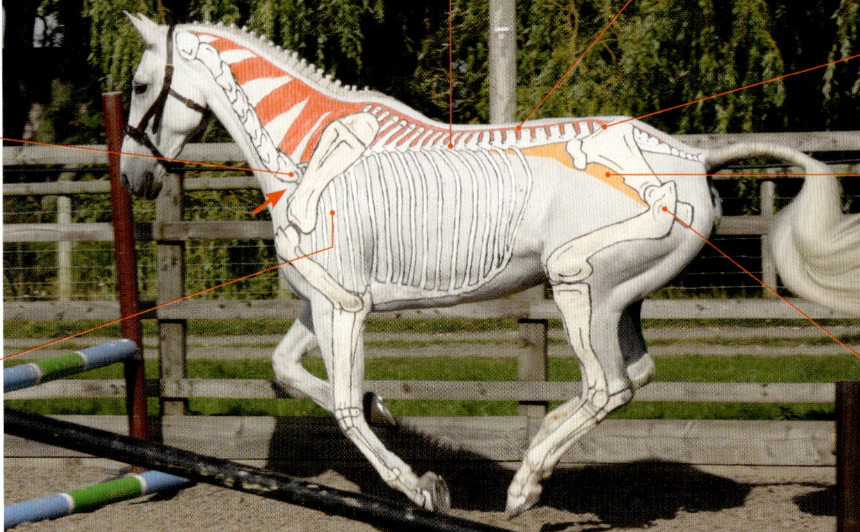


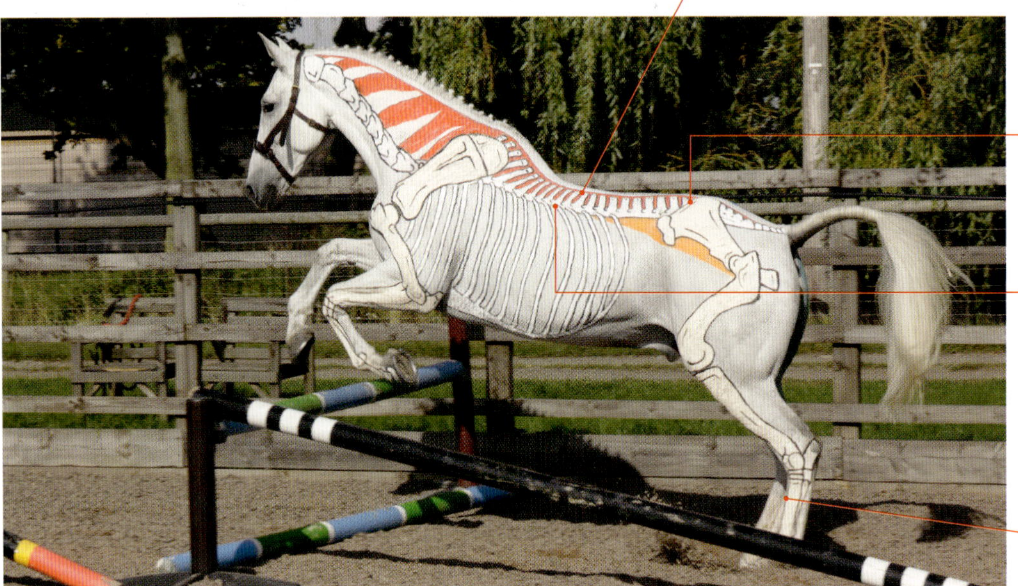

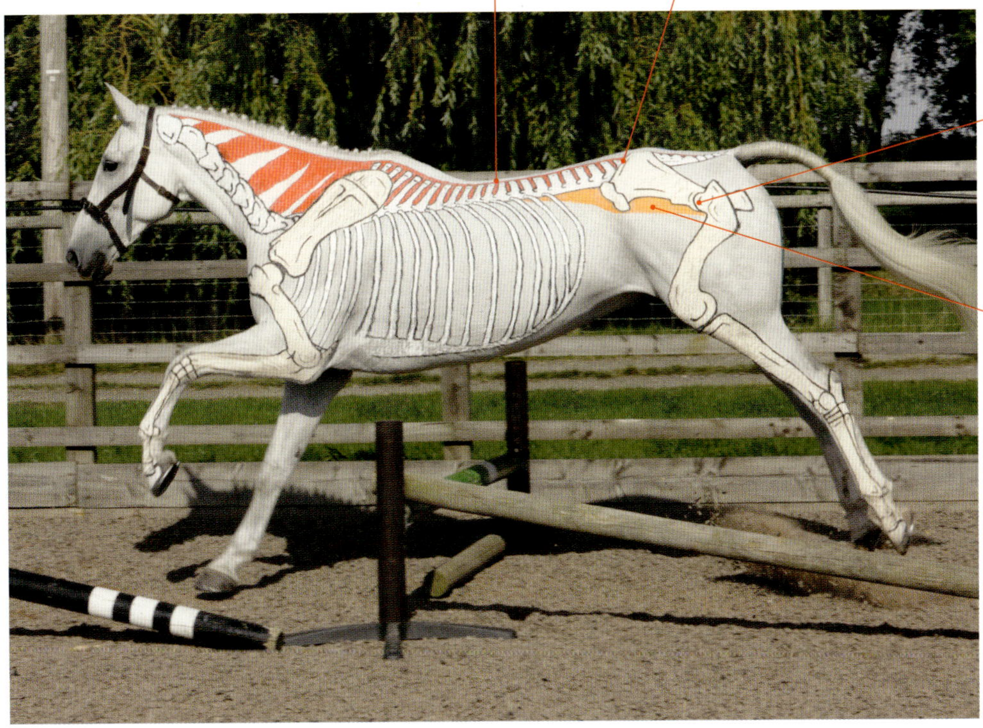
Spinous spaces reducded
Lumbosacral junction extended
Hip joint extended
Iliopsoas muscle elongated

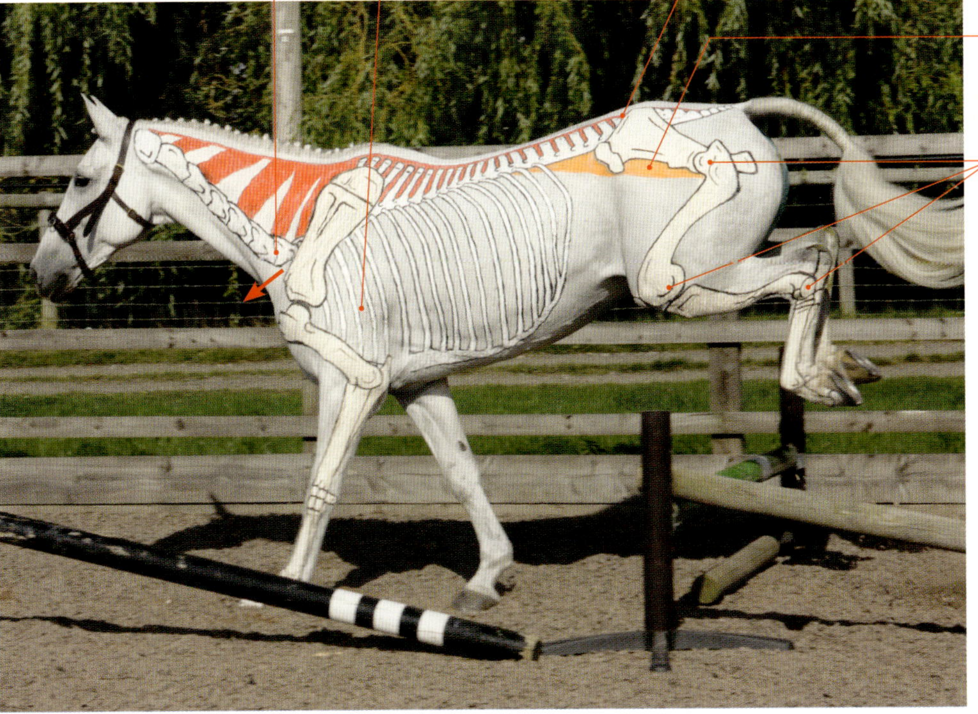
Base of the neck protracts
Thorax lowers relative to scapulas
Lumbosacral junction flexing
Iliopsoas muscle shortened
Hip, stifle and hock flexing

# How Bounces Affect the Muscular System

When jumping a bounce the limb load increases as downward landing forces are converted into upward take off forces as the muscles contract and lengthen in rapid succession. Bounces are a suppling, gymnastic activity which take all the muscles through their full range of movement. They require the muscles to exert maximum force swiftly, powerfully and efficiently. This provides an invaluable strengthening and conditioning exercise which uses eccentric, concentric and isometric muscle contractions and contributes to the horse's ability to perform in any discipline.

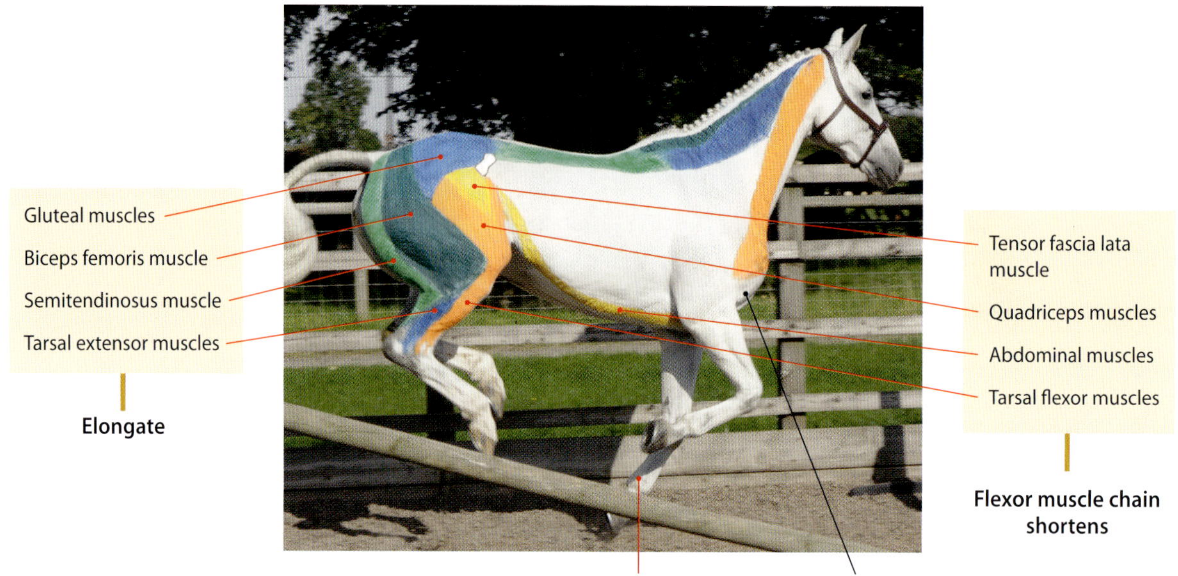


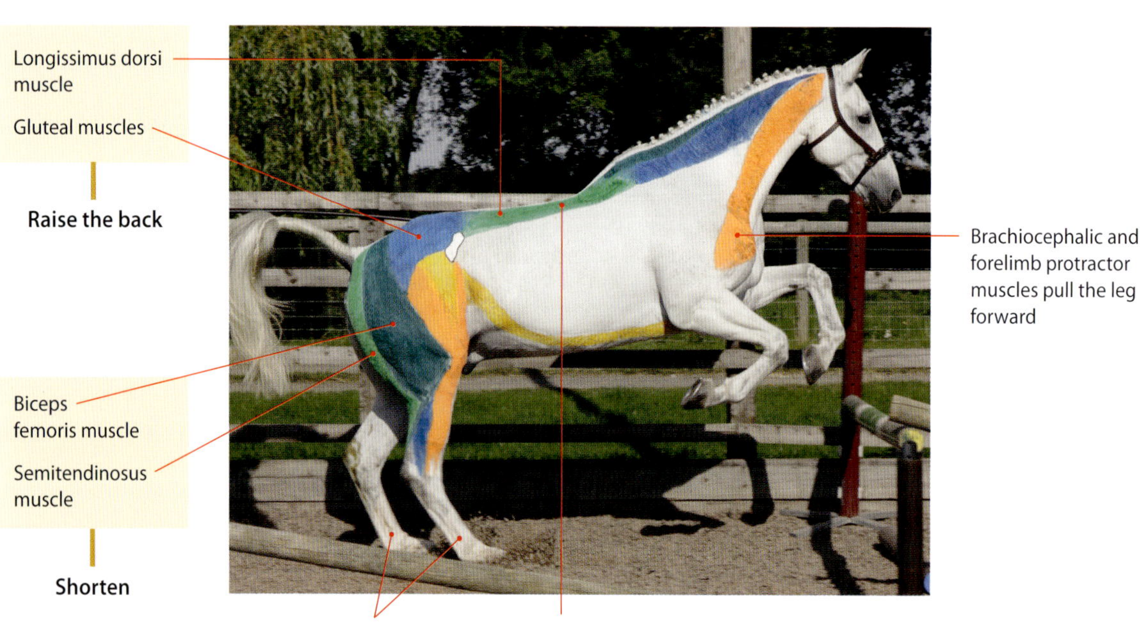

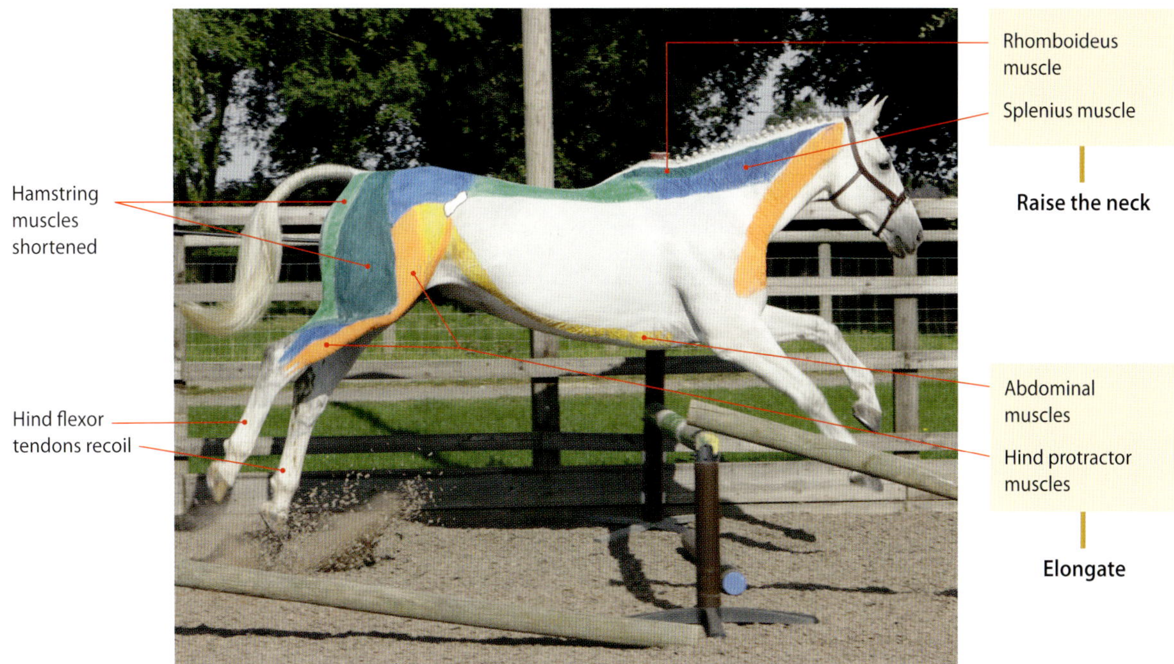

Rhomboideus muscle
Splenius muscle
Raise the neck
Hamstring muscles shortened
Abdominal muscles
Hind protractor muscles
Elongate
Hind flexor tendons recoil


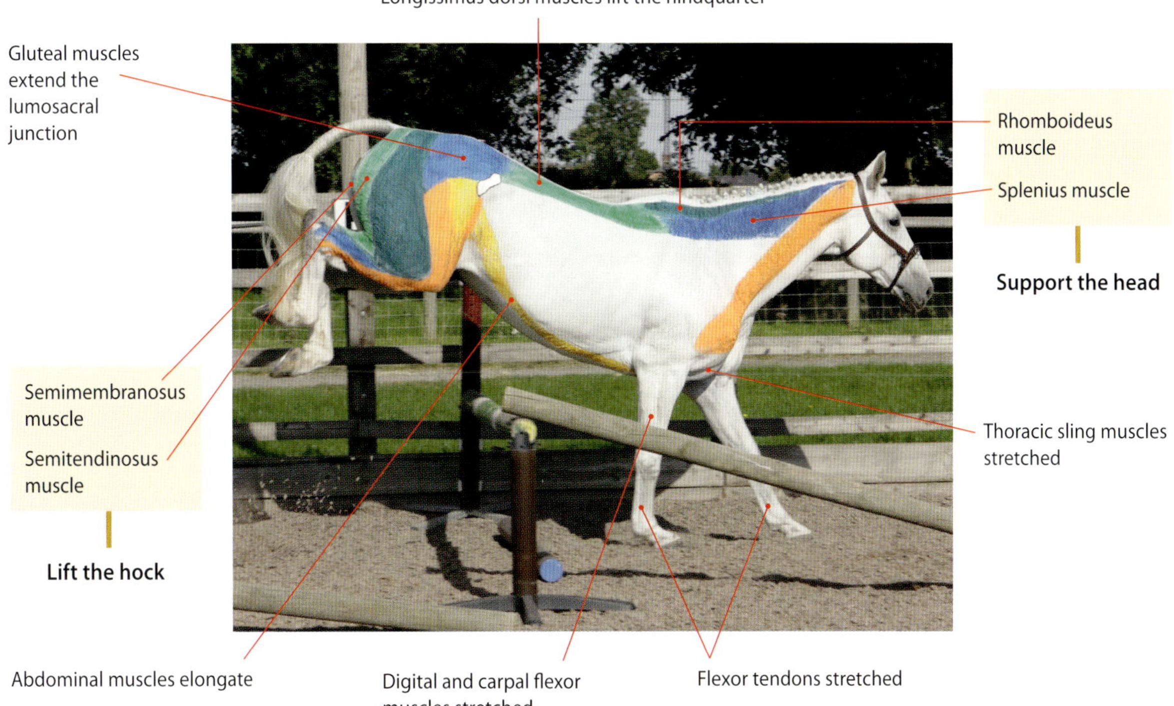

Longissimus dorsi muscles lift the hindquarter
Gluteal muscles extend the lumosacral junction
Rhomboideus muscle
Splenius muscle
Support the head
Semimembranosus muscle
Semitendinosus muscle
Thoracic sling muscles stretched
Lift the hock
Abdominal muscles elongate
Digital and carpal flexor muscles stretched
Flexor tendons stretched

# Gymnastic Grid Work Exercises

Grid work exercises combine the biomechanical and musculoskeletal advantages of jumping bounces, uprights and wide fences. Grids, which should be designed with a clear purpose in mind, can be arranged in a variety of configurations including different types of fence, distance and inclusion of ground poles. They should cater for musculoskeletal strengths and weaknesses, take account of age, stage and skeletal maturity, be planned to give confidence and meet the needs of each individual combination of horse and rider.

Short distances within the grid put the horse closer to the fence at take off, encourage a short, bouncy canter, a steep jump trajectory and will help to develop cadence and power. Longer distances, where the horse takes off further away from the fence, encourages an extended canter stride and elongation of the frame.

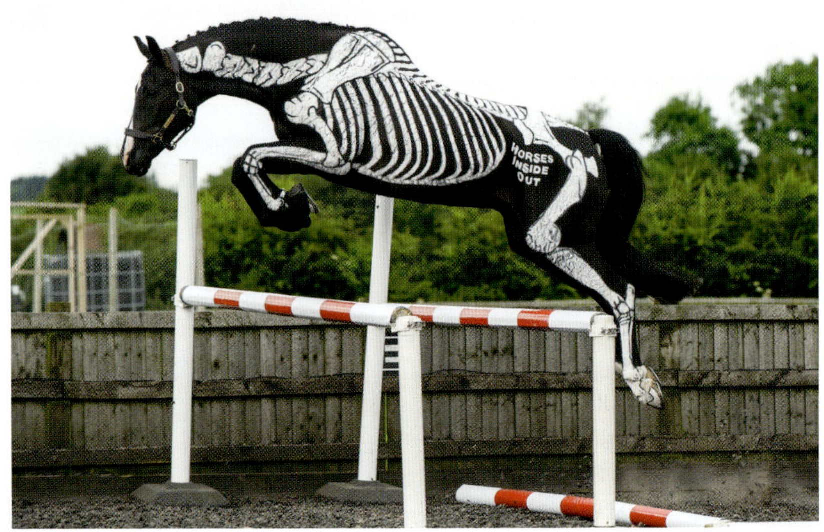


*This horse is jumping the last fence in a short-distance grid designed to encourage him to compress, elongate, develop musculoskeletal control and produce a powerful jump. The grid consisted of a placing pole to a bounce for compression and back flexibility, one short stride to an upright to develop shoulder action and finally one short stride to the parallel for strength and power.*

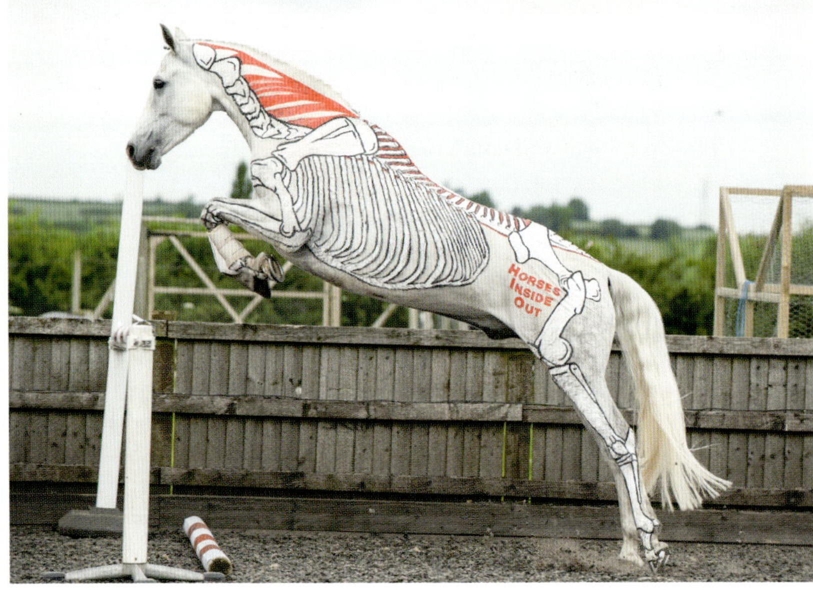


*This horse is jumping the last element in a line of three fences on longer related distances designed to encourage him to cover more ground and develop forward thrust. The exercise consisted of an upright, three forward-going strides to a parallel, followed by three forward-going strides to another upright.*

Gymnastic jumping in the form of grids constructed in a variety of configurations can:

- Improve quality and adjustability of the canter
- Encourage collection, cadence and control
- Develop stride length, reach and power
- Improve technique
- Supple, strengthen and condition the thoracolumbar spine, lumbosacral junction and flexor and extensor muscle chains
- Improve fore and hindlimb flexion
- Condition the muscles through isometric, concentric and eccentric contractions
- Increase impulsion
- Contribute to lateral suppleness, bend, balance, strength, core stability adjustability and control
- Contribute to versatility and safe jumping.

Jumping fences on an angle or approaching a jumping exercise in leg-yield, shoulder-in or travers improves horse and rider focus. As well as being a valuable suppling exercise, improving the quality of lateral work, it tests and enhances straightness and the quality of the canter.

## SUMMARY

As with all the exercises in part 2, the exercises suggested in the pole work and gymnastic jumping chapters are only starting points for considering the impact that Training Horses for Posture and Performance has, not only the musculoskeletal, cardiovascular respiratory but all the systems of the horse. With imagination, either alone or with the help of an experienced coach, all the exercises in this book can be extended, customized, developed, adjusted and fine-tuned to fit the age, circumstance, ability and fitness of each and every individual horse. Riding and training in this sympathetic, patient and empathic manner with posture, anatomy and welfare in mind will give the horse the best possible chance of a successful, happy healthy life and give us as riders the pleasure and satisfaction of a job well done.

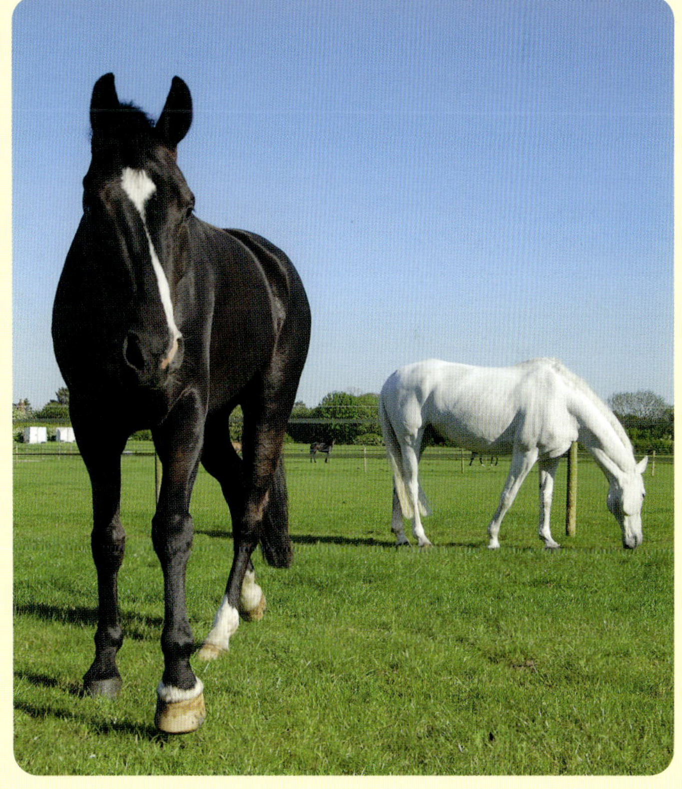

# Index